Managing *Multiple Sclerosis* Naturally

A SELF-HELP GUIDE TO LIVING WITH MS

Judy Graham

Healing Arts Press
Rochester, Vermont • Toronto, Canada

Healing Arts Press
One Park Street
Rochester, Vermont 05767
www.HealingArtsPress.com

Healing Arts Press is a division of Inner Traditions International

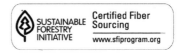

Text paper is SFI certified

Originally published in 1989 by Healing Arts Press under the title *Multiple Sclerosis: A Self-Help Guide to Its Management*

Note to the reader: This book is intended as an informational guide. The remedies, approaches, and techniques described herein are meant to supplement, and not to be a substitute for, professional medical care or treatment. They should not be used to treat a serious ailment without prior consultation with a qualified health care professional. Any products or specific brands recommended in the context of this book have been found useful in the author's individual experience. Please consult with your health care professional on what specific products might be best suited for your unique situation.

Library of Congress Cataloging-in-Publication Data
Graham, Judy.
  Managing multiple sclerosis naturally : a self-help guide to living with MS / Judy Graham. — [Rev. and updated ed.]
      p. cm.
  Originally published under the title: Multiple sclerosis: a self-help guide to Its management, 1989.
  Includes bibliographical references and index.
  Summary: "A totally revised and updated edition of the first book to offer a holistic approach to slowing the progression of MS"—Provided by publisher.
  ISBN 978-1-59477-290-0 (pbk.)
  1. Multiple sclerosis—Popular works. 2. Multiple sclerosis—Alternative treatment—Popular works. 3. Multiple sclerosis—Diet therapy—Popular works. I. Graham, Judy. Multiple sclerosis. II. Title.
  RC377.G65 2010
  616.8'340654—dc22

                                                                                    2010018207

Printed and bound in the United States by Lake Book Manufacturing

10 9 8 7 6 5 4 3 2 1

Text design and layout by Priscilla Baker
This book was typeset in Garamond Premier Pro with Avant Garde used as a display typeface

Contents

PART THREE

Physical and Complementary Therapies

PART FOUR

Living a Healthy Life

Foreword

A WEEK AFTER MY SON was diagnosed with MS in 1995 a friend gave us a book on managing multiple sclerosis by Judy Graham. Up to that time my wife and I were feeling very helpless and full of despair because it seemed there was nothing to be done about MS except hope it didn't progress too fast. The neurologist who had diagnosed my son had not given us any words of encouragement. The best he could muster was to say to my son, "Don't buy some bricks and jump off the Bowness Bridge yet."

I literally devoured Judy's book, which was clearly written and a wonderful mix of science and practical advice. This was exactly the type of information I was looking for to help guide a course of action to fight our son's MS. Our mood of hopelessness was immediately replaced by one of confidence that MS could be successfully managed.

Ever since that day, Judy Graham has been an icon in our home, and I am most pleased that I have this opportunity to introduce the latest edition of her book on the many ways to fight back against this insidious disease.

Much has changed in the world of multiple sclerosis since 1995, the biggest transformation being the introduction of various drug therapies. Multiple sclerosis is now big business, and drug therapy is essentially the only type of treatment option that is discussed by neurologists and national MS societies. Unfortunately, the drugs have a modest effect at best and only slightly slow progression for most. They also come with a host of semi-toxic side effects.

A person with MS should not rely solely on one of the current drug therapies to ensure they will not progress to severe disabilities. It is fine to use a drug therapy, but it is essential to use additional therapies as well.

In this new edition Judy Graham provides a comprehensive compilation of all the various therapies that have been proposed to help slow MS progression and to relieve symptoms associated with the disease. Notably Judy does not push one therapy over another but objectively describes each one and provides appropriate scientific data and references for many. This is exactly what every person with MS needs in order to make an informed decision as to what therapies exist, which might be worth trying, and which ones might be tried first.

Often experiential accounts are provided with the description of the therapies, and these are always enlightening. I have always believed that if one person with MS has found value in a therapy then there is a chance it may well help another person who tries it. In most cases, one has much to gain and little to lose in trying the various therapies that Judy has chosen to include.

There is no doubt that this book is by far the most comprehensive, objective, and scientifically sound overview of all the options a person with MS has to help keep the MS disease process well controlled.

Judy has done all persons with MS a great service by taking the time and energy to write such a wonderful book. I have no doubt it will help innumerable people lead healthier, much more satisfying lives than if they only listen to what their neurologist has to offer.

Thanks, Judy. Your iconic status remains intact.

ASHTON EMBRY, PH.D.

Ashton Embry, Ph.D., a research scientist for more than forty years, plunged into the scientific literature on MS following his son's diagnosis. Together with his wife and a group of others affected by MS, Embry founded the charity DIRECT-MS to make the information he discovered freely available to all those in need of it. Their website, www.direct-ms.org, provides reliable, science-based information on the role that nutritional factors play in MS. Today, Embry's son, Matt, is in excellent health with no MS symptoms.

Preface to the
New Edition

I WAS DIAGNOSED with multiple sclerosis (MS) in 1974 at age twenty-six, and I am writing this in 2010—thirty-six years later and sixty-three years old! During the intervening years I have had a full-time career as a TV producer, radio broadcaster, and print journalist. I also raised a wonderful son, Pascal. For the past ten years, I have been editing a progressive magazine on MS called *New Pathways,* published in the United Kingdom by the Multiple Sclerosis Resource Centre.

Back then I didn't think I would last this long, let alone still be walking and working hard. Indeed, thirty-five years is the average life expectancy of someone who has been diagnosed with MS, yet here I am, far from dead.

Perhaps it is a testament to the many things I've been doing—watching my diet, taking nutritional supplements, avoiding foods to which I have intolerance, practicing Pilates, and being treated with many complementary therapies.

In those thirty-six years, an enormous amount has happened in the self-help management of MS, and this book reflects those many changes. In the 1970s, the emphasis in MS healing was very much on fats and oils, and while fats are still important, other things have since emerged in the natural treatment of MS: food sensitivities; the Best Bet Diet (BBD); Dr. Wahls's

Brain Nutrient Diet; the importance of vitamin D, antioxidants, and other nutrients; exercise; detox; and also dealing with emotional pain.

In that same period of time, some of the people who inspired me have died, some of the charity groups have morphed into new entities, and new ones have emerged. A new group, informally known as The Best Bet Diet group, sprang up thanks to Ashton Embry, Ph.D., whose son was diagnosed with MS. Embry, a Canadian geologist, did extensive research of the medical literature and came up with scientific data to support a particular treatment for MS. This methodology was used to treat his son, Matt, who has been in good health ever since. Embry has written many excellent essays about MS, which can be found at www.msrc.co.uk or www.direct-ms.org.

Each MS "guru" who has come along has had firm ideas about how to self-manage MS, and each has disagreed to some extent with the others, emphasizing some unique angle, such as a particular diet, detox, or emotional healing.

However, this book is an ecumenical church and takes a wide overview of all possible solutions. No one has suggested that anything in this book constitutes a cure, but you'll find many suggestions that may help you to improve on several levels. There's no risk of harm, and a great potential for benefit.

This book also provides information about specific exciting products that have been personally tried and tested by people with MS, including me. However, even though we name particular brands of products, there are always other brands and options available, and readers are advised to do their own additional research.

The non-drug approach to MS is still derided by most neurologists, who tend to say, "There's no scientific evidence; don't waste your time and money." However, there is plenty of scientific evidence and you'll find references to this inserted throughout the book. Interestingly, when physicians themselves get MS, they are as likely to turn to the health alternatives described here as to disease-modifying drugs.

I'm also heartened by the increasing number of neurologists who support their MS patients who do well with the techniques described in this book. They offer encouragement by saying, "Whatever you're doing, carry on doing it!"

❧ GETTING BETTER AND NOT WORSE

Total recovery from MS is a lofty aim, and I take my hat off to those who achieve it. Recovery may be the ultimate goal, but many people diagnosed with MS would be quite happy to stabilize their condition and improve their health, rather than have it deteriorate. The intention of this book is to assist anyone with MS in being as healthy and stable as possible.

Recovering from MS, or at least improving and not getting worse, *has* been achieved by many MS sufferers, including such high-profile people as Ann Boroch; Ann Sawyer; Judith Bachrach; Sue Ellen Dickinson; Montel Williams; Gina Kopera, M.H.; Professor George Jelinek; Terry Wahls, M.D.; Dermot O'Connor; and, the now late, Roger MacDougall. There are also countless ordinary people who have gotten better, rather than worse, by following this kind of self-help program. Not all have totally recovered from MS, but they are able to lead productive, useful, "normal" lives.

We can say with confidence that there *are* ways to control, or manage, the disease. There is a huge amount of agreement worldwide on the effectiveness of a holistic approach, and I can personally attest to it. Some of these therapies, then, probably deserve to be called "treatment" for MS.

❧ MY STORY

My first symptoms started when I was about nineteen, or earlier. By the time my MS was diagnosed at the age of twenty-six, I had a range of typical MS symptoms: My feet and legs were often like blocks of ice or felt like cotton wool or Jell-O. I sometimes went numb along my left hand and arm, all the way up my face. At other times both hands tingled and were weak, I had tight banding around my middle, and electric shocks jolted me when I moved my neck. Sometimes my walking was horribly stiff and I had to hold on to walls and furniture to keep my balance when crossing a room.

I remember sometimes coming home from work and collapsing on the sofa, not knowing why I felt so lifeless. After one nightmarish day shooting on location for a TV documentary (I was working as a researcher in BBC Television at the time), I was faced with a flight of stairs that had no handrails, and I knew the only way I could possibly get down them would be on my bottom or on someone's arm.

Thirty-six years later, I still have MS symptoms, but not very badly, and many people who meet me wouldn't even know I have the illness. But I can't wear high-heeled shoes, can't run, and use a mobility scooter for long distances or shopping at the mall. Even so, after thirty-six years, many people with MS would be quite happy to be as mildly disabled as I remain.

So what have I done to help control my MS? Every four months I see a nutritional doctor (Dr. Georges Mouton) who checks me for food sensitivities, measures my body's biochemistry, and prescribes supplements specially formulated for my particular case. I have given up eating eggs, dairy, bananas, and chocolate, and I try to go easy on sugar.

Over the years I have been on (and off) the Best Bet Diet, and always feel better when I'm on it. I have also incorporated some of the elements of Terry Wahls's diet, such as eating more kale, cabbage, and salad greens.

I have been taking evening primrose oil and fish oil capsules every day since 1974, plus a variety of vitamin and mineral supplements (for the full list, see chapter 8). I have also recently started taking the nutrients—both in food and supplements—recommended by Dr. Terry Wahls's Brain Nutrient Diet.

I take a Pilates class once a week and also practice at home, and I'm convinced that sticking to a regular exercise program—and stopping before I get tired—is beneficial in terms of fitness, strength, suppleness, muscle tone, and increased stamina. In the past, I had a course of hyperbaric oxygen, which gave me a boost of energy. For much of the time since my diagnosis I've been treated by an acupuncturist, who also administers reflexology. I have seen an osteopath and a homeopath, have had deep massage treatments, and currently have shiatsu massage every Friday.

I think there can be no doubt (although some neurologists might disagree) that my high-level functioning can be credited to these various programs and treatments.

Acknowledgments

THIS BOOK COULD NOT HAVE BEEN WRITTEN without the help of a great many people. Very little in it is original material—I have simply gathered into one place a number of various bits and pieces researched and written by others about the management of MS. To credit all of those people would fill several pages. Many doctors—both M.D. and Ph.D.—have written papers and books of their own, or given verbal advice. Others, such as Ashton Embry, Ph.D., offer goldmines of information on their websites, listed in the Resources chapter at the back of the book.

Personal thanks are due to Professor Michael Crawford, the late Professor Roy Swank, Professor E. J. Field, the late Dr. David F. Horrobin, Dr. Jurgen Mertin, Dr. John Mansfield, Dr. Patrick Kingsley, Dr. Tom Gilhooly, Dr. Bob Lawrence, Professor George Jelinek, Ashton Embry, Ph.D., and Dr. Terry Wahls, most of whom I have had the privilege to meet or otherwise connect with personally. Two enlightened dentists also belong on this list—Drs. Vicky Lee and Jack Levenson.

People with MS who have inspired me by their own personal recovery include the late Roger MacDougall, Dubliner Dermot O'Connor, Professor George Jelinek from Australia, Terry Wahls, M.D., Sue Ellen Dickinson, and Gina Kopera, M.H.

I would also like to thank Ann D. Sawyer and Judith E. Bachrach, authors of *The MS Recovery Diet,* for picking up the ball and running with it so brilliantly after reading the first edition of this book in the 1980s.

I also thank the U.K. Multiple Sclerosis Resource Centre (www .msrc.co.uk) for having such an excellent and informative website, and its predecessor, Action for Research into Multiple Sclerosis, for initiating some of the research mentioned.

I also wish to extend my gratitude to the many people with MS who so kindly allowed me to use their stories.* Nearly all of these first appeared in *New Pathways,* the magazine I edit, which is published by the Multiple Sclerosis Resource Centre. I wish to thank the MSRC and Helen Yates, its chief executive, in particular, for supporting me in writing this book.

I would also like to thank my Pilates teachers, especially Clare Lennard and Adina Thomas, for teaching me so much and helping to keep my body toned; my shiatsu practitioner Michael Rose, who is a genius at what he does; and all the holistic practitioners I have seen over the years, all of whom have helped me, including Functional Medicine expert Dr. Georges Mouton and the Belgian laboratory that routinely tests my blood and urine, Dr. Patrick Kingsley, Dr. Tamara Voronina, and osteopath/ reflexologist/acupuncturist Byron Spiers.

Also, many thanks to my editors, Jamaica Burns and Abigail Lewis, for knocking this completely revised and expanded edition into shape.

---

*Names have been changed in some instances.

PART ONE

Understanding MS

1

MS Can Be Controlled

IF YOU ARE READING THIS, chances are your life is affected by MS in some way. Maybe you've been told you have MS, or perhaps someone close to you has it. The good news is that MS can be controlled. Far from being all doom and gloom, the future can be joyous and productive.

A natural, drug-free way of self-treating is to use an all-embracing approach covering every aspect of your life and lifestyle—food, exercise, thoughts, and emotions. In brief, it involves:

- Getting tested for food sensitivities and giving up the offending foods
- Dealing with gut problems, such as leaky gut and candida
- Switching to the Best Bet Diet
- Eating a diet high in nutrients for the brain
- Taking many nutritional supplements—vitamins, minerals, trace elements, antioxidants, amino acids, enzymes, and essential fatty acids
- Exercising regularly
- Cleansing your body of environmental toxins
- De-stressing and rebalancing your life, and dealing with emotional and psychological hurts
- Avoiding fatigue, resting as needed, and getting sufficient sleep
- Shifting your thought patterns from negative to positive and making a decision to live life to the fullest

- Having satisfying relationships
- Maintaining your self-esteem

It may also mean receiving some complementary treatments, such as acu-puncture, ayurveda, reflexology, shiatsu, or Reiki, all of which have been shown to help MS. You'll find alphabetized information in chapter 13.

THE BEST TIME TO START IS NOW

The earlier you start this program, the better. Studies have shown that the people who benefit most from this self-help regimen are those who have been recently diagnosed. Don't wait until you get worse before you decide to try this program. Use it as an insurance policy to help prevent you from getting worse.

However, all is not lost if your illness has progressed. Some people have reversed their MS symptoms several years after diagnosis, and even in the secondary progressive stage of the disease.

It is not a cure, nor is it recognized as a treatment by the medical establishment (although there are elements in it that have had so much, and such good, scientific research that they deserve to be recognized as treatments for MS). This program can help you manage your illness. It gives you an opportunity to enjoy life fully—even with MS.

PRESCRIPTION MEDICATION

Most neurologists wonder why anyone would want to go on such a rigor-ous program as this when there are drugs to treat MS. Part of the answer is that the pharmaceuticals that have been used so far—the "disease-modifying" drugs—can help somewhat in reducing relapses but can't stop disease progression. Also, some people don't like having injections or the flu-like side effects of some of these drugs. Also, we don't really know the long-term effects of these drugs.

The next generation of drugs includes Tysabri, which is used to slow the progression of aggressive MS and is usually only prescribed for severe cases. Some people definitely do benefit from this drug. However, as of November 2009, there had been twenty-four cases of a brain infection called progressive multifocal leukoencephalopathy (PML) and four subsequent deaths linked to Tysabri. Because of this, Tysabri was temporarily withdrawn from the market in 2005, but was reintroduced in July 2006 with stricter safety warnings.

In the pipeline are "immune modulating" drugs, such as alemtuzumab (Campath), which has had dramatically good results in trials, but also carries risks. It has been shown to stop MS in its tracks and is hailed as the most effective treatment yet for early relapsing/remitting MS, reducing attacks by 74 percent, reducing sustained disability by 71 percent, and in many cases restoring lost function. However, any benefits need to be weighed against the associated risks; doctors are hesitant to prescribe this drug except in patients in the early stages of the disease, not yet disabled, who have frequent bad attacks.

During the trials for this drug, three patients contracted a condition called idiopathic thrombocytopenic purpura, in which low blood platelet counts can lead to abnormal bleeding. This was fatal in one case. Also, nearly a quarter of the patients on alemtuzumab suffered from a thyroid autoimmune condition, with a very high prevalence of Graves' disease. In addition, because alemtuzumab suppresses the immune system by seriously depleting white blood cells called T-lymphocytes, vital for fighting infection, patients on this drug have an increased risk of serious bacterial, fungal, and viral infections.

All pharmaceutical drugs have side effects, and you have to weigh whether taking them is worth it; the choice is yours. Some people do both—they take drugs for MS *and* follow this book's management program. However, one of the benefits of the program outlined in this book is the treatments do not have unpleasant side effects. Also, unlike many of the drugs for MS, they are intended to do the exact opposite of suppressing the immune system; they are designed to actually boost, or normalize, the immune system.

As to taking certain drugs for specific MS symptoms, such as pain or bladder urgency, that, again, is up to you. Many people with MS favor a natural approach to healing, yet swear by certain drugs for specific individual symptoms.

Personally, I have never taken any disease-modifying or immune suppressant drugs to treat my MS. On the other hand, I do take ibuprofen for pain and HRT for estrogen (see chapter 15, Hormones and MS), and I would not be opposed to taking tolterodine (Detrol or Detrusitol) or Botox injections if my bladder were to worsen.

ᐒ A DARK CLOUD LIFTS

Many people with MS have successfully managed to control or even recover from MS by using techniques described in this book. When you see how effective these strategies can be, a great dark cloud lifts from your shoulders as you realize that MS doesn't have to be a life sentence, or a death sentence.

However, care is needed. This is *not* a cure, it is an ongoing, life-long treatment. If you go back to your old diet, lifestyle, and negative thought patterns, MS is likely to come back. The treatments, or management programs, may not all have been rigorously tested by scientific method, but there are enough studies to suggest strongly that the progression of MS can be slowed, halted, or even reversed. In addition to the scientific studies, there is also a huge amount of anecdotal evidence.

At the very least, this book suggests healthier ways to live your life.

2

What Exactly Is MS?

IF YOU KNOW what is happening in MS, it's easier to understand why the self-help management program is relevant.

MS is described as an autoimmune, degenerative disease. The prevailing wisdom is that the body mistakenly attacks part of itself as if it were a foreign body. In MS, the myelin sheath—the insulating layer that protects the nerves—is targeted and attacked by rogue cells in the immune system.

ROGUE T CELLS

In a healthy immune system, white blood cells called lymphocytes are the crack troops that defend the body against attack from foreign invaders. Lymphocytes are made up of three types of cells: T cells, B cells, and NK (natural killer) cells.

Receptors on T cells are normally able to differentiate between antigens—those invaders that cause your body to produce antibodies, such as bacteria or viruses—and your own body. Once an antigen is identified, certain T cells, called helper T cells, trigger the B cells to release those antibodies. These are molecules designed to attach to, and destroy, the chosen target antigen, or foreign body.

In MS, the T cells in the immune system have a hard time distinguishing between a foreign invader and self. The T cells mistake the body's own myelin as foreign and target it in the same way they would target a bacteria or virus.

In response, the deranged T cells set off a cascade of immune events, including the release of B lymphocytes, to rid the body of the perceived threat. These B lymphocytes fire off antibodies, and this destructive process perpetuates through a cascading series of events in which the B and T cells continue to interact, creating numerous different self-antigens.

Once the lymphocytes have launched a response to an antigen, they also release masses of other white blood cells to gather at the injured or infected site. The major players in this destructive process are called leukocytes, in particular, ones called cytokines. When too many are produced, it causes inflammation and damage.

∿ MALFUNCTIONING NK CELLS

In September 2009, scientists at the prestigious Imperial College, University of London, published a paper in which they put forward the hypothesis that MS (among other diseases) is caused by malfunctioning NK cells that turn on the body, attacking healthy cells.

They also identified the master gene—E4bp4—that causes blood stem cells to turn into natural killer cells; and they have succeeded in putting this gene out of action in a mouse model. This breakthrough should help solve the mystery of NK cells in diseases such as MS. Clarifying NK cells' role could lead to new ways of treating MS and other similar conditions.

∿ MYELIN

Myelin is an insulating material that wraps many times around nerve fibers to form what looks a bit like a Swiss roll.

The function of myelin is similar to that of insulating material surrounding an electrical cable—it allows impulses to travel along the cable. Myelin helps messages to be delivered quickly and smoothly between the brain and various parts of the body.

Myelin Damage and MS

If myelin gets damaged, the nerve signals travel more slowly, get distorted, follow the wrong path, or don't get properly transmitted.

When myelin is attacked, there is inflammation that leaves a scar, or sclerosis (from the Greek word *skleros*, for hard). Several attacks leave multiple scars, or multiple sclerosis, and increasing disability.

The usual course of MS is to get progressively worse. In the later stages of MS both the axons (nerve fibers) and the cells that make myelin (oligodendrocytes) are damaged by the MS disease process, causing progressive disability. Other nerve cells may also be involved.

Myelin Can Regenerate

Whatever the reason or reasons for myelin breaking down, the heartening thing to know is that it can regenerate. Until the mid 1990s it was thought that myelin could not regenerate, but now there has been sufficient research to show that it can. Although myelin is a relatively stable structure, old components break down and—under the right circumstances—are replaced with newly formed components.

This means that some of the damage sustained by the nervous system is, in principle, capable of recovery. It may be that MS plaque sites do not represent permanent damage, but are areas in which damaged tissues are attempting self-repair. The challenge is to know exactly what conditions support that recovery.

Some of the therapies featured in this book, alone or in combination, may provide the conditions that aid myelin regeneration. Researchers have long said that if only they could find out what makes myelin regenerate, they could solve the puzzle of MS, and intensive research continues in this area. (In fact, some of the new generation of drugs for MS aim to regenerate myelin.)

VASCULAR ABNORMALITIES—CHRONIC CEREBROSPINAL VENOUS INSUFFICIENCY

Recently, an Italian vascular surgeon named Paolo Zamboni discovered that every single MS patient he saw had an abnormality in the veins from the brain to the heart. Dr. Zamboni called this defect chronic cerebrospinal venous insufficiency (CCSVI).

CCSVI is a condition in which certain veins in the head and neck become narrowed. This narrowing restricts the normal outflow of blood from the brain, causing alterations in the blood flow within the brain and a reflux of blood back into the brain—something that eventually causes injury to brain tissue and degeneration of neurons.

Blood that refluxes into the brain contains iron and, according to

Zamboni, many neurologists consider iron dangerous because it is linked to neurodegeneration, MS progression, and disability. CCSVI was found to be strongly associated with MS, increasing the risk of developing MS by forty-three fold. CCSVI appears to be peculiar to MS and has not been found in other neurodegenerative conditions. At the time of writing, further research into CCSVI and MS was being carried out at the University of Buffalo, the State University of New York. Principal investigator on the study, Robert Zivadinov, M.D., Ph.D., said: "If we can prove our hypothesis, that cerebrospinal venous insufficiency is the underlying cause of MS, it is going to change the face of how we understand MS." (See chapter 14, page 208, for further information on this condition.)

⤲ IS MS JUST A NEUROLOGICAL DISEASE?

MS is classified as a neurological disease, mainly affecting the nervous system, which is the brain and spinal cord. But it also affects the immune system, the digestive system, and the vascular system.

From an allopathic medical perspective, the elements that comprise MS are ever more complex. However, practitioners of alternative medicine do not see things in the same way at all. Their holistic viewpoint doesn't fragment the body into bits and systems, but considers the whole organism—body and mind—as one entity.

Holistic practitioners see each person as an individual, and are willing to try therapies that haven't been submitted to carefully controlled trials. Rather than applying a particular disease label, each patient's unique needs are addressed.

There is a huge amount of anecdotal evidence that presents a very hopeful picture for treating MS, and it's discouraging to see it dismissed so disparagingly by most orthodox doctors. Medical doctors are quite happy to use anecdotal evidence when it suits them, and there's a good argument to be made for listening to anecdotal evidence in regard to MS.

⤲ SIGNS AND SYMPTOMS OF MS

Symptoms may include any or all of the following, and generally are worse during an attack.

- Tingling, prickling, or a sensation of pins and needles anywhere in the body
- Numbness—you can hardly feel a needle stuck in your skin
- Heavy legs, as if wearing thick boots and trudging through mud
- Difficulty walking
- Difficulty using arms and hands
- Weakness in any limb
- Paralysis—you cannot move a limb
- Dragging either foot, or dropped foot, where you have difficulty lifting a foot off the floor
- Overwhelming fatigue
- Poor coordination
- Poor balance
- Loss of sensation or distorted sensation anywhere in the body. Feeling as though the body is made of cotton wool, rubber, or Jell-O
- Electric shock sensations on lowering the head
- Clumsiness—often dropping things
- Double or blurred vision, or temporary blindness in an eye
- Slurred speech
- Urgency to urinate and/or frequency, or hesitancy in passing urine; incontinence
- Fecal incontinence
- Constipation
- A feeling of tight bands around the trunk or lower limbs (the "MS hug"), which can be itchy
- Pain anywhere
- Vertigo—dizziness; the room spins
- Vomiting
- Tremors in the hands and arms
- Spasticity—tight, stiff limbs
- A feeling of extreme cold, like frostbite, in the extremities; or the opposite—burning feet
- Abnormal sensitivity to heat and cold
- Feeling like a wet rag in humid weather
- Abnormal sensitivity to light

- Cognitive impairment, from mild to severe, with short-term memory problems
- Emotional volatility—get upset and cry easily

TYPES OF MS

There are two major types of MS. The most common is relapsing/remitting, which is characterized by symptoms that flare up (an attack, or relapse), followed by a period of remission during which the person's condition returns to what it was, or slightly worse than it was, before the attack. Attacks, also known as relapses, can range from mild—you're able to carry on daily activities without hindrance—to so severe that you must be hospitalized. Attacks can involve just one symptom or several. Scientists are trying to discover what triggers the switch into remission, which some believe may be a critical link in the treatment of MS.

In the second type, progressive MS, there are no clear-cut attacks and the person just gets progressively worse. Within this category are primary progressive—the person has never been subject to attacks; and secondary progressive—the person first develops relapsing/remitting MS, but after a certain period it becomes progressive. This latter form is the most common course.

Although there are rare cases of a galloping form of the severest type of MS, in which the person degenerates rapidly and dies within a few years, sometimes a person will have just one attack of MS and never have another. Those who don't get worse are said to have a "benign" course, though it may become less benign some years later. How you are at the end of your first five years is sometimes used as a predictor for what is likely to happen later in the course of the disease.

WHO GETS MS?

MS mostly affects young adults between the ages of twenty and forty, but it is increasingly being diagnosed in children younger than sixteen, and it's not uncommon for people in their fifties and sixties to get MS. The mean age for a first attack of MS is about thirty. It is almost twice as common in women as in men.

MS is twenty times more common in northern Europe and America than in Africa. The further from the equator, the higher the incidence. It is practically unknown in equatorial countries.

Those who get MS invariably have a genetic predisposition. There also has to be one or more environmental triggers.

Studies show that, in adult MS, the risk of MS is determined by exposure to an environmental factor or factors during or before adolescence. People who emigrate before the age of fifteen run the same risk of getting MS as the local inhabitants of the place to which they move. (See chapter 3 for more about environmental factors.)

3

Possible Causes of MS

IT'S HELPFUL TO HAVE AN IDEA of the possible causes of MS in order to treat it. Orthodox neurologists generally say that MS is caused by an unknown environmental agent interacting with genetic predisposition. However, common sense suggests the likelihood that MS has more than one cause, with one or several environmental factors interacting with genes.

It is also possible that the exact same causes don't apply to everyone with MS. For example, although the Epstein-Barr virus, which causes infectious mononucleosis (commonly known as mono, or glandular fever), can precipitate MS, not everyone with MS has been infected with it.

Different people have different views on what the various causes of MS might be. Each of the predominant theories is dealt with more thoroughly later in this chapter. This list includes:

- Genetic predisposition
- Environmental factors: lack of sunlight (and therefore lack of vitamin D), geographical distribution
- Infection: viral, bacterial, or parasitic
- Oxidative stress
- Dietary factors: modern diet—gluten and dairy, food sensitivities, nutrient deficiencies
- Digestive problems: leaky gut and candida, anomalous fat processing, inability to handle saturated fats

- Problematic proteins and molecular mimicry
- Chronic cerebrospinal venous insufficiency (CCSVI)
- Breach of the blood-brain barrier
- Hormones and gender
- Toxic overload, including mercury poisoning
- Physical or emotional stress, or negative mindset
- Childhood events

☙ GENETIC PREDISPOSITION

Specific genes are definitely implicated in MS. A cluster of genes on chromosome 6 plays a significant role in multiple sclerosis, according to the most complete genetic study to date.[1] The genes pinpointed on chromosome 6 are known as "major histocompatibility complex" genes. One particular gene on chromosome 6, known as HLA-DRB1*1501, indicates heightened risk. There is also a gene—HLA-DRB*14—which decreases risk for MS. Other genes associated with susceptibility to MS include those on chromosomes 5q33, 17q23, and 19p13. There are additional gene indicators for those who contract MS, and specific genes may also determine the severity of the disease.

You are more likely to get MS if it runs in your family; however, these genes implicated in MS are also common in the general population and their presence doesn't necessarily indicate that someone will get MS. Countless healthy people are walking around with the suspect genes, but do not have MS and will never get it. Other factors must be involved.

☙ ENVIRONMENTAL FACTORS

You can't do anything to change the genes you were born with, but you can sometimes do things to change the environmental and lifestyle factors that interact with genetic factors to cause MS. That's why this book focuses on the things you *can* do something about, rather than those you can't.

Lack of Sunlight (and Vitamin D!)

More and more evidence is pointing to vitamin D deficiency as a likely cause of MS. Vitamin D primarily comes from sunlight, which may explain why MS is so prevalent in the sun-deprived latitudes of Scotland, Canada, and Norway, whereas in tropical countries MS is virtually unknown.[2] (More information under Epidemiology—Geographical Distribution, below.)

Professor George Ebers, a world-renowned epidemiologist at Oxford University, is convinced that lack of vitamin D is an environmental factor in MS. Ashton Embry goes so far as to say that MS is a disease of vitamin D deficiency. (See chapter 9 for more on Vitamin D.)

Epidemiology—Geographical Distribution of MS

One of the most marked features of MS is its geographical distribution. It is five times more prevalent in northern latitudes and almost unknown in tropical areas. Research increasingly indicates this may have to do with how much vitamin D a population gets from sunlight.

Scotland has the highest rate of MS in the world. The incidence of MS varies sharply within certain countries, partly depending on latitude. For example, in Canada, the incidence varies from a high of 340 cases for every 100,000 people in the Prairies to a low of 180 cases per 100,000 in Quebec, according to a 2005 study by researchers at the University of Calgary.[3]

There are also sharp differences in the United States: The prevalence of MS is lowest in the southern and highest in the northern states. For example, in Texas, at a latitude of 33°30' N, the prevalence is low at 47.2 cases for every 100,000 people. In the Missouri area, at 39°07' N, the rate is intermediate at 86.3 cases per 100,000. In Ohio, at 41°24' N, the prevalence is high at 109.5 cases per 100,000.[4]

Although the variations in incidence may have to do with the varying amounts of vitamin D from sunlight, geography also determines what kinds of food people eat.[5] Where MS is most prevalent, people consume considerable amounts of dairy products. In places where MS occurrence is lowest, the general diet consists of more fish and vegetable oils. The difference between an area of high MS and low MS can be as little as a few miles. Some of the starkest contrasts in MS occurrence are within Norway, comparing inland dairy farming areas (where MS is high) with coastal fishing areas (where MS is low).

Similarly, in some of the Scottish islands, the incidence of MS can vary from very high to very low, according to the primary diet of the local people. Again, it's elevated in areas of dairy farming and low in fishing areas.

One of the first doctors to look at the world map of MS was neurologist Roy Swank, a professor at the Oregon Health & Science University in Portland. Swank noticed that the amount of saturated fat in the typical American diet was rising dramatically, due to several factors: improvements in the processing of dairy foods; advanced techniques for fattening beef, providing gourmands with coveted marbling of their beef and a better income for stock farmers; and hydrogenation of vegetable oils, changing them from their natural states into saturated fat margarines.

As the consumption of saturated fat increased, so, too, did the incidence of certain diseases, particularly multiple sclerosis, heart disease, and stroke. A link between a high fat diet and these diseases seemed probable, and when Swank observed this correlation, he devised his now-famous MS Diet in 1948.

During the Second World War, fat consumption in occupied Norway fell by 50 percent, due to food shortages. At the same time, there were significant reductions in death rates from heart attacks and in the incidence of multiple sclerosis. After the war, however, as fat intake went back up, so did the rates of heart disease and MS.

✑ INFECTION

Multiple Sclerosis is associated with viral infections, especially the Epstein-Barr virus (which causes infectious mononucleosis), human herpes virus 6, herpes simplex, varicella zoster (causes chicken pox), and retroviruses. A new theory links canine distemper virus and MS. Bacterial infections include *Chlamydia pneumoniae*. Some people believe that parasites are a cause of MS. Any of these can infect the body from early childhood onward.

- *Epstein-Barr virus.* The Epstein-Barr virus causes infectious mononucleosis. It is very common for people with MS to have had such a childhood infection, also known as mono, or glandular fever. This infection can rob the body of essential nutrients, such as zinc and essential fatty acids, and seriously upset the immune system so that it cannot tell the difference between self and non-self.

- *Herpes.* Human herpes virus 6 (HHV-6), human herpes virus 7, human herpes virus 8, and herpes simplex viruses 1 and 2 have all been linked to MS. Several studies have found higher levels of the human herpes viruses in MS patients than in controls and also evidence of active herpes infection more often than in controls. Some think the HHV-6 virus may be a cause of MS but this is disputed by others. A theory has also been put forth that MS may be a sexually transmitted disease. Herpes simplex virus 2 (HSV-2) is the strain that causes genital herpes.

- *Varicella-zoster virus.* Chickenpox is caused by the varicella-zoster virus (VZV), and along with childhood eczema, it has been linked with later MS. Mexican researchers found that the link between VZV infection and MS was particularly strong among people with the relapsing/remitting forms of MS.[6] In a controlled study of nearly three hundred people, VZV infection was found in 42 percent of controls, but in 66 percent of people with MS. People with relapsing/remitting MS had four times the risk of VZV infection, and those with secondary progressive MS had a threefold increase in risk, when compared with control patients. Overall, patients with a history of VZV infection had triple the risk of MS.

- *Retroviruses.* Some retroviruses are also implicated in MS. Retroviruses are viruses that turn their RNA into DNA for integration into the host's genome and can be passed to the next generation and persist for long periods in the host's genome. However, they are generally only infectious for a short time.

- *Canine distemper virus.* A link between the canine distemper virus and MS was put forward by Dr. J. A. Lincoln and his associates in the August 2008 issue of *Neurologic Clinics*. Adult exposure to canine distemper virus and also the Epstein Barr virus could lead to an immune response, which could subsequently cause symptoms of MS.[7]

- *Chlamydia pneumoniae.* Another school of thought points the finger at this bacterial infection (see page 200). In 2002, researchers at the Vanderbilt School of Medicine in Nashville, Tennessee, found a specific type of bacterium—*Chlamydia pneumoniae*—in each of the thirty-seven MS patients they studied. A relationship between risk for multiple sclerosis and infection with Chlamydia pneumoniae was also shown in a study published in the March 2003 issue of *Epidemiology*.[8] In that study, Harvard researcher Kassandra Munger found a 70 percent increased incidence of multiple sclerosis in women who tested positive for the presence of C. pneumoniae antibodies.

- *Parasites.* The late Dr. Hulda Clark, author of *The Cure for All Diseases,* believed that MS is caused by any of the four common fluke parasites reaching the brain or spinal cord and attempting to multiply there. These parasites can come from undercooked meat, other people, and pets. Toxic substances, such as the solvents xylene and toluene, may accumulate in the brain, attracting parasites. Clark said that in every MS case she saw, there was evidence of the Shigella bacteria, which comes from dairy products, in the brain and spinal cord. Clark believed parasites can be killed using a device she invented called the Zapper. (For more information, see page 290.)

⟡ OXIDATIVE STRESS

Leading American nutritional doctor Ray Strand thinks that oxidative stress is the cause of MS. Oxidative stress occurs when the body has insufficient antioxidants to neutralize the free radicals (unstable molecules that create abnormal cells) that result primarily from "bad" fat metabolism and environmental pollution. Several studies support this thesis. Strand, who sees many MS patients in his clinic, reports, "I see the most amazing results using antioxidants."

Strand's theory about MS concurs that the immune system attacks the myelin sheath around the nerve and causes an inflammatory response. However, he believes it is actually the oxidative stress caused by this inflammatory response that damages the myelin sheath. A tremendous number of harmful free radicals are being produced.

Oxidative stress plays an important role in the progression of neurodegenerative and age-related diseases, causing damage to proteins, DNA, and lipids. Since Strand believes that oxidative stress is the cause of multiple sclerosis, he recommends putting patients on powerful antioxidants as soon after diagnosis as possible. (His website is www.raystrand.com.)

Ashton Embry agrees that oxidation is a key component of inflammation and damage to the myelin. People with MS have low levels of antioxidants and increased oxidative stress, which is more apparent during attacks.

❧ DIETARY FACTORS

Some theorists believe that "wrong diet" is the main cause of MS and its progression, noting that diet correlates to the geographic distribution of MS around the world. Wrong diet refers to damaging foods and beverages, usually consumed over a long period of time. The typical modern Western diet—high in refined sugar, refined carbohydrates, carbonated drinks, saturated fat, and trans-fats—paves the way for a host of chronic diseases. But a wrong diet may also include foods that are accepted by most people as perfectly healthy, but which are harmful to your particular body.

Modern Diet—Gluten and Dairy

One strong theory is that human beings are not designed to eat certain foods, such as gluten grains (found in wheat, barley, and rye) and dairy, which were introduced relatively recently into our diets, compliments of modern agriculture. Perhaps we would be healthier on a Stone Age or Paleolithic diet. Without a doubt, MS is most common in places where gluten grains, dairy, sugar, and a large amount of saturated and trans-fats are a major part of the diet.

Food Sensitivities

It is very common for an individual with MS to have food sensitivities. The theory is that these food sensitivities trigger the immune system to attack the body in an autoimmune response.

Food sensitivities can be to absolutely anything, no matter how nutritious, so you're just as likely to have an immune reaction to broccoli, bell peppers, bananas, or eggs as to milk, wheat, or soy. However, someone else with MS may be fine with these, but react to kiwi, eggs, or lemons, for example.

Food sensitivities are a very individual thing, so it's important to determine which foods cause a reaction in your particular body. There are various tests to detect and measure food sensitivities. Food sensitivities may be a cause, as well as an effect, of leaky gut (see below).

Nutrient Deficiencies

Sometimes nutrient deficiencies occur, either because a person isn't eating a proper diet, or because the nutrients aren't being properly absorbed from the gut, due to leaky gut syndrome. These nutrients can cover a broad spectrum.

∽ DIGESTIVE PROBLEMS

Leaky Gut and Candida

In the condition known as leaky gut, the gut wall is perforated by the long spiky tentacles of the *Candida albicans* fungus, exacerbated by the puncturing effects of certain food sensitivities, such as gluten. The lining becomes like a sieve, allowing intact food proteins into the bloodstream where they are perceived as foreign invaders, thus activating the immune system. Leaky gut means nutrients are not absorbed properly, triggering a cascade of negative consequences.

People who have MS often experience gut disorders. Possible explanations include:

- Certain foods, gluten grains in particular, can damage the lining of the gut, leading to leaky gut.
- Food sensitivities can cause the gut to become irritated.
- Overuse of antibiotics and other drugs to treat infections can cause dysbiosis in the gut, where unhealthy intestinal flora outnumber the healthy flora (probiotics), leading to the fungal condition candidiasis. This is very common in MS.
- Overgrowth of *Candida albicans,* whether caused by wrong diet, drugs, or both, can lead to leaky gut, otherwise known as intestinal permeability.

Anomalous Fat Processing

The theory of an inborn mishandling of essential fatty acids, called "Thompson's anomaly," was put forward by British scientist R. H. S. Thompson in the 1960s.[9] The significance of this anomaly is that the conditions are ripe for the development of MS. Because of this mishandling of essential fatty adds, *all* cells in the body are abnormal, and myelin is built in such a weak way that it is prone to degeneration and crumbles like a poorly built wall.

Taking Thompson's work a step further, scientist Professor E. J. Field confirmed that it is not only the red blood cells in people with MS that are subtly different, but also the lymphocytes (white blood cells), which play a part in the body's immune system.[10]

One of the implications of this hypothesis is that certain people—those with anomalous cell membranes lacking in essential fatty acids—have a predisposition to MS. In other words, they are probably born with this abnormality that lends itself to development of MS later in life. Either some "X factor" comes along to bring on the MS in "fertile ground," or the myelin is so flawed that in due course it simply falls apart.

Inability to Handle Saturated Fats

Roy Swank, champion of the low-fat diet, believed that a diet high in saturated fats causes platelets to bunch together, thereby stretching the blood vessel walls. This leads to a loss of integrity of the vessel walls, and in time, toxic materials are able to seep through the blood-brain barrier into the brain. In Swank's theory, MS is primarily due to an unstable blood emulsion from excess intake of fat in susceptible people.[11] This susceptibility might be a defect in the red blood cell membrane or a plasma abnormality.

PROBLEMATIC PROTEINS AND MOLECULAR MIMICRY

According to a hypothesis championed by Ashton Embry, in MS the myelin-sensitive immune cells are activated by fragments of foreign proteins that closely resemble fragments of myelin proteins. In other words, the molecular structure of an alien cell and that of "self" are so similar that the immune cells get confused and respond inappropriately. This is known as "molecular mimicry."

There is some scientific evidence to suggest that food proteins in dairy products, gluten grains, and legumes may be playing a role in the activation of auto-aggressive immune cells in MS. If this is so, then avoiding these foods might help to decrease the activation of myelin-sensitive immune cells, and therefore help to control MS.

Dairy

Immunological studies have shown that protein fragments from milk closely resemble sections of proteins associated with myelin, and that these "mimicking" milk proteins can activate auto-aggressive immune cells that are sensitive to myelin. People with MS have much higher amounts of milk-sensitive T cells than do healthy control subjects. Scientists have shown that when laboratory mice are injected with a milk protein, they get *experimental autoimmune encephalomyelitis (EAE)*, an animal neurological disease that closely resembles MS. So it appears that milk proteins have the potential to activate auto-aggressive immune cells that attack myelin.[12]

Gluten Grains

Other sources of potentially problematic proteins are the grains wheat, rye, and barley, all of which contain a complex mix of proteins known as glutens. An animal study found that EAE-afflicted mice on a gluten-free diet had much less disability than those on a regular diet.[13]

Until there are studies to determine whether or not proteins in gluten grains are "molecular mimics" of myelin proteins, this question will remain open.

Legumes

Another food group suspected of contributing to MS and other autoimmune diseases is legumes, including peas, beans, soybeans, and peanuts. Like gluten and dairy, legumes have protein fragments that closely resemble self-proteins in the pancreas and in joints.

However, no studies have been done on legumes and MS, and Embry cautions, "At this stage of scientific knowledge, we do not know for sure if milk products, gluten grains, and legumes are contributing to the MS disease process by activating auto-aggressive immune cells. All we can say is that there is a reasonable chance that they are. Each person with MS has to weigh the scientific evidence and decide whether or not to take a chance and eat such foods, or play it safe and avoid them until science decides the issue."

∾ CHRONIC CEREBROSPINAL VENOUS INSUFFICIENCY (CCSVI)

Chronic cerebrospinal venous insufficiency (CCSVI), in which blood from the brain and spine has trouble getting back to the heart, may be a cause of MS symptoms. CCSVI is caused by a narrowing of the veins (stenosis) that drain the brain and the spine. Blood takes longer to return to the heart, and it can reflux back into the brain and spine or cause edema and leakage of red blood cells and fluids into the tissues of the brain and spine.

Blood that remains in the brain too long creates a delay in deoxyginated blood leaving the head, causing hypoxia (a lack of oxygen in the brain). Plasma and iron from blood deposited in the brain tissue can also be very damaging, leading to iron and other unwelcome cells crossing the crucial brain-blood barrier (see below). MS *symptoms* may be a result of the narrowing of the primary veins outside the skull. Neurologists at the University of Buffalo are conducting more research into this. At the time of writing, more research was being planned elsewhere in the United States and in Canada, the United Kingdom, and Europe.

∾ BREACH OF THE BLOOD-BRAIN BARRIER

Several researchers working in the field of MS have come to the conclusion that the primary event in MS is the breach of the blood-brain barrier, and is, therefore, the first event that should be stopped. Other events known to occur in MS, such as the breakdown of myelin or rogue macrophages on the rampage, seem to happen only after the blood-brain barrier has been broken.

Normally impenetrable, the breached blood-brain barrier allows toxic substances into the brain, where they can cause damage. This may be due to hypersensitivity to certain foods, weak blood vessel walls, or both. (See also under Physical or Emotional Stress, or Negative Mind-set, page 25.)

Dr. Philip James, a champion of hyperbaric oxygen treatment for MS, believes that fat embolism is responsible for the breach in the blood-brain barrier.[14] Broadly speaking, several theories agree that fat is to blame for damaging vessel walls.

Blood is not supposed to cross over into the brain. Potentially harmful substances carried in the blood must be kept away from the central nervous system. If blood does get across the barrier, it is toxic to nerve tissue.

A breach in the blood-brain barrier is followed by local swelling, breakdown of myelin, an inflammatory macrophage response, and the formation of a central hardened zone of fibrous material, called plaque.

There is now widespread agreement that MS plaques are associated with, and form around, very small veins—or venules—within the central nervous system. These perivenular (in the surrounding connective tissue) plaques form when the blood-brain barrier is breached. There is consensus among neurologists that the blood-brain barrier is breached in MS patients, and new drugs have been designed to address this. Some of the non-drug strategies described in this book, such as taking powerful antioxidant foods and supplements, also aim to stop any breaches in the blood-brain barrier. (See Strengthening the Blood-Brain Barrier in chapter 5, page 43.)

OTHER MECHANISMS POSSIBLY INVOLVED IN MS

Although none of these theories have been proven, there is strong anecdotal support for all of them.

Hormones and Gender

MS occurs almost twice as frequently in women, and MS symptoms can sometimes virtually disappear when a woman becomes pregnant. (See chapter 15 for further information on hormones and MS.)

Toxic Overload

Some people believe that the toxic effects of mercury poisoning are a causal factor in MS. Areas of high MS correspond with areas of high dental caries, which suggests not only that people are eating a lot of sugar, but also that they are likely to have mercury amalgam fillings in their teeth (see chapter 18). The accumulation of airborne toxins, additives in foodstuffs, drugs, and so on may also be a factor.

Physical or Emotional Stress, or Negative Mind-set

Many theorists believe that some emotional or physical trauma triggers clinical symptoms of the disease. Often people with MS say that some devastating event or accident preceded their diagnosis, such as divorce, a car crash, or some other type of accident, particularly one involving a neck injury. Also, negative thought patterns are known to depress the immune system.

Believing that your life is over once you are diagnosed with MS will only lead to depression and lethargy, which can aggravate symptoms and possibly lead to additional problems. Those who give up hope, or make MS the focus of all their energy, may experience many more physical and emotional problems than those who get on with their lives.

There is also some evidence that factors such as trauma or stress can weaken the blood-brain barrier intermittently and thus allow substances in the blood to leak through to the brain (as previously discussed). These factors include:

- Stressful events
- Overdoing things, leading to fatigue
- Fever
- Emotional upsets
- Heat
- Injury—trauma to the body

All events such as these provoke a physiological coping response, which includes the release of adrenaline (epinephrine). This brings about arousal and mobilization of bodily resources, part of which involves an increase in blood supply to the central nervous system.

Childhood Events

Childhood events that have been linked to MS include stress, traumatic experiences, negative attitude, lack of love and joy, lack of physical activity, poor diet with nutritional deficiencies, poor detoxification, medications, vaccinations, intolerance to mother's milk, formula feeding, viruses, bacteria, yeast, parasites, and environmental toxins, including mercury amalgam fillings. (See www.curezone.com for a full explanation of each of these.)

PART TWO

Nutrition for MS

4

Food Sensitivities

FOOD IS A KEY ISSUE in handling MS. For best results you are likely to have to change your diet and exclude foods to which you show sensitivity. You can't plan your diet until you know your sensitivities. These sensitivities trigger your immune system to launch an attack against your own body.

Food sensitivities can be to absolutely anything—however "healthy" the food may be—and are not limited to just the usual suspects in MS, which are gluten grains, dairy, and legumes. In my case, I'm sensitive to eggs, dairy products, bananas, kiwi, broccoli, and chocolate (cocoa). How convenient it would be if everyone with MS suffered from the same food sensitivities, but they don't. You have to find out what foods *you* are sensitive to. It is vital to get yourself properly tested for food sensitivities so you can eliminate the foods that cause you problems.

SYMPTOMS OF FOOD SENSITIVITY

Symptoms of food sensitivity can range from very subtle to blatantly obvious. At the mild end, you may feel slightly off-color. More obvious symptoms include fatigue (especially immediately after eating), brain fog, bloating, digestive problems, skin problems, depression, behavioral and mood changes, muscle aches and pains, general malaise, and feeling distinctly unwell. You may not immediately attribute these symptoms to the food you've eaten.

Specific MS symptoms, such as brain fog, extreme lack of energy, blurred vision, numbness, tingling, can also be brought on or exacerbated by eating harmful foods. Many people find a dramatic improvement in these symptoms when they give up the offending foods.

LINK WITH LEAKY GUT AND CANDIDA

Leaky gut—or increased gut permeability—has various causes, including eating foods to which you are sensitive, candida overgrowth, drinking too much alcohol, infection, parasites, trauma, and taking too many non-steroidal anti-inflammatory drugs. Lectin, a type of protein found in grains and legumes, also increases gut permeability.

Intestinal candidiasis is a major cause of food sensitivity. Once this is treated, food allergies often diminish. The link between candida and MS was explored by William G. Crook, M.D., in his book, *The Yeast Connection*.[1] Included are several cases of patients with MS who, based on their medical history, seemed to be good candidates for anti-candida treatment. In all of the cases described in his book, MS symptoms improved when candidiasis was treated.

Crook was not the first to suspect this link. Clinical ecologist Dr. Orian Truss recognized the problem of candidiasis as far back as 1953.[2]

What Can Make Someone Sensitive to Candida?

- *Antibiotics.* The story can usually be traced to the patient's childhood, when there may have been recurrent infections—such as urinary tract infections or sinusitis—that were treated with antibiotics. Antibiotics are very nonselective about which bacteria they kill; they destroy all of them, good and bad. This upsets the delicate balance of bacteria in the body.
- *Oral contraceptives.* The artificial hormones in contraceptive pills disturb many processes in the body. The known metabolic abnormalities produced by the pill include zinc deficiency, excess copper, altered liver function, changes in hormonal levels, and gross changes in the function of many enzymes. Many women with MS who have candidiasis also take birth control pills, which alter and depress the immune system and change the acidity of vaginal secretions. This often results in thrush.

- *Sulfonamide drugs.* These drugs are described for conditions such as cystitis, a urinary tract infection. Again, MS patients who have candida sensitivity are frequently found to have taken sulfonamide drugs.
- *Steroid drugs.* Candidiasis is more likely in patients who have been given large doses of steroids, which is a common prescription when patients have an attack of MS. The contraceptive pill is also a steroid drug. It is not unusual for someone with MS, especially if it's a woman, to have been treated with both antibiotics and sulfonamide drugs, and to have been on oral contraceptives in the years before the diagnosis of MS.

Signs and Symptoms of Chronic Candidiasis

The most common sign of candida overgrowth is thrush. In children it can occur in the mouth and gastrointestinal tract. In men it can show up as a sore penis. In women it is a sore vagina, with a white discharge. Thrush can result when a course of antibiotics kills off all bacteria, both good and bad.

With chronic candidiasis, the possible symptoms are extensive. They range from vaginal irritation to malaise to headache. Once the body has chronic candidiasis, it is unbalanced and predisposed to food and other sensitivities. You can find out whether you are sensitive to candida by the same techniques used to detect food sensitivities. (See Testing for Food Sensitivities, page 31.)

Treatment for Chronic Candidiasis

Candida, like all forms of yeast, loves sugar and moist places. The common recommended treatment is to eliminate from your diet all yeast, sugars, white flour, coffee, alcohol, tea, mushrooms, cheese, fruit, and fermented products, such as vinegar and soy sauce. Also, do not eat anything showing signs of mold, such as in grapes or soft fruits like blueberries or raspberries.

An antifungal drug called Nystatin* is sometimes prescribed.

---

*Dr. Stephen Davies, co-author of *Nutritional Medicine,* offers a note of caution about Nystatin. He says: "In some situations, anticandida treatment with Nystatin can cause an acute exacerbation of the condition, so one should progress very cautiously in MS."[3]

Doctors who specialize in nutritional medicine would probably also recommend vitamin and mineral supplements, acidophilus, and evening primrose oil.

ꙮ TESTING FOR FOOD SENSITIVITIES

There are various ways of testing for food sensitivities. One is to get a blood test analyzed by a laboratory that specializes in this field. Other methods include a skin test, a special device called a Vega machine that detects sensitivities when you hold certain substances in your hand, and applied kinesiology, or muscle testing. Another method is to test foods yourself, one by one, and see what reaction you get.

The ELISA Test

ELISA, which stands for Enzyme-Linked Immunosorbent Assay, is a fast and scientific way to identify food intolerances. It's one of the most widely used methods but is said to be only 80 percent accurate.

You'll receive a simple home kit that comes with a lancet (medical needle used to prick your finger) and a swab on a little wand, for collecting a small amount of blood. The most difficult part is squeezing enough blood out of the tiny hole in your skin made by the lancet. The entire swab must be covered with blood or the lab won't have enough blood to complete the tests. You'll then seal the bloodied swab and used lancet in the plastic box provided, and mail it back to the laboratory within two days.

What Does The ELISA Test Detect?

When food is digested, the many proteins that it contains are broken down into smaller fragments, known as peptides. Sometimes the immune system recognizes these as foreign, and produces IgG (immunoglobulin) antibodies against them. The ELISA test detects food intolerances by looking for IgG antibodies that indicate your body is unable to digest certain proteins correctly, and measuring them. Each protein can be traced to a particular food. The presence of IgG antibodies aimed against certain foods suggests the immune system is involved and that body has become intolerant of those foods.

What Foods Are Tested?

A company in England, called YorkTest, offers a choice of two tests, for either 42 or 113 common foods.* In the United States, Optimum Health Resource Laboratories uses a similar method and offers several levels of panels, from the basic four most common suspects (egg, gluten, milk, and soy) to ninety-six foods. Meridian Valley Laboratory in Washington state offers two levels—ninety-five foods or double that. And another U.K. company, Cambridge Nutritional Sciences, offers tests for forty to two hundred foods, with vegan and vegetarian options available. (See Resources for more information.)

Jules: Dairy Was My Downfall

I have had an ELISA test twice. The first was in June 2001—a few months after I started the Best Bet Diet (BBD). I was *very* strict about the diet at that time and so was surprised to find that the highest food sensitivity for me was cow's milk, as I had not had *any* dairy for quite some time.

My second test after at least eighteen months on a stringent BBD again showed my most dramatic result to cow's milk! I do know without any doubt that dairy exacerbates my symptoms noticeably, and within about ten or fifteen minutes of eating anything containing it I become dramatically weaker, my left side goes numb, and I become almost unable to use my left hand to manipulate things (like a fork or keyboard, for example). It also seems to affect me cognitively and I am likely to become irritable and distressed.

Wheat also affects me and causes an almost instant plummeting mood and depression. (My husband always knows when I've had wheat!) The consumption of either dairy or wheat makes me tired for days afterward, and it takes days of dedicated avoidance of both of these to regain my normal energy.

---

*To give you an idea of the scope of these tests, YorkTest's test of 42 foods includes: barley, corn, oats, rice, wheat, cow's milk, whole egg, chicken/turkey, pork/beef, cod/haddock, shellfish mix, nuts (almonds, brazils, cashews, hazelnut), legume mix (haricot, pea, peanut, soy), mustard mix (broccoli, brussels sprouts, cabbage, cauliflower), potato, apple/pear, berry mix (raspberry, blackberry, strawberry), citrus mix (grapefruit, lemon, lime, orange), spice mix (chili, pepper, garlic, ginger), yeast (brewer's and baker's). The 113 foods test includes a wider range of foods, including gliadin (gluten).

The ALCAT Test

The ALCAT test utilizes electronic, state of the art, hematological instrumentation to measure leukocyte cellular reactivity in whole blood, which is a final common pathway of all mechanisms.

Cell Science Systems, provider of the ALCAT test, says that standard allergy tests, such as skin testing or RAST (radioallergosorbent test), are not accurate for delayed type reactions to foods and chemicals. "The ALCAT test reproducibly measures the final common pathway of all pathogenic mechanism; whether immune, non-immune, or toxic. It is the only test shown to correlate with clinical symptoms by double blind oral challenges, the gold standard."[4]

The ALCAT tests for more than three hundred foods, food additives, food colorings, environmental chemicals, and molds. (See Resources for more information.)

✑ INTERPRETING LAB TEST RESULTS

Test results may be shown in the order of how badly you react to particular foods. You will likely be advised to avoid the worst foods, rotate other foods, and go easy on the mildest culprits.

Your test results may not include foods you have been avoiding. Les Rowley from YorkTest reports: "An intolerance will not show up on the test if you have not eaten it at all or not for the last three months. Patients who have a high intolerance to a particular food might need up to nine months without eating the food for it not to show up." However, some anecdotal reports say ELISA tests have shown results for foods that subjects had stopped eating for some time.

You are more likely to show a reaction to foods you eat quite frequently. Yeast, milk, wheat, and eggs often appear in the results because generally we eat more of those foods than anything else.

....

Lucy: Food Sensitivity Surprises

My ALCAT test showed a severe reaction to wheat (which I hadn't eaten for nine months prior to the test), casein (which I haven't eaten in years), and brussels sprouts (which I've *never* eaten as an adult), as well as to some foods I was eating frequently at the time of the test (chicken, pork, potatoes, and tomatoes).

....

➢ DO-IT-YOURSELF TESTING

An inexpensive process for finding out which foods you are sensitive to begins with a strict cleansing fast, to clear impurities from the body. Some doctors recommend a complete fast, but others think it safe to start with a cleansing diet of low-risk foods. For five to seven days, eat only low-risk foods, such as lamb, pears, cod, trout, flounder, carrots, zucchini, avocados, string beans, parsnips, rutabagas, and turnips. These foods can be eaten in any quantity.

While you are casting off toxins into your bloodstream, you will probably not feel very well. That will pass by the fifth day. On the sixth day, you should feel better.

Testing Foods, One by One

At the end of the five to seven days, when you start to feel better, you can begin testing other foods, one by one. This is not as arduous as it sounds. Once you have passed a food as safe, you can continue to eat it, together with your new food. So you could be eating large and varied meals within a matter of days. There is no limit on quantity.

Begin with foods that don't cause a reaction in most people. This list includes broccoli, beef, rice, melon, pineapple, lettuce, apples, grapes, and chicken. Introduce these at the rate of one per meal. Separate the meals by five to six hours. Watch for a reaction, which can normally be expected to happen during this period of time. Allow two days to test wheat, corn, oats, and rye, as they can have a delayed reaction. Foods from the same food family should be spaced out. For example, if you are testing tomatoes, wait four days before testing eggplant, also in the nightshade family. Same family foods should not be introduced within four days of each other.

By testing new foods one at a time, you should be able to see if a food gives you any symptoms. If you get no reaction, you can add that food to the next meal. For example, if you had tested lamb safely and rice safely, you could eat lamb, rice, and leeks on the next day for lunch. You would be testing only the leeks at that time, so if you got any reaction, you would know it must be the leeks.

If you do get a reaction, you should not test another new food until you feel well again, to avoid confusing the whole test. You might have to wait as long as three days. If you do get a certain reaction, it is wise to retest that food, but not for at least another five days or more.

If you break the diet once, you might have to start all over again. You should stick to each day's foods rigidly and eat nothing else—no sauces, flavorings, or embellishments.

This do-it-yourself food allergy test could contain many foods high in saturated fat. You may think it worthwhile to include them in the test to see what kind of reaction you have. Cut the fat off the lamb during the first five days. If you are taking dietary supplements, watch out for additives, such as sugar or yeast. Gelatin-covered capsules can be taken throughout the test.

Isolating the Allergen

Testing foods one by one is useful because it isolates individual ingredients. You may, for example, feel ill after eating a piece of cake—but what in the cake is making you feel bad? It could be the eggs, sugar, wheat flour, butter, or any other ingredient.

With bread, you could find that you are allergic to the yeast, rather than the wheat. Be particularly careful about sugar. Beet sugar and cane sugar are not the same thing, and you could react differently to each.

Do not think that foods must be safe because they are "natural." It is possible to have a sensitivity to things like bananas, almonds, peanuts, or the nightshade plants, even though they are not refined, processed, or in any way adulterated.

Needless to say, the process of testing for food allergies is very difficult socially. If you go anywhere for a meal, it is safest to take a picnic of "safe" foods with you, and explain the reason to your host or hostess. Be very careful when eating at restaurants. You must also avoid all alcoholic drinks and tobacco.

Once you have avoided a troublemaker food for several days, you will react much more strongly to it when you do eat it again. This is a good way of double-testing the suspect foods. Even though these foods give you a bad time, do not be surprised if you also long for them—the two together are a sure sign. Once you have isolated the foods to which you are allergic, you should ideally give them up completely. If this is impossible, you could try being "desensitized." (See page 38.)

∝ ADDITIONAL WAYS OF TESTING FOR FOOD SENSITIVITIES

Although the ELISA and ALCAT blood tests are the most common, there are other ways of testing for food sensitivities without taking blood. Although not always as reliable, these tests can serve to confirm results of a blood test.

Vega Test

The Vega test works on the principles of bioenergetic regulatory medicine. It looks at the body in an electrical (bioenergetic) context, and combines aspects of both acupuncture and homeopathy.

The Vega testing machine is about the size of a CD-player amplifier. It has buttons, an indicator, and a wire connected to a handheld electrode and a measuring stylus.

Glass vials containing homeopathic doses of substances (possibly offending foods and chemicals) are placed in the machine and the patient is given a handheld cylinder to complete the electrical circuit. As each substance is placed in the machine, one at a time, the operator applies a tiny electrical current via an electrode to a point on the end of the patient's finger or toe. This point corresponds with a known acupuncture point.

A bleep emits from the machine. An abnormal bleep indicates that the substance is having a negative effect on the patient's condition. If the bleep sound is normal and the reading on the indicator dial is normal, then the person does not have an allergic response to that particular substance. This is a relatively fast and painless way of pinpointing substances that are toxic to you.

Applied Kinesiology

Applied kinesiology is logically difficult to explain, but it really does seem to work. This bioenergetic method tests the reactions of muscles as a way of detecting food allergies and nutrient imbalances.

The practitioner of applied kinesiology gives the patient a succession of glass vials to hold in his left hand, each containing a different substance. (Sometimes the vials may be placed on the stomach.) The practitioner then asks the patient to raise his right arm into the air and resist any pressure put on it.

If the patient is not sensitive to the substance in a particular vial, he will be able to resist the pressure on his right arm from the practitioner. The muscles in his arm will remain strong and resistant, and he will have no trouble keeping his arm up in the air.

However, if the substance given to the patient to hold is toxic to him, he will be unable to resist the pressure of the practitioner on his right arm, the arm will feel weak, and he will give way under the pressure.

Many doctors give no credence to applied kinesiology and consider it to be more of a magic show than real medicine. Even so, many who were once skeptical have now had to admit that, crazy as it sounds, it does work.

In addition to being a way of testing for food allergies, applied kinesiology can also be a treatment. (See also section in chapter 13, page 153.)

Cytotoxic Testing

This type of testing exposes live white blood cells to a variety of foods and chemicals in succession. If the cells are damaged by any one of them, it indicates sensitivity. If there is no damage to the white blood cells, the substance being tested is harmless to that individual.

Intradermal Injection Techniques

Intradermal techniques, which have been practiced for half a century, involve injecting tiny amounts of a potential allergen just beneath the skin surface. A wheal—a small, round bump—appears. If the wheal gets bigger, this suggests an allergy to the substance. If the wheal stays the same size, there is no allergy.

Nutritional Profile

Practitioners of nutritional medicine often use both blood tests and hair analysis to determine a patient's nutritional profile.

Hair analysis can show nutrient status over a period of time. The hair is cut from close to the scalp, not using dyed or processed hair, and sent to a lab for analysis, after which remedial supplements are prescribed. Testing is available from www.DoctorsData.com (and elsewhere) for around $100, but any U.S. lab that doesn't offer an on-site doctor for counseling will require that tests be ordered through a health professional.

Some doctors also use the sweat test, a very sophisticated test that detects the nutritional status of a patient extremely accurately.

☙ OTHER WAYS OF DEALING WITH FOOD ALLERGIES

Desensitization

The principle of desensitization is to find a dilution of the food to which the person is sensitive that will switch off the allergic reaction to that particular food. Generally speaking, practitioners of clinical ecology—specialists in environmental medicine—prefer that MS patients exercise self-control and avoid the offending foods completely. However, desensitization is a possibility in certain cases.

Rotation Dieting

Giving up all foods to which you are sensitive is not quite enough. You also need to vary the remaining foods, making sure you don't always eat the same things every day. This is called rotation dieting. By not eating the same food twice within a three-day period, you minimize the chance of developing a sensitivity to a new food.

Some nutritional medicine doctors will allow a prohibited food to be carefully reintroduced after it has been avoided for six to nine months, with the proviso that it be eaten only as part of a rotation diet, and not with daily repetition. If you go back to old, addictive eating habits, you could develop masked sensitivity.

5

The Best Bet Diet

WHILE THERE ARE GENERAL GUIDELINES for controlling MS, the specific diet you choose will be based on your own needs and challenges. For most people, however, the Best Bet Diet (BBD) is exactly that—your best bet for controlling MS.

The aim of the Best Bet Diet, devised by Ashton Embry, Ph.D., is to minimize the chance of inflammation and autoimmunity in MS by avoiding foods containing proteins that could ignite these reactions. The science behind this is explained later in this chapter. (For an even more complete explanation, read Embry's essay, "Multiple Sclerosis—Best Bet Treatment," on the Direct-MS website, www.direct-ms.org.)

In a nutshell, the Best Bet Diet involves completely giving up:

- Gluten
- Dairy
- Legumes
- Refined Sugar
- Foods to which you show a sensitivity

Other foods should be reduced and others need to be added to the diet. Taking supplements and doing a food sensitivity test are also integral parts of the Best Bet Diet. Full details are provided later in this chapter.

ᴥ ASHTON EMBRY AND THE BEST BET DIET

Ashton Embry, Ph.D., is a Canadian geologist whose son, Matt, was diagnosed with MS in his early twenties. Spurred into action to stop his son from getting worse, Embry scoured the medical literature to see what methods to treat MS had a solid basis in science.

After extensive research, Embry came to the conclusion that dietary factors are the main cause of MS onset and progression, and devised the Best Bet Treatment. It's also referred to as the Best Bet Diet, although it encompasses more than diet alone. It is similar to the Roger MacDougall Diet (see page 47) but goes further and has a more extensive scientific basis.

ᴥ FOOD RECOMMENDATIONS FOR THE BEST BET DIET

The Best Bet Diet is essentially the diet of our ancestors in the Paleolithic period, or Stone Age, consisting mostly of lean meats, fish, vegetables, and fruits. This period lasted around 2.5 million years, ending around 10,000 years ago with the introduction of agriculture and "new" foods such as grains, dairy, legumes, potatoes, and sugar, for which we are not genetically designed. Ten thousand years may seem like a long time but in fact is quite recent in terms of human evolution.

In following this diet, some foods need to be eliminated completely, others can be reduced, and others are important to include.

Foods to Eliminate

The following foods should be given up completely:

- Gluten: found in *all* wheat, rye, and barley, and *all* products containing them. Although there is no gluten in oats, it is a modern grain with increased chances of creating an autoimmune reaction, and thus should be avoided. Gluten contamination can also be an issue with oats that are sometimes processed in the same facility as gluten grains.
- Dairy: found in *all* animal milk; *all* butters, cheeses, and yogurts made from any animal milk; and *all* products that contain any of these. This means milk not just from cows but also from sheep and goats.

- Legumes: beans, peas, and edible seeds—especially soy—and all products containing them. All other vegetables are fine, unless you show an intolerance on an ELISA or ALCAT test.
- Refined sugar: found in sweets, soft drinks, and many other foods. Sugar alters the intestinal flora, which can make a leaky gut worse and can also have a deleterious effect on the immune system. High glycemic carbohydrates should also be avoided.
- Foods to which you show a sensitivity. Particular foods can cause increased gut permeability (leaky gut) and increased immune reactions in individuals. You should have an ELISA or ALCAT blood test done to find out if you have a sensitivity to any foods. Give these up, however beneficial they may seem.

Eggs, yeast, and tomatoes are allowed in limited quantities on the Best Bet Diet, so long as the individual shows no specific allergic reaction to them.

Foods to Reduce
The following foods should be consumed only in moderate amounts:

- Saturated Fat: Eat lean meat only once a week.
- Omega-6, found in many baked goods, margarine, salad oils, and so on. There is plenty in the diet anyway.
- Non-gluten grains, such as corn and oats.
- Alcohol: Completely avoid beer. Wine is okay in moderation if you show no sensitivity.

So What Can You Eat?
As long as you show no sensitivity, you can eat as much as you like of:

- Fish: especially oily fish like salmon, mackerel, tuna, sardines. Also skinless chicken or turkey breast, and game meats.
- All fruits and vegetables except legumes and any to which you show a sensitivity (paying special care to be sure you aren't sensitive to the nightshade family—eggplant, tomatoes, potatoes, and so on).

- Nuts and seeds (remembering that peanuts are not really nuts, but legumes).
- Extra virgin olive oil.
- Gluten grains can be replaced with quinoa or buckwheat (both of which are actually in the fruit family), rice, or a whole range of other grains and flours that are gluten-free and widely available.
- Replace dairy with rice, nut, or hemp milk, or low fat coconut milk, all of which are available in supermarkets.
- Acceptable alternatives to sugar are honey, maple syrup, fruit sugar (fructose), and stevia.

Isabelle: Previously, the Pasta Princess

For the year before my first MS attack, my diet consisted mainly of pasta, pasta, and pasta! Why? Because I was managing an Italian restaurant and my salary package included a pasta meal for lunch, and I took lunch leftovers home for dinner. I was living by myself, rarely cooked, and ate no fruit and minimal vegetables.

I was also smoking and drinking two cups of strong coffee daily. No wonder I was tired most of the time! I had been feeling quite nauseous for two weeks and then started "walking funny," so my GP sent me to the hospital for tests that diagnosed me with MS.

On the day I was discharged from the hospital it was a huge effort to walk up the three steps to my home, and for many months I walked more slowly than an old woman. My right arm felt as if it were wrapped in cotton wool. Many things made me feel teary and apprehensive.

Much of the time my cognitive processes were really slow; I'd just go blank and not be able to think of the words to explain a thought, memory, or feeling. And I felt pretty useless for the next two years, not being well enough to work much.

However, I went on the Best Bet Diet straight away and stuck to it rigidly. In the early months I was often tempted by chocolate, cheese-cake, or a piece of pizza, but I resisted the urge by thinking: "Shall I eat this or continue to be able to dance with my partner, and run and play games with my little nephews?" The choice was simple.

Now, I no longer crave cakes and bread, chocolate, coffee, spaghetti, and so on. Just smelling other people's toast gives me the wheat experience without actually eating it.

Of course I fall off the wagon every now and then, but I reckon it's important to make my own decisions about what I eat and when, and not be ruled by fear. As I've become more in tune with my body over the past few years, I'm better able to listen to its messages and respect what it tells me.

....

THE SCIENCE BEHIND THE BEST BET DIET

The problem that occurs when people with MS eat certain foods is that intact food proteins escape into the bloodstream via a leaky gut. These then activate the immune system against tissue in the central nervous system. This may be happening because the molecular similarities between the food proteins and the self-proteins in the central nervous system confuse the immune system. The aim of the Best Bet Diet is to halt the activation of the immune system, reduce inflammation, strengthen the blood-brain barrier, and heal a leaky gut.

Halting Activation of the Immune System

One way of halting activation of the immune system is by healing a leaky gut, thus preventing intact food proteins from entering the circulatory system. The other way is to stop eating foods containing certain proteins that can potentially mimic self-proteins in the central nervous system. This includes lectins (a type of protein) found in grains and legumes that increase gut permeability. The entire Best Bet Diet treatment is aimed at strengthening the immune system.

Strengthening the Blood-Brain Barrier

The most effective way to strengthen the blood-brain barrier is by eating foods or taking supplements that contain the powerful antioxidants anthocyanosides, proanthocyanidins, and procyanidolic oligomers. These are found in blueberries, cherries, blackberries, grapes, and the bark and needles of certain pine trees. In supplements they are called bilberry, grape seed extract, and pycnogenol. Less powerful antioxidants include vitamin A (cod liver oil), vitamin C (with bioflavonoids), and vitamin E. These, along with vitamin B complex and vitamin D$_3$, should be taken daily.

Eliminating Autoimmune Potential

Strict adherents to the Best Bet Diet insist that you *must* give up gluten grains, dairy, saturated fat, and legumes, *even if* your ELISA or ALCAT test gives them the all-clear. Their reason for this is as follows: Although the ELISA or ALCAT test can detect IgG (immunoglobulin) antibodies, indicating delayed food sensitivity, some people with MS will show little or *no* IgG reaction to proteins in gluten (gliadin), dairy, or legumes. However, the proteins from these foods will still activate myelin-sensitive T cells when they meet the immune system.

As there is no test to determine what food proteins are stimulating myelin-sensitive T cells, those with MS are ill-advised to continue consuming foods with the potential to provoke such autoimmune reactions simply because their ELISA test failed to detect the presence of IgG antibodies. It is well known that a sensitivity or intolerance to gluten (gliadin) cannot always be detected by the presence of IgG antibodies, and there is every indication that continued consumption of gluten will interfere with efforts to heal leaky gut.

This might happen in one of two ways. Either the large gliadin molecules will embed themselves between the tight joints of the gastrointestinal tract, or gluten consumption could increase production of the protein zonulin, which regulates the permeability of both the gut wall and blood-brain barrier. Either way, the passage through the gut wall remains open, allowing other large food particles to find their way into the bloodstream and leaving the individual at increased risk of both allergic and autoimmune reactions.

❧ SUPPLEMENTS FOR THE BEST BET DIET

Strengthening the immune system, healing the blood-brain barrier, minimizing inflammation, and healing a leaky gut are also helped by taking certain supplements, which should include vitamins, minerals, trace elements, and oils. (See also chapters 8, 9, and 10.) The latest list also takes account of vein problems in MS—chronic cerebrospinal venous insufficiency, or CCSVI.

Essential Supplements

Even if you take no other supplements, these are essential:

- Vitamin D_3: 6,000–8,000 IU (International Units) per day for most. (Also see chapter 9.) Avoid products containing vitamin A.
- Omega-3 fish oil: 5 g of DHA and EPA per day. Salmon oil is good.
- Calcium: 1,000–1,200 mg per day.
- Magnesium: 500–600 mg per day.
- Calcium and magnesium *must* be taken with vitamin D_3.

Recommended Vitamins

The following vitamin supplements are recommended daily:

- Vitamin A: 5,000 IU
- Vitamin B-100 complex: 100 mg
- No-flush niacin (vitamin B_3): 2 g
- Folic acid: 400 mcg
- Vitamin B_{12}: 1–2 mg
- Vitamin C: 1 g
- Vitamin E (natural): 400 IU

Minerals and Trace Elements

The following mineral supplements should be taken daily:

- Zinc: 25–50 mg
- Copper: 1–2 mg
- Selenium: 200 mcg
- Manganese: 20 mg
- Iodine: 200 mcg

Antioxidants

All of the following should be taken daily:

- Grape seed extract: 2–4 capsules (up to 300 mg per capsule)
- Ginkgo biloba: 120 mg

- Alpha lipoic acid: 500 mg
- Coenzyme Q_{10}: 60–90 mg
- EGCG max (epigallocatechin-3-gallate—the primary antioxidant, or catechin, in green tea): two 700 mg capsules
- Quercetin: 400 mg
- Bromelain: 400 mg

Probiotics

Probiotics are recommended for maintaining beneficial bacteria in the gut. The term *acidophilus* usually refers to *Lactobacillus acidophilus* combined with other beneficial bacteria such as *Bifidobacterium Bb12, Lactobacillus rhamnosus, L. casei,* and *L. bulgaricus.*

- Acidophilus: 4–8 capsules daily, 2–3 with each meal, each containing at least 10 billion live probiotic bacteria

⤳ THE BEST BET DIET PLUS

The latest version of the Best Bet Diet incorporates the main points of the Brain Nutrient Diet, devised by Terry Wahls, M.D. (see chapter 6).

You'll find the most up-to-date information at www.msrc.co.uk and www.direct-ms.org. The Best Bet Diet is regularly featured in the magazine *New Pathways,* published by the U.K.'s Multiple Sclerosis Resource Centre, and there are also numerous websites, books, and magazines that offer Best Bet Diet advice and recipes (see Resources).

....

Janet: Best Bet Diet Helped More Than Anything Else

Since I've had MS, the Best Bet Diet and its supplements have helped me more than anything else. If only I'd found them sooner, I might not be in this wheelchair now. It wasn't until I began to follow the Best Bet Diet 100 percent that I saw improvements in my MS.

Breaking myself in slowly, I eliminated foods gradually and wouldn't move on until I was sure I wouldn't cheat on that one.

Gluten was the first to go. Within just five weeks my brain fog lifted. It was like a weather front had passed and I woke up one morning and shrieked, "I'm back!"

Encouraged, I then eliminated dairy, which was hard for me. But every time I craved dairy, I would re-read the information on why it is potentially harmful for people with MS. As a result of giving up dairy, lots of little symptoms disappeared: blurred vision, aches behind the eyes, tinnitus, neuralgia, some swallowing difficulties, and my balance improved slightly.

Next I tackled legumes. Having been a vegetarian on and off, this was a big change for me. I had always eaten healthily (or so I thought) with masses of fresh fruit and vegetables . . . and soy products. A week into it, I kidded myself that giving up legumes wasn't going to help and ate a Japanese meal riddled with legumes (miso soup, fermented black beans, tempeh, and tofu). Boy was I ill! Since that day I have never eaten anything but Best Bet Diet foods. The removal of legumes from my diet stopped slurred speech, "banding" in the neck and legs, the MS bear hug, and the numb bum.

Tomatoes were then declared suspect by Dr. Loren Cordain of Colorado State University in his essay "The Paleo Diet and Multiple Sclerosis." An ELISA food allergy test showed me to be intolerant of tomatoes anyway. This test also showed sensitivity to corn, pulses, egg white, Brazil nuts, cashews, sunflower seeds, and melon. Once I'd removed all of these foods, my neck (where most of my lesions are) ached less, sore throats went away, and I had even more energy.

Refined sugar was the next thing I gave up. As a result, the vestiges of fatigue went, along with all numbness except on the soles of my feet. My eyesight was sharper and my writing no longer looked like a spider had crawled across the page.

My attitude toward the Best Bet Diet is to focus on what symptoms it is eradicating. I see it as a long-term insurance policy. The benefits of these dietary approaches to MS take time. It has taken me three years to get where I am today—no disease progression and the disappearance of one lesion.

❧ THE ROGER MACDOUGALL DIET

A forerunner of the Best Bet Diet was the Roger MacDougall Diet, which became popular in the 1970s. It is similar to the Best Bet Diet but does not have the same scientific rationale in terms of preventing autoimmune reactions and inflammation, strengthening the blood-brain barrier, and healing leaky gut. Roger MacDougall died many years ago, so his protocol is not as up-to-date as the Best Bet Diet, but his work was very influential in the field of diet and MS.

In 1953 MacDougall was diagnosed as having MS and showed many of the classic symptoms. Within a few years his eyesight, legs, fingers, and speech were badly affected. Before long, he was in a wheelchair.

Without any medical training (he was a playwright and professor in the University of California's theater department), MacDougall set about finding ways to treat his degenerative condition. By a mixture of inspiration, guesswork, research, and borrowing from other dietary regimens, MacDougall devised his own diet for MS.*

To come up with his diet, MacDougall did a great deal of reading about many degenerative and autoimmune diseases, such as celiac disease, diabetes, and heart disease, to see if he could find any similarities with his own illness and learn any lessons.

Celiac disease causes inflammation of the lining of the small intestine and can also cause complications in various organs. Those with celiac disease have an allergy to gluten, the elastic-type component in dough; gluten damages the mucosal lining of the bowel, making it difficult to absorb nutrients. Patients with celiac disease can also have central nervous system and brain white matter abnormalities similar to the brain lesions in MS.

MacDougall wondered if people with MS were experiencing something similar to those with celiac disease—that foods containing gluten damage the lining of the small intestine in such a way that the nutrients required to keep renewing the myelin sheath are prevented from reaching the bloodstream.

MacDougall's research into other diseases, such as diabetes and heart

---

*Roger MacDougall's own account can be read at www.direct-ms.org; search on the site for his name.

disease, led him to think that people with MS should also restrict their sugar and saturated fat intake.

The Roger MacDougall Diet was best known as being gluten-free, but it was much more than that. It was a Paleolithic, or Stone Age diet, consisting almost exclusively of lean meats, fish, vegetables, and fruits, and excluding such "modern" foods as grains and dairy.

Progressive versions of the MacDougall Diet were also high in poly-unsaturated fats and low in saturated fats, excluded foods that caused individual allergic responses, and recommended a long list of vitamin, mineral, trace element, and other supplements. In its final form, the Roger MacDougall Diet had five main tenets:

- No gluten or dairy
- No foods to which you are sensitive
- Low sugars
- Low animal fats/high unsaturated fats
- Several supplements

By following this regimen MacDougall experienced an impressive recovery and could be witnessed leaping down stairs two at a time. Anyone with MS will appreciate that this is indeed some feat. The fact that MacDougall was able to get out of his wheelchair and resume an active life made his diet extremely popular, as everyone hoped it would do the same for them.

MacDougall, a genial fellow, happened to live near me in Hampstead, northwest London, and when I went to meet him soon after my diagnosis, he convinced me to follow his protocol.

Over the past thirty-six years, I have been on and off the Roger MacDougall protocol and the Best Bet Diet and have *always* felt better when I've been on it (which I am at the time of writing), with less fatigue; more energy; fewer MS symptoms; and improved walking, balance, and coordination.

6

Feed Your Body,
Feed Your Brain

THE BRAIN NUTRIENT DIET was devised by Terry Wahls, M.D., associate professor of medicine at the University of Iowa who has had secondary progressive MS since 2003. Soon after the onset, she couldn't walk and needed a wheelchair.

Wahls researched medical literature on MS and other diseases—Parkinson's and Alzheimer's—in which brain cells die prematurely. The common threads she found among these conditions were excito-toxicity and mitochondrial failure. Some of the literature specifically talked about mitochondrial performance and the food supplements creatine, carnitine, lipoic acid, coenzyme Q_{10}, and B complex vitamins.

After intensive scientific research, Wahls came up with a diet rich in nutrients that specifically target the brain. She began taking these supplements and a few weeks later her energy improved. As a test, she stopped taking the supplements, but after three days her fatigue had worsened so she went back to her new regimen and again improved. Wahls became convinced that nutrients were critically important in treating MS.

She recovered from MS by following this diet, and also using an electro-stimulation machine and doing regular exercise to strengthen her muscles. She is now able to walk, cycle five miles a day, cross-country ski, and teach.

ᴥ MITOCHONDRIA AND MS

Mitochondria are the energy factory in cells. They convert the food we eat into ATP (adenosine triphosphate) the molecule that stores energy for the cell. If the mitochondria don't make ATP, the brain cells don't have the energy to do their work; they can't make myelin, make few neurotransmitters, and are unable to repair damage to the myelin sheath. In someone with MS, the mitochondria are not healthy, and if the mitochondria aren't healthy, the brain isn't healthy.

In the course of her studies, Wahls discovered that if there were not enough co-factors or antioxidants in cells, a lot of free radicals were generated, causing oxidative stress. If not neutralized quickly, those free radicals could harm the mitochondria or the cellular DNA. Wahls's diet is intended to increase the health of the mitochondria by giving the body foods that contain the specific nutrients needed by the mitochondria in order to maintain health.

When the mitochondria are deficient in B vitamins and coenzyme Q_{10}, more free radicals are created; and when there aren't sufficient antioxidants, free radicals are not neutralized and instead begin to damage the brain cells. Cells need a good supply of antioxidants, most of which are found in *fruits and vegetables.*

A diet very rich in green leafy and cruciferous vegetables also helps the body maintain healthy detoxification systems, and can help the body process mercury from amalgam fillings. (For more on mercury fillings, see chapter 18.)

ᴥ NUTRIENTS FOR THE BRAIN

There are specific nutrients that brain cells need in order to communicate with each other, and to make myelin and neurotransmitters work properly. These nutrients include omega-3 fatty acids (to make brain cells and myelin), organic sulfur (to make GABA—gamma-aminobutyric acid— the chief inhibitory neurotransmitter that regulates neuronal excitability), and serotonin (the "happiness molecule").

The full list of nutrients Wahls considers essential to healthy brain cells includes:

- Thiamine (vitamin B_1)

- Riboflavin (vitamin B_2)
- Niacinamide (vitamin B_3)
- Cyanocobalamin (vitamin B_{12})
- Ubiquinone (coenzyme Q_{10})
- Lipoic acid
- Omega-3 fatty acids
- Magnesium
- Organic sulfur (glutathione, N-acetyl cysteine, methionine)
- L-carnitine (from the amino acids lysine and methionine) and the amino acids taurine and creatine.

✖ RECOMMENDED BRAIN FOODS

Using the book *The World's Healthiest Foods,* by George Mateljan, as her primary source, Wahls investigated which foods contained these nutrients.

Fruits and Vegetables

Wahls recommends a wide variety of fruits and vegetables across the color spectrum, including those that are green, red, blue, purple, yellow, orange, and black. Gradually increase the number of daily servings until you reach at least *nine* cups of fruits and vegetables every day.

- Three of these should be dark green vegetables, which are rich in B vitamins and coenzyme Q_{10}, such as spinach, chard, and mustard greens.
- Three should be rich in organic sulfur, including kale, collards, cabbage, broccoli, onions, and garlic.
- The final three should be rich in antioxidants, such as raspberries, blueberries, black currants, carrots, and red cabbage. Wahls also eats mushrooms every other day.

Once you have eaten your nine cups of the above, you can eat starchy vegetables such as corn, potatoes, turnips, parsnips, kohlrabi, and rutabaga, as well as rice and other grains.

Fish, Shellfish, and Meat

Wahls recommends eating fish, ideally oily fish, such as salmon, mackerel, sardines, or shellfish two to three times a week; and organ meats, such as liver, kidneys, and brains (for coenzyme Q_{10} and B vitamins) once a week. Wheat germ should be taken daily for its coenzyme Q_{10}. An alternative to fish is eggs enriched with omega-3 essential fatty acids. Other sources of omega-3 include fish oil, flaxseed oil, and hemp oil, one to two tablespoons (or capsules, up to 4 g) a day.

Wahls also encourages eating seeds, such as sesame, pumpkin, and pignoli; nuts, particularly almonds; and instant greens—packets or bottles said to contain antioxidants equal to five servings of fruits and vegetables—to mix with juice or water and drink several times daily.

All the food you eat should be high in nutrients, and not empty calories. If you think you might be sensitive to gluten or other substances, try giving them up for a month to see if there is any difference in your symptoms.

The order of priority is to have the three cups of fruit and vegetables first, then the protein, then whatever else you'd like to include that doesn't cause a sensitive reaction.

◌ COOKED OR RAW

Wahls believes that eating food uncooked may be somewhat preferable. Frying food converts many of the valuable antioxidants into less useful oxidized forms, so second choice would be steamed or poached.

> The whole food is superior to the juice, although smoothies made from the entire fruit or vegetables are fine. Foods which are rich in nutrients provide a greater synergy of vitamins, minerals and trace elements than single nutrient supplements. For example, it is better to eat sesame or pumpkin seeds than to make a magnesium supplement, or to get the amino acid taurine from shellfish rather than a supplement, or to get organic sulfur from the cabbage or garlic family rather than a supplement. Drinking several glasses of instant greens will likely provide more usable sulfur, mineral, and anitoxidant activity than single nutrient supplements.

It's also important to consume any cooking water, because this is where all the water-soluble nutrients have gone. If you cook below boiling point and drink all the liquid, food is more digestible and retains most of its micronutrients.

❧ SUPPLEMENTS

Terry Wahls's philosophy is, "If you have a sick brain, eat the food *and* take the supplements. If you're healthy, just eat the food." In general, Wahls is clear that supplements cannot replace the micronutrients from nine cups of fruits and vegetables. However, fish oil or flaxseed oil supplements are fine if you cannot eat fish, and if you cannot eat organ meats once a week, take coenzyme Q_{10} tablets. Dr. Wahls also takes vitamin B supplements.

Wahls also recommends some daily supplements, including a multivitamin/mineral that has all the trace elements, milk thistle for liver support, *Lithium orotate* to help stimulate growth factors, and 4,000 IU of vitamin D.

❧ RECOVERY TIME

Dr. Wahls cautions that this is a slow process, and that nobody should expect instant results. Her estimate is that it generally takes three months to replace the cells in a solid organ. It took three months before she could see any improvements in her own condition. For more about Dr. Wahls's complete protocol, visit www.terrywahls.com.

7

The Body's Delicate Balance

SOME PEOPLE WITH MS have improved by going on a diet that favors alkaline-forming foods over acid-forming foods. This makes for the ideal pH in the body, with an alkaline environment that allows the body to heal.

In order to function properly, your body needs to maintain equilibrium. It is most important for your blood to have the right acid-alkaline balance. The pH of human blood should be slightly alkaline: 7.35 to 7.45. Neutral is 7; below 7 is acidic. When this is out of kilter, your body is more susceptible to inner malfunctioning and external agressors, making it easier for disease to take hold. In an acid environment, the microzyma found in every living cell can switch to an unhealthy form and become a yeast, fungus, or mold.

Microbiologist and nutritional scientist Robert O. Young, Ph.D., who, with his wife Shelley Redford Young, wrote *The pH Miracle,* believes that disease is caused by a diet and lifestyle that is too acidic. He posits that a diet high in acid-producing foods, such as dairy, sugar, and animal protein, causes acid waste to build up in the body, eventually transforming it into a toxic wasteland. He believes that this is the root cause of MS and many other diseases. Fatigue is one of the most common symptoms of an over-acidic body.

Young says that the primary way to regain health is to:

1. Eat a diet that is 80 percent alkaline and 20 percent acid
2. Drink juiced vegetables and green drinks
3. Drink alkalized water

GETTING THE ACID-ALKALINE BALANCE RIGHT

You can test the pH of your urine or saliva by buying special testing kits from a pharmacy or online. The strips change color according to the acidity of the substance tested.

The Western diet is heavily weighted toward acid-producing foods. If your body has become too acidic, you need to address this imbalance by ingesting more food and drinks that are alkalizing: vegetables—particularly green vegetables, sprouted and soaked nuts and seeds, essential oils, and low sugar fruits.

At the same time, you need to avoid acidic foods. In general, animal foods (meat, eggs, dairy), processed and refined foods, yeast products, fermented foods, grains, artificial sweeteners, fruit, sugars, alcohol, coffee, chocolate, black tea, and fizzy drinks are acidifying.

To help reverse the over-acidification of the blood and tissues, Young says that you also need to drink liberal amounts of alkaline water. Typically alkaline ionized water has a pH between 8 and 10. There are several water ionizing products on the market, including alkaline jug filters; undersink alkaline water ionizers; fixed countertop or wall units that hook up to a faucet; drops; and cartridges that you add to ordinary water.

ACID- AND ALKALINE-FORMING FOODS

There is some controversy among experts as to which foods are acid-forming, which are alkaline-forming, and which are neutral. The following information is taken from the book *The pH Miracle*.[1]

Common Alkalizing Foods

The most alkalizing foods are fresh vegetables: artichokes, asparagus, broccoli, brussels sprouts, all kinds of cabbage, carrots, cauliflower, celery, chives, cucumbers, eggplant, garlic, green beans, kohlrabi, leeks, greens of all kinds (lettuce, spinach, mustard greens, collards, kale, watercress,

Swiss chard), okra, onions, parsley, parsnips, peas, peppers (red, yellow, or green), potatoes, radishes, rhubarb, tomatoes, turnips, and zucchini. Sprouted grains, beans, and seeds are also alkalizing, as are the following fruits: banana, sour cherry, coconut, and lemon.

Common Acid-Forming Foods

The following foods are acid-forming: dairy and fats (butter, cheese, cream, margarine, milk); meat, poultry, and fish; bread products; nuts (cashews, macadamias, pistachios, as well as peanuts—technically a legume); sweets and desserts (artificial sweeteners, beet and cane sugar, chocolate, honey, molasses); condiments (ketchup, mayonnaise, mustard, soy sauce, vinegar); many beverages (beer, black tea, coffee, fruit juice, spirits, wine); and corn.

Potentially Neutral Foods

There is a great deal of conflicting information about neutral foods. However, the *Mayo Clinic Diet Manual* (7th edition) categorizes the following foods as neutral (neither acid nor alkaline), and not acid-forming: butter, margarine, cooking fats and oils, plain candies, sugar, syrup, honey, arrowroot, corn, coffee, and tea. You may need to do some testing to determine what causes acid in your individual body.

❧ MAKING THE TRANSITION TO AN 80 PERCENT ALKALINE/20 PERCENT ACID DIET

Unless you are very ill, Young suggests that the transition be made gradually—over the course of up to two years—rather than all at once. The basic outline for Young's program is as follows:

Step 1: Transition. For twelve weeks, gradually eliminate acidifying foods, substituting alkalizing foods.

Step 2: Cleanse. For one week take some supplements and mild, natural laxatives.

Step 3: Eat *only* 100 percent alkaline foods for seven weeks, with additional supplements, including probiotics. This means eating mainly green vegetables with high water content—raw, as much as possible. Young states that raw food is more alkalizing than cooked food.[2]

Step 4: You may now proceed to a diet that is 70–80 percent alkaline, and the rest acid. You may introduce fish, grains, and starchy vegetables, as well as a full range of supplements. Switching to a primarily alkaline diet usually means completely changing what you eat for each meal—especially breakfast, for which Young recommends soup or salad.

In addition to transitioning to an 80 percent alkaline/20 percent acid diet, Young also recommends chewing food very well, as this is an important part of the digestion process, and food combining. (*Food combining* is the practice of eating foods that complement each other for digestion. One of the basic rules of food combining is not to mix carbohydrate-rich foods such as breads and cereals with protein-rich foods such as meat, milk, and eggs in the same meal.)

⁓ BLOOD SUGAR BALANCE

It's crucial to keep the blood sugar balanced, not allowing it to get too high or too low, which is directly related to the acid-alkaline balance. If your blood sugar gets high, you can bet that you have too much acid.

Cake, biscuits, bread, and bakery items impart a rapid burst of sugar energy, the pancreas secretes a lot of insulin, and too much sugar gets into the bloodstream very quickly. However, this is just as quickly followed by a drop in blood sugar levels, causing a drop in energy accompanied by dizziness, fatigue, and shakiness.

You can keep your blood sugar balanced by eating complex carbohydrate foods, which give a slow release of energy.

....

Alan: Sick and Tired of Being Sick and Tired

From the time of my MS diagnosis in 1986, I have believed that MS is related to what we eat. My belief is that it is caused by an over-acidic body, coupled with trauma as the catalyst or trigger. My body became acidic at an early age when I was given cow's milk after weaning from my mother's milk. I had many head injuries as a child, which may have been the trauma, and also was given many vaccinations and inoculations that are traumatic to the body.

In 1999, I eliminated sugars and white flour and began to eat more balanced meals. Even so, the slow decline continued and I had to start using a wheelchair and give up driving.

In my search for answers I read *Sick and Tired* by Robert O. Young, Ph.D. The concept of acid versus alkaline had puzzled me for some time, and that book gave me the scientific explanation I was seeking. I have since read more than thirty books on acid-alkaline balance.

My wife and I started on a raw vegetable regimen that includes limited raw fruits, such as lemons, limes, avocadoes, and tomatoes. In effect it is an alkaline-forming diet and eliminates acid-forming foods. It also eliminates an acid lifestyle.

I noticed several changes within two weeks: my muscle spasms and cramps were almost gone; I could turn over on my left side in bed, which I hadn't been able to do for years; my bladder was functioning better; my facial acne was clearing; bowel movements became more regular; and I had no underarm odor.

Today most of the muscle spasms and cramps are gone and I can more easily exercise my legs. I went to a physical therapist and began walking again with a walker, improving from 75 feet to 225 feet in two months.

MACROBIOTICS

The health and lives of many people with MS have improved after switching to a strict macrobiotic diet and way of life. Followers of the macrobiotic diet believe that this is the best diet for MS, as it is said to protect against chronic diseases. According to the theories behind macrobiotics, in multiple sclerosis the immune system is damaged from a chronic acidic blood condition caused by eating unbalanced, or "extreme," foods such as meat, eggs, poultry, dairy, sugar, chocolate, and salt. There have not been any scientific studies into this.

The Eastern concepts of yin and yang are at the basis of a macrobiotic diet, which literally means "great life." Yin and yang represent opposing and complementary polarities, like male/female, day/night, sun/moon, hot/cold, acid/alkaline. To achieve a Zen-like balance, you need to have both yin and yang in what you eat. Foods are classified as being sour, sharp, sweet, or bitter. Yin foods are cold, sweet, and passive while yang foods are hot, salty, and aggressive.

A macrobiotic diet is not as bleak as some people might think. It is not just brown rice and vegetables. It is quite varied, and, as a modified vegetarian plan, it includes plenty of grains, vegetables, fermented soy, and soups, supplemented with small amounts of fish, nuts, seeds, and fruits in season. Foods should be eaten slowly and chewed thoroughly. The macrobiotic diet is part of a whole lifestyle and needs to be tailored according to the season, climate, activity, age, sex, and individual health condition.

All foods eaten need to be natural, locally and organically grown, wholesome, nutritious, and in harmony with the seasons. It does not have to be totally vegetarian or vegan; this depends on where you live. In most of North America and Europe the traditional staple is whole grains: wheat, rice, oats, barley, millet, and rye, eaten together with beans such as red kidney, aduki, chick peas, and black-eyed peas.

A typical macrobiotic diet consists of:

- 50–60 percent whole grains, especially brown rice
- 25–30 percent vegetables and seaweed
- 5–10 percent beans
- 5–20 percent fish, nuts, seeds, fruits, miso
- Soup made from the above ingredients: 1–2 cups a day

Foods *not* allowed on a macrobiotic diet are fatty red meat, most dairy, all processed and refined foods, all forms of refined sugar and foods containing them (such as chocolate, candies, and cakes), tomato sauce, very hot spices, poultry, potatoes, and zucchini. Tea and coffee are not allowed; they are substituted with herb teas and drinks such as Barleycup. Cigarettes, alcohol, and all additives are also prohibited.

Followers of the macrobiotic diet strongly believe that food and food quality impact health, happiness, and well-being. Eating natural food that is closer to the earth and less processed is healthier for the body and soul. One of the objectives is to become more sensitive to the food you eat and how it affects your life.

Erica: Finding Harmony with Macrobiotics

It wasn't until I had had MS for a few years that I found out about macrobiotics. At that time my MS symptoms, which would come and go, included slurred speech, problems with walking, and double vision.

Michio Kushi, the Japanese guru of macrobiotics, inspired me. Hearing the clarity of his thoughts was like seeing the light at the end of the tunnel. It was as if I'd been in a dark cave.

From the first day I went macrobiotic I felt much better, though it took me four years to fully recover. In addition to the diet, I did yoga and t'ai chi. I also included macrobiotic home remedies such as special dishes that clean out and strengthen the system, certain drinks, moxibustion, and ginger compresses.

I am attracted to the philosophy of a macrobiotic way of life. If we can create peace and harmony within ourselves physically, mentally, emotionally, and spiritually, then everything else follows.

8

Nutritional Supplements

MS PATIENTS ALMOST ALWAYS have nutritional deficiencies. Common ones include vitamin D, zinc, magnesium, selenium, and essential fatty acids, but it can be anything.

You may be deficient in certain nutrients because your diet isn't providing enough, you need more than the average person because you have a chronic illness, and/or you may not be assimilating all the nutrients you are eating. Whatever the reason for your being deficient, you need nutrients at their optimum level in order to have normal biochemistry and a properly functioning body. The more normal your biochemistry, the more likely things will work in your body as they should.

My own nutrient and biochemical status has been regularly tested over the decades by doctors specializing in nutritional medicine. I currently have my blood and urine checked in a London clinic every six months by Belgian doctor and nutritional expert Georges Mouton, author of two books in French on functional medicine, *Les méthodes du Docteur Mouton* and *Ecosystème intestinal et santé optimale*. He is a great believer in getting your biochemistry back to normal.

When Dr. Mouton gets the computer printout of my results back from the lab, it's easy to see if a particular nutrient needs to be adjusted or if a biochemical is out of kilter. In my own case, the nutrients and other things Dr. Mouton prescribes are formulated for my specific nutrient and biochemical status. Though expensive, this is ideal.

〜 GETTING YOUR BODY'S BIOCHEMISTRY BACK TO NORMAL

In my own case, tests showed I had a sensitivity to eggs, dairy, bananas, chocolate, and kiwi fruit, which meant giving them up. Dr. Mouton also advised me to keep sugar to a minimum, as this interferes with the amount of insulin released from the pancreas.

My tests also showed I had slightly low thyroid function, so Dr. Mouton put me on Armour Thyroid (pig thyroid supplement), and also L-thyroxine (pharmaceutical thyroid hormone). He also prescribed pregnenolone, which is claimed to have anti-degenerative properties.

Pregnenolone is made from cholesterol and is the master hormone from which all the steroid hormones are derived—estrogen, progesterone, testosterone, DHEA (dehydroepiandrosterone), aldosterone, cortisol, and so on. Pregnenolone has been reported to help slow the aging process, increase energy, enhance memory, stimulate the immune system, detoxify the body, and improve the body's response to stress. On the down side, pregnenolone can cause side effects, such as too much of a particular hormone (for example, testosterone), irritability, anxiety, hair loss, heart palpitations, insomnia, headaches, and acne. DHEA is also controversial. Long-term use use can increase possible risk for breast, ovarian, and prostate cancer. Either of these should be taken only when prescribed by a health professional, and under close supervision.

A great believer in probiotics, Dr. Mouton also prescribed Probactiol Plus (see Probiotics, page 71), an excellent product that has the added benefit of keeping me very regular. I take it every day on an empty stomach before breakfast. Dr. Mouton also advises high doses of vitamin D_3 for people who have MS, as well as omega-3 and omega-6 essential fatty acids. You can learn more about Dr. Mouton's protocol at his website, www.gmouton.com.

The full list of supplements I take is as follows:

- Multivitamin and minerals (Lamberts Multi-Guard), one daily
- EPA/DHA fish oils (Pure Encapsulations), 300 mg EPA and 200 mg DHA, two daily
- Evening primrose oil (Lamberts), 1,000 mg, two daily
- Vitamin D_3 (Pure Encapsulations), 5,000 IU, one daily

- Calcium magnesium citrate/malate (Pure Encapsulations), 75 mg, one daily
- Calcium citrate/malate (Pure Encapsulations), 150 mg, one daily
- Zinc (Lamberts), 15 mg, one daily
- Vitamin B-50 complex (Lamberts), one daily
- Resveratrol Extra (Pure Encapsulations), 500 mg, one daily
- Probactiol Plus (Biodynamics), one daily
- Serotone 5HTP (Higher Nature), 100 mg, one daily
- Glucofunction (Pure Encapsulations), one daily
- Optiferin (Pure Encapsulations), one daily
- Flaxseed oil (Jarrow Formulas), one daily
- Alpha lipoic acid (Lamberts), 250 mg, one daily
- Pycnogenol (Lamberts), 40 mg, one daily
- Coenzyme Q_{10} (Lamberts), 200 mg, one daily
- Ginkgo biloba (Lamberts), 6,000 mg, one daily
- Serrapeptase (Nature's Aid), 60,000 IU, one daily
- Yaemama Chlorella, 250 mg, six daily
- Aloe (BodyTech), one daily
- Kelp plus greens (Vega Vitamins), one daily
- Turmeric (Lamberts), 10,000 mg, one daily
- Ibibsene artichoke extract (Lamberts), 8,000 mg, one daily
- Shark Cartilage, 750 mg, one daily
- B_{12} injections, monthly
- Pregnenolone 40 mg/Calcium citrate 560 mg (made by a compounding pharmacist), one daily
- L-Thyroxine, 100 mcg, one daily
- Armour Thyroid, ½ grain, one daily*

Taking all these things helps keep MS fatigue and other symptoms to a minimum.

---

*This equates to 32.4 mg natural thyroid. The amount you take is completely individual and determined by a blood test.

❧ HOW NUTRITIONAL SUPPLEMENTS WORK IN MS

Nutritional supplements have seven main functions in MS:

1. Strengthen the immune system
2. Reduce inflammation
3. Strengthen the blood-brain barrier
4. Provide antioxidants to fight free radicals
5. Help heal a leaky gut so nutrients from food are better absorbed
6. Improve nerve signals
7. Reduce fatigue and give you more energy

Supplements to Strengthen the Immune System

Vitamin D_3, zinc, selenium, fish oil, and flaxseed oil all help to strengthen the immune system. Many of these supplements serve other functions as well, including reducing inflammation.

Vitamin D_3

There is mounting evidence that a lack of vitamin D_3 is a cause of MS.[1] Vitamin D_3 can suppress autoimmune reactions and slow relapse and progression in MS. It increases levels of TGF1 (beta) in the bloodstream, associated with MS remission. The main source of vitamin D_3 is sunlight. In countries where MS is rampant, such as Scotland and Norway, the scarcity of winter sunlight can affect individuals from birth.

D_3 is the most active form of the vitamin, far more so than D_2. For vitamin D_3 supplementation to be effective, it *must* be taken with adequate calcium and magnesium. (See chapter 9 about the crucial importance of vitamin D_3.)

Zinc

Zinc is a vital trace element involved in hundreds of processes in the body. It plays an essential role in maintaining a robust immune system and metabolizing essential fatty acids. It also helps in coping with stress. Certain foods, such as cow's milk, cheese, coffee, and bran, can inhibit the absorption of zinc. Also, viral infections, such as glandular fever, can cause a loss of zinc. During an MS relapse, zinc levels in red blood cells decrease dramatically.

Selenium

The trace element selenium is needed to make the important enzyme gluta-thione peroxidase, which helps fight against free radicals and damage from lipid peroxidation. The prevalence of multiple sclerosis may be inversely related to selenium levels in the soil. For example, MS is high in a district of Finland where the selenium levels are low. The prevalence of MS is low in nearby Lapland, where the selenium level is high.

One study reported that supplementation of eighteen patients with high doses of selenium, vitamin C, and vitamin E for five weeks increased levels of the enzyme glutathione peroxidase fivefold.[2] Good natural sources include seafood and sesame seeds.

Fish Oil

Fish oil is able to soothe inflammation. Fish and fish oil supplements are high in essential fatty acids from the omega-3 family, called eicosa-pentaenoic acid (EPA) and docosahexaenoic acid (DHA), which are important in maintaining normal function of the nervous system and the production of myelin.[3] They are incorporated into the myelin sheath, where they may increase fluidity and improve nerve transmission.

Throughout the world, MS is lower in places where fish consumption is significant. For example, there is a relatively low incidence of MS in the Faroe Islands, northwest of Scotland, compared to the Shetlands.[4] They share the same Danish genetic background and similar latitude. But in the Faroe Islands they eat a lot of fish, whereas in the Shetlands, not far away, they have adopted British agriculture and eat more meat and dairy products. Similar contrasts are apparent in Scandinavia.

The best kind of fish for MS is oily cold water fish such as mackerel, herring, sardines, salmon, tuna. Seafood is also good.[5] White fish, such as plaice (similar to sole) and cod, are fine, but oily fish is better. You should eat oily fish at least three times a week. Make sure the fish is not fished in waters contaminated by mercury.

In addition, take fish oil supplements every day. When purchasing fish oil supplements, look for EPA and DHA on the label, along with the amount they contain, as different brands can vary significantly. Buy the very highest quality, purest supplements, which have had the least amount of processing. Also, be aware of contaminants and toxins. Cod liver oil and other fish liver oils risk having these. Buy only high quality brands and read the labels carefully.

Flaxseed Oil

Flaxseed oil (also known as linseed oil) contains a good balance of both families of essential fatty acids—20 percent omega-6 (linoleic acid) and 60 percent omega-3 (alpha-linolenic acid). These support the nervous system and are essential in forming normal myelin.

Epidemiological studies indicate that dietary deficiency of alpha-linolenic acid (omega-3) is a greater causal factor than deficiency of linoleic acid (omega-6) in MS patients. Alpha-linolenic was found to be 19 percent lower in MS patients.

Flaxseed oil is a good alternative to fish oil because it is suitable for vegetarians and you can buy organic flaxseed oil, whereas fish might have contaminants. It is a simple process to make high quality flaxseed oil. It is more stable than fish oil, giving it a better shelf life, and includes several minor ingredients missing in fish oil. In addition to being one of the richest sources of essential fatty acids, flaxseeds are also very rich in lignans, an anti-cancer substance found only in high-fiber foods. Lignans also have antiviral, antifungal, and antibacterial properties.

However, in studies comparing fish and flaxseed oil, fish produces better results. Fish oil is faster acting, and you need ten times more flaxseed oil to get the same results you'd get from fish oil. Dr. Udo Erasmus recommends two to five tablespoons of flaxseed oil a day.[6] If you can, buy organic flaxseed oil in a dark bottle and keep it in the fridge once opened, as flaxseed oil can go bad.

Also recommended is a good source of gamma-linolenic acid, such as evening primrose or borage oil (see page 69).

Antioxidants: Strengthening the Blood-Brain Barrier

Antioxidants combat free radicals—reactive, unstable compounds that damage cell membranes—that are implicated in degenerative illnesses such as MS.

Antioxidants are found in such things as grape seed extract, anthocyanosides, and oligomeric proanthocyanidins (OPCs) found in pycnogenol (pine bark extract), bilberries, blueberries, blackberries, and cherries.

In MS, OPCs help maintain the integrity of the blood-brain barrier, which prevents immune cells from reaching the brain and spinal cord.

OPCs also bind to collagen, a protein in connective tissue, to maintain and restore its flexibility and integrity. Collagen is a primary component of the skin, blood vessels, joint tissues, respiratory tract, and intestinal tract. OPCs are also anti-inflammatory, anti-allergic, enhance the effect of vitamin C, and protect capillaries.

Less powerful antioxidants that also help maintain the blood-brain barrier are vitamins C, E, and A; alpha-lipoic acid; coenzyme Q_{10}; and ginkgo biloba.

Vitamin C

Vitamin C is involved in at least three hundred biochemical pathways in the body. It is needed for a healthy immune system, repair of tissue, and production of collagen. You can safely take 1,000 mg a day, but most modern diets provide only a tenth of this. Take a vitamin C capsule with bioflavonoids, as they assist in the absorption and use of vitamin C and the maintenance of healthy capillaries.

Vitamin E

Vitamin E protects unsaturated fatty acids in cell membranes. It enhances the immune response, slows down the degenerative process, and regulates platelet aggregation.

Alpha-lipoic Acid

This is a very potent antioxidant that can travel across cell membranes and scavenge free radicals, both inside and outside of the cells.

Coenzyme Q_{10}

Coenzyme Q_{10} is made by the human body, but diminishes as we age. It is involved in producing adenosine triphosphate (ATP), which is the cell's primary energy source and produces protein. Is is fat soluble, so for best absorption, it should be taken with a meal that contains fat.

Ginkgo Biloba

Ginkgo biloba helps maintain healthy peripheral circulation, including blood to the brain, so it can help maintain cognitive functions. It helps keep blood vessels dilated, allowing blood to flow more freely to the extremities, including the brain. Blood carries oxygen and essential nutrients as it circulates, and these are especially important to the brain, which demands high levels of oxygen and glucose for its many functions. It also works as an antioxidant and has positive effects on platelet function.

The active constituents of ginkgo are natural substances called ginkgo flavone glycosides, ginkgolides, and bilobalide. These play a beneficial role in scavenging free radicals and in preventing platelets from clumping.

Nutrients to Help Heal a Leaky Gut

Leaky gut is a simpler way of describing damage to the intestinal lining, which allows semi-digested particles into the bloodstream where they are toxic. The cells of the intestine, or gut, are the fastest growing cells in our bodies. They form a very thin (one-cell thick) barrier between the digestive tract and the rest of the body, and have to be replenished constantly. When gaps open between these cells, the result is leaky gut.

Evening Primrose and Borage Oil

Among the nutrients that can help heal a leaky gut are evening primrose oil and borage oil.[7] They do this mainly by maintaining the integrity of cell membranes and by strengthening blood vessel walls so there are no gaps in the fragile gut wall.

However, evening primrose and borage oils are involved in more functions than just healing a leaky gut. They are both high in gamma-linolenic acid (GLA), a more biologically active substance than linoleic acid. GLA converts into an anti-inflammatory molecule called an eicosanoid, which helps regulate the immune system. GLA also has antiviral properties. GLA is able to bypass all the blocking agents in the metabolic conversion process of linoleic acid.

For evening primrose and borage oils to work effectively, they need to be taken with zinc, magnesium, and vitamin C. Also, you need to eat a low saturated fat diet and take vitamin E.

There are various ways in which evening primrose and borage oil might alleviate the symptoms of MS. They:

- Stimulate the T lymphocytes, boosting the immune system.

- Make prostaglandin E1, which stimulates the normal function of T suppressor lymphocytes (the white blood cells that control the immune system and ensure that the body's defenses attack foreign materials, and not the body's own tissues).
- Keep the platelets from clumping together. Platelets are small, plate-like particles in the blood that help the blood clot. In people with MS, the platelets clump together in an abnormal way. Prostaglandin PGE1 regulates the platelets and keeps them from bunching up and sticking to each other and to blood vessel walls.
- Make faulty red blood cells return to normal. In people with MS, red blood cells are not only very low in essential fatty acids but are also much bigger than they ought to be, and have a poor ability to regulate the passage of fluids through cell membranes. Evening primrose oil and borage oil can correct this defect within a matter of months (through the actions described below).
- Correct the defect in the mobility of red blood cells. Electrophoretic mobility tests have shown that the red blood cells of people with MS move more slowly than those of healthy people. This was first identified by Professor E. J. Field and coworkers in 1977, and confirmed in 1980.[8] After several months of evening primrose or borage oil supplements, these red blood cells have been shown to behave normally.
- Strengthen blood vessel walls. In the microcirculation of people with MS, the blood vessel walls are breached so that blood—which is toxic to nerve tissue—seeps into the brain. When the blood vessel walls are strengthened, they are also better able to keep platelets and cholesterol from clumping and sticking to them. In addition to keeping the blood-brain barrier intact, it also helps prevent leaky gut by strengthening the walls of the intestines.
- May act as antiviral agents.
- Affect nerve conduction. PGE1 has strong regulating effects on the release of neurotransmitters at nerve endings, and also on the postsynaptic actions of the released transmitters. These effects can produce profound changes in the workings of both the central and peripheral nervous systems.
- Maintain a healthy balance between series 1 and 2 prostaglandins. If the body is very low in essential fatty acids, there is a sharp rise in

the inflammatory series 2 PGs, which are made from arachidonic acid. A high level of the series 2 PGs is a feature of various inflammatory disorders, such as rheumatoid arthritis and probably multiple sclerosis. It has recently been shown that the cerebrospinal fluid from MS patients contains high levels of PGF2a, one of the 2 series prostaglandins that is inflammatory.

Fish or Flaxseed Oil

See page 66 and 67.

Probiotics

Probiotics (literally, "for life") have many beneficial effects in MS. They reinforce the barrier effect in the gut and help the body resist infections and inflammation that can cause leaky gut. Probiotics also support the body's acid-alkaline balance. Good health requires trillions of beneficial bacteria—100 billion to 1,000 billion per milliliter—from one end to the other of your digestive system, mouth to anus. These friendly bacteria help restore proper balance by crowding out the harmful bacteria.

MS oftens brings about the decline of beneficial bacteria and disrupts the natural acid-alkaline balance in the gut, allowing harmful viral and fungal organisms, such as candida, to flourish. Probiotics promote proper functioning of the intestinal tract and immune system, helping the body to defend against invaders. They also help protect against food intolerances, particularly lactose and casein; aid digestion and absorption of nutrients; and produce significant amounts of B vitamins and enzymes, which help enormously in keeping you regular.

Many researchers now believe that declining levels of friendly bacteria in the intestinal tract may actually mark the onset of chronic degenerative disease and a suppressed immune system.

Personally, I take a high-quality probiotic every day. If I miss one for any reason, I immediately feel worse. A good probiotic needs to contain many billions of the recognized super strains of beneficial bacteria, L-acidophilus and bifidobacterium. The one I take, Probactiol Plus, is made by Metagenics. There are similarly high-quality products available in the United States and Canada as well as the United Kingdom. Good brands include BioCare, Solgar, Winning Team, Optibac, Cytoplan, and Savant.

Digestive Enzymes

Enzymes help the digestion and assimilation of food and prevent toxic buildup of undigested food. The digestive enzymes are lipase, amylase, lactase, cellulose, and protease. Digestive enzymes found in raw foods work together with those made in the mouth, stomach, and small intestine to make nutrients absorbable. It's useful to take supplements in case you're not making enough of your own.

You can take capsules between meals but you'll get better results taking enzymes with food, so that they can help with digestion. How much should be taken each day depends on the person and how much food is prepared, since cooking at high heat destroys enzymes. Some people do fine on two capsules; others need six or more. Signs of improvement are less gas and bloating, and fewer food sensitivities, allergies, and immune problems. You may have to try out a few different enzyme products to determine which one works best for you.

Research shows that pancreatic enzyme preparations, including bromelain and papain, effectively reduce the severity and frequency of MS attacks.[9] They particularly help with visual and sensory disturbances, and problems with the bladder, bowel, and gut.

NUTRIENTS THAT WORK IN COMBINATION WITH OTHERS

Some nutrients cannot function alone, or function minimally as individual supplements. These require other nutrients to optimize their benefit.

- *Zinc.* Needed for the metabolic conversion process of evening primrose oil and borage oil. (See page 69.)
- *Magnesium.* Necessary for the metabolic conversion process of evening primrose and borage oils, helps absorption of calcium, and helps metabolize B vitamins and essential fatty acids. Magnesium (and calcium) must be taken with vitamin D. Almost every metabolic system is dependent on magnesium. It helps produce cellular energy and is needed for nerve impulse transmission. A magnesium deficiency is common in MS, and spasticity can often be traced to low levels. This deficiency may be caused by a diet high in refined and processed foods and saturated fat, by

bran added to the diet, and by diuretics. Magnesium helps relax muscles; reduce tremor, spasticity, fatigue, cramps, numbness, and tingling; increase energy levels; and improve circulation to warm up cold extremities. It can be taken orally or in higher doses by intravenous infusion or injection into a muscle.

- *Calcium.* Calcium is needed for B_{12} absorption, and works together with magnesium for the healthy function of nerves and muscles. Calcium absorption is improved by taking vitamin D_3 and hampered by lead (from car exhaust), alcohol, coffee, tea, and lack of hydrochloric acid in the stomach. Calcium and magnesium need to be taken together. Calcium supplements are essential if you give up dairy products.

  There is a theory that deficiency of calcium and vitamin D during puberty causes predisposition to multiple sclerosis. Demyelination in MS results from a breakdown due to abnormal lipid composition and structure produced during the period of brain development. There are deficiencies in enzymes that govern myelin synthesis. This can happen due to inadequate supplies of vitamin D and calcium at times of rapid myelination and growth, especially adolescence. If this theory is correct, it may be possible to help control the disease by dietary supplementation with vitamin D and calcium during puberty.[10]

- *Manganese.* Manganese is involved in the production of the enzyme superoxide dismutase, and protects cells from free radical damage. It also helps the body absorb vitamin C and some of the B vitamins.

∾ B COMPLEX VITAMINS

The B vitamins work together to release energy from food, regulate functioning of the brain and nerves, regenerate the liver, and maintain the health of the digestive system. The most important B vitamins for MS are:

- *B_1 (thiamine).* Vitamin B_1 is uniquely important for nerves. It plays a crucial role in the release of energy from food and helps convert blood sugar into energy in muscles and nerves. Certain foods, beverages, and substances, such as tea, coffee, alcohol, and oral contraceptives, rob the body of B_1.* People who eat refined foods may also be low in B_1. Vitamin B_1 helps improve mood, memory, muscle strength, sensory symptoms, and fatigue. You need around 10–50 mg daily.

- B_2 *(riboflavin)*. Helps to repair and maintain soft tissue and membranes.
- B_3 *(niacin or nicotinamide)*. Involved in more than fifty different processes in the body.
- B_5 *(pantothenic acid)*. Supports the adrenal glands as they prepare the body and nervous system to meet everyday challenges. Steps up the release of energy from food and the rate of fat metabolism, and is necessary for the production of natural antibodies that help combat allergic reactions.
- B_6 *(pyridoxine)*. This is the prime B vitamin. It is vital for the health of the nervous and immune systems, and for the production of serotonin, the brain and mood hormone. Vitamin B_6 plays a major role in the metabolism of protein, sugar, essential fatty acids, and magnesium. B_6 also helps maintain the body's water balance. A deficiency can hamper the absorption of zinc and impair enzyme activity. Smoking, certain pharmaceutical drugs, carbon monoxide, and junk food can increase the need for B_6. If you take a dose higher than 50 mg, the other B complex vitamins must also be taken at that level dose.
- *Choline and inositol*. These are involved in fat metabolism, efficient transmission of nerve impulses, and metabolism of cholesterol and fat in the liver. Lecithin is a rich source of choline and inositol.
- *Folic acid*. Essential for many bodily functions, including the production of healthy red cells. Abundant in green leafy vegetables.

Special Importance of Vitamin B_{12}

Even though vitamin B_{12} is part of the B complex, it is advisable to take additional B_{12}. Vitamin B_{12} is needed for a healthy myelin sheath and

---

*In fact, the hormones in oral contraceptives may create certain nutrient deficiencies, and most of the B vitamins, particularly pyridoxine (B_6) and folic acid, are needed in higher amounts when birth control pills are taken. The copper level usually rises, and zinc levels often fall. Thus, more zinc is needed as well. An increased need for vitamins C, E, and K may also result from the use of birth control pills.[11]

axons, which are very important in healing MS. Lack of B,
the functioning of the immune system. People with MS m
in B_{12} due to poor absorption in the gut or to a disorder in
transport of the vitamin.

When there is B_{12} deficiency, toxic fatty acids destroy the myelin
sheath. However, sufficiently high doses of B_{12} can repair it. Vitamin B_{12}
usually helps people with MS to have more energy, less fatigue, a reduction
in pins and needles and tingling sensations, improvement in neurological
symptoms, less depression, and better sleep. Eyesight and hearing may also
improve. Since B_{12} deficiency can mimic MS symptoms, remediating the
deficiency can result in overall reduced symptoms.

Vitamin B_{12} is found in meat, especially beef, as well as in eggs, fish,
and dairy, which means that vegetarians and vegans are at great risk of
being deficient in dietary B_{12}. Also, vitamin B_{12} is not assimilated very
well via the gut, so best results are from injections into the muscle of the
arm or buttock. Try to get a weekly injection of 1,000 mcg from your
doctor or nurse. Some private doctors specializing in MS administer several times more B_{12} than this. Alternatively, you can take B_{12} under the
tongue in liquid or tablet form.

There is conflicting evidence as to whether people with MS have a
deficiency of B_{12}. However, it is probably a good idea to have B_{12} injections
to be on the safe side.

Studies on B_{12} and MS

Some studies have reported a significantly higher rate of vitamin B_{12} deficiency in people with MS, which is suspected to be due to problems with
binding and transport of vitamin B_{12} (meaning that the body does not
process vitamin B_{12} efficiently, which makes it difficult to maintain normal levels without supplementation). One study found low B_{12} levels in
the cerebrospinal fluid of people with MS, although their blood levels of
the vitamin were normal.[12]

Dr. E. H. Reynolds, from King's College Hospital in London, was
one of the first doctors to observe a B_{12} deficiency as well as abnormally
large blood cells in several patients with MS. Measuring the B_{12} and folic
acid levels in twenty-nine MS patients, Reynolds found that compared to
normal, healthy controls, all of them had abnormally low levels of B_{12} and

nine had extremely low levels of folic acid. Reynolds raised the question of whether this B_{12} deficiency was aggravating MS or impairing recovery. Writing about this in the *Archives of Neurology,* Reynolds says:

> Our observations suggest there is a significant association between MS and vitamin B_{12} deficiency, and that vitamin B_{12} deficiency should always be looked for in MS. . . . In neurology and hematology text-books, multiple sclerosis is not listed among the neurological compli-cations of vitamin B_{12} deficiency. Vitamin B_{12} deficiency is not even recognized as being associated with multiple sclerosis. There is no men-tion of vitamin B_{12} in the index of textbooks devoted to multiple scle-rosis. It is relevant that for some thirty years, there has been a tendency to treat multiple sclerosis with injections of vitamin B_{12}. . . . Although this is done for placebo purposes, this was not the original intention, and some patients are impressed with their neurologic benefit . . . the subject should be reawakened.[13]

After giving an account of his findings to a meeting of the Association of British Neurologists, doctors referred ten MS patients with B_{12} deficiencies to Dr. Reynolds.[14] Of these seven women and three men, eight of the patients were less than forty years old—unusually young to have a deficiency of B_{12}.

However, Donald W. Jacobsen, Ph.D., director of the Department of Cell Biology at Ohio's Cleveland Clinic, did not find as many B_{12}-deficient MS patients as in the British study. He said, "Researchers at the Cleveland Clinic, using tests that measure blood levels of B_{12} and two B_{12}-related compounds, homocysteine and methylmalonic acid, found fewer B_{12}-deficient people than did the British. At this point, we just don't know what to make of all of this." Dr. Jacobsen continued, "We still feel like we are missing major pieces of the puzzle. It's still an open question whether true, functional vitamin B_{12} deficiency exists in MS."[15]

Another study on B_{12} and MS showed vitamin B_{12} levels that were normal in the blood, but lower than usual in the cerebrospinal fluid, sug-gesting that people with MS might not be able to metabolize vitamin B_{12} in the same way as others.[16]

Another study on B_{12}, together with the antidepressant Lofepramine and L-phenylalanine (the Cari Loder treatment), did not find that B_{12} had any statistically significant effect on MS.[17]

However, Sarah Myhill, a medical doctor practicing in Wales said: "High dose vitamin B_{12} is of proven benefit in multiple sclerosis. I use this routinely in my MS patients and many report improvements in energy levels and well-being, and improvement of their neurological symptoms. The joy of B_{12} is that it has no known toxicity. It probably works because it is a very efficient scavenger of peroxynitrite, which is a free radical produced when superoxides combine with nitric oxide. I suggest initial injections of ½ mg (500 mcgms) daily subcutaneously, and adjust according to clinical response. B_{12} provides 'instant' antioxidant cover."

Dr. Britt Ahlrot-Westerlund in Sweden treated MS with methylcobalamin (the most active form of B_{12} and the form most frequently used as a treatment), selenium, and vitamin E. Vitamin B_{12} comes in many different forms, which freely transform into each other in the body. However, the brain and central nervous system utilize the methylcobalamin form of B_{12}. Cyanocobalamin, the form of B_{12} found in foods such as meat, fish, eggs, and dairy, is converted by the liver into methylcobalamin.

Although many doctors around the world use B_{12} as a vital part of their treatment for MS, few have written about it in the medical literature.

❧ OTHER ESSENTIAL NUTRITIONAL SUPPLEMENTS
These lesser known nutrients are essential for optimal body functioning. If you're not getting them from your diet, you may want to supplement.

MSM (Methyl Sulfonyl Methane)
MSM, or methyl sulfonyl methane, is a naturally occurring organic sulfur found in the tissues of all plants and animals, and is the fourth most abundant mineral in the body. The proper acid-alkaline balance of the body cannot be maintained without it. Sulfur is vital to the creation and regeneration of the body's tissues and is needed in the body for immune function, repair of damaged tissue and myelin, relief of muscle cramps, bowel regularity, supple joints, strong hair and nails, healthy skin, and collagen. Sulfur is also antibacterial, antiparasitic, helps remove toxins from cells, reduces inflammation, and promotes healing. Symptoms associated with sulfur deficiency include a poorly functioning immune system, gastrointestinal

problems, allergies, arthritis, and nail, hair, and skin problems. If the body is not receiving enough sulfur it produces weak, dysfunctional cells. MSM is virtually nontoxic and has no side effects. The body uses vitamin C with bioflavonoids to metabolize MSM to sulfur.

MSM is suggested to be effective in restoring the integrity of the blood-brain barrier in MS patients, thus reducing the invasion of CD4 T cells into the brain and diminishing the process of autoimmune attack. The substance also appears to be effective in reducing the incidence of muscle spasm. The dose is one or two grams each day.

Many people are deficient in organic sulfur because the sulfur present in foods, such as in milk, meat, seafood, grains, beans, onions, garlic, eggs, fruits, and vegetables (including broccoli and brussels sprouts) is often destroyed during cooking, refining, or processing.

Lecithin

Lecithin helps in fat metabolism. It is a precursor of acetylcholine, a neurotransmitter necessary for the transmission of messages between brain cells.

Amino Acids

Amino acids are the building blocks of all proteins, including all cells, membranes, and tissue. Amino acids are found in good quality proteins, such as fish, lean meat, poultry, and eggs. Eight of the amino acids are considered essential because you cannot make them in your body, but have to get them from foods. A lack of these essential amino acids may be due to faulty digestion or absorption, which then disrupts metabolic processes and creates general symptoms of weakness, fatigue, and lethargy.

At the Tahoma Clinic in Seattle, it was found that in nearly 100 percent of MS cases, the amino acid blood levels were abnormally low. By improving metabolism, amino acid supplements alleviate weakness and fatigue, and contribute to greater energy and well-being. You'll find more reports from the Tahoma Clinic at www.tahoma-clinic.com.

ADDITIONAL SUPPLEMENTS THAT CAN HELP MS

There have been enough positive anecdotal reports regarding all of the following supplements to warrant giving them a try.

Padma 28

This Swiss product, derived from an ancient Tibetan herbal formula, contains twenty-two powerful herbs that promote antioxidant activity. It helps regulate the immune system and promotes the body's own interferon. Research in Poland showed that MS patients improved by 44 percent when taking Padma 28.[18] They experienced release of tight banding around the middle, alleviation of paralysis, and improvements in muscle strength, bladder and bowel control, coordination, eyesight, and hearing.

Chlorella and Spirulina

These are blue-green sea algae very rich in protein, minerals, and trace elements, and therefore called superfoods. They both have properties that help to rebuild nerve tissue. Chlorella contains 60 percent protein—including all the essential amino acids—and high levels of chlorophyll and beta-carotene. It has more chlorophyll than any other plant, making chlorella a powerful detoxifying agent that helps to eliminate mercury. Spirulina is the most digestible form of protein, and one particular strain is high in gamma-linolenic acid (the key substance in evening primrose oil), vitamin B_{12}, and friendly bacteria for the gut. There are claims that spirulina is good for fatigue.

ENADA

ENADA, or NADH (nicotinamide adenine dinucleotide), is the active coenzyme form of vitamin B_3. It boosts energy and the immune system.

Bee Pollen, Royal Jelly, and Propolis

Bee pollen boosts energy and endurance, strengthens the immune system, helps build resistance to allergies, and assists in coping with stress. It contains ninety-six different nutrients and is considered by some to be the perfect food. Bee pollen contains twenty-two amino acids, vitamin C, B complex (including a high level of folic acid), polyunsaturated fatty acids, enzymes, and carotene—all of the known major antioxidants.

Propolis is a resinous substance used by bees to build their hives. It helps regulate hormones, has antibiotic properties, stimulates the formation of cells and tissue, and boosts the immune system. It also contains protein, amino acids, vitamins, minerals, and flavonoids.

Royal jelly, also known as royal cells, is the thick, creamy, extremely nutritious substance produced by bees to feed the queen bee, who lives forty times longer than all the other bees and produces one and a half times her weight in eggs. There are two hormones in royal jelly, called juveille and ecdyson. It contains proteins, carbohydrates, at least seventeen amino acids, fatty acids, sugars, sterols, phosphorous compounds, and acetylcholine, which is needed to help transmit messages from cell to cell. It also contains the vitamins A, C, D, and E, and is particularly useful for its B complex content, including B_1, B_2, B_6, B_{12}, biotin, folic acid, inositol, and pantothenic acid (B_5). On top of all that, this power-packed substance contains the minerals calcium, copper, iron, phosphorous, potassium, silicone, and sulfur. It is claimed to be good for the immune system.

A Greek company named Royal Cells did a three-year pilot study in 2001 to find out whether royal jelly mixed with other natural substances can slow the progress of MS. This study involved 140 MS patients from Greece, the United Kingdom, Israel, and Canada who were treated for one to forty-two months with increasing daily doses. There was no control group, and patients were asked for their own evaluation of results, so this is not strictly scientific. However, the company reports that the results were positive and in some cases the royal jelly not only slowed the progress of MS but improved the clinical condition. Of the 140, 120 responded favorably, and twenty not at all. None reacted negatively. Of the 84 percent who responded positively, improvements were reported in the areas of vision, swallowing, mobility, fatigue, coordination, trigeminal neuralgia, speech, mood, sexual dysfunction, and numbness. Relapses were reduced by 50 percent.

Royal Cells subsequently improved their product by adding additional nutrients. This new product, Nectar M, is a mixture of 80 percent royal jelly, 18 percent thyme honey, and 2 percent thyme propolis. Thyme honey has high levels of antioxidants, amino acids, vitamin B_6, riboflavin, and pantothenic acid; and trace amounts of calcium, copper, iron, magnesium, manganese, phosphorus, potassium, sodium, and zinc.

Nectar M arrives from Greece in single-dose pots to be taken before breakfast on an empty stomach. It has no side effects. I take this brand myself every morning, but there are many others available in the marketplace. One caution would be that if you are allergic to bee stings, you may want to be tested for sensitivity to royal jelly.

Aloe Vera

(See also Glyconutrients, page 83.)

Aloe vera is an immune system tonic that soothes the digestive tract and helps heal a leaky gut. It contains three glyconutrients—glucose, mannose, and xylose—and is an excellent dietary source of fructo-oligosaccharides, which attract beneficial bacteria to inhabit the gut. It also helps with constipation, increasing the frequency of bowel movements and softening stools.

Aloe vera contains a wide range of vitamins, the most important being the antioxidants C, E, and beta-carotene. It is one of the few plants in the world to contain vitamin B_{12}, and also contains the minerals magnesium, manganese, zinc, copper, chromium, calcium, sodium, potassium, and iron. Aloe vera provides twenty out of the twenty-two amino acids the human body requires, and provides seven of the eight essential amino acids the human body requires but cannot manufacture. Other components are enzymes (break down food and aid digestion), anti-inflammatory plant sterols, and saponins, soapy substances that exert a powerful antimicrobial effect against bacteria, viruses, fungi, and yeast.[19]

Bottled aloe is available in natural food stores, but if you have an aloe plant at home, you can just peel a stalk and add a piece to a fruit or vegetable shake, without changing the flavor or texture.

....

Betsy: More Energy with Aloe Vera

After taking aloe vera for about two months, I began to notice small benefits. Then, after altering the dosage, I found I was experiencing significant improvements. I used to suffer numbing fatigue, malaise, and anxiety. Now I am less stressed and have loads more energy and a feeling of well-being. Continence has improved. So have the spasms and tremors in my hands and legs, which had been very bad. My hands are a lot steadier and I am able to do some drawing again.

Aloe vera is not to everyone's taste. Personally, I don't mix it with anything but you can add fruit juice if you like, or buy it already mixed with juice. The suggested dose is between 60–100 mls (about one-third of a cup) a day. However, I take 150 mls (nearly two-thirds of a cup) a day, as I have found that this amount suits me best. If I am particularly tired, I take a little more; you can't overdose on aloe vera. It's best taken on an empty stomach, so I drink it slowly about an hour and a half before breakfast.

....

Calcium EAP2

Calcium EAP2 stands for calcium 2-aminoethylphosphate, sometimes called vitamin M_1, and in some places sold under the brand name Mynax. It was made famous as a treatment for MS in 1960 by German doctor Hans Nieper, who died in 1999. It's been approved in Germany as a therapy for MS since 1966, and has since been adopted by other doctors in both Europe and the United States. EAP2 helps with neurotransmission, is an important transporter of minerals in the body, and maintains the integrity of cell walls, keeping out toxins.

Nieper believed that in MS there is cell membrane damage throughout the body. Calcium EAP is claimed to gradually repair areas of demyelination, sealing areas of damaged cell membrane. Calcium EAP2 works best with a nutritional diet and supplements. Some doctors inject calcium EAP so it goes straight into the bloodstream, but it can also be taken in capsule form, 300–500 mg daily with food.

Nieper wrote many papers on calcium EAP during the 1960s and '70s, and in 1992 wrote "Mineral Transporters," published in *Let's Live* magazine. This is available from the Brewer Science Library.

D-Mannose

D-mannose is a natural glyconutrient that is used to prevent and treat bladder infections in MS. It flushes away *E. coli* bacteria but without causing thrush, as antibiotics can do. It goes virtually straight through you, passing very quickly into the urine with hardly any metabolizing, making it a fast and natural way to treat urinary tract infections. Brands include Waterfall D-mannose and D-Mannose.

The founders of Waterfall D-mannose, Anna Sawkins and John Bremner, who run the company Sweet Cures of York, came up with D-mannose after Anna suffered from serious repeat bladder and kidney infections. They found some research that suggested that the way that *E. coli* with fimbriae (the only variations that cause bladder infections) attached to cells in the body was mainly by attaching to the mannose in cells. They thought that by filling those receptors with an innocuous form of mannose with the correct optical orientation to fit the *E. coli* receptors precisely, the bug's receptors would be filled, and they would slip out of the bladder with normal urination.

D-mannose is an essential glyconutrient and a natural component of every cell in our bodies.[20] It should not be confused with Mannitol, which does not attach itself to *E. coli.* and has completely different properties. In simple terms, D-mannose fools *E. coli* into believing that it is attaching to body cells.

Glyconutrients

Glyconutrients are simple sugars composed of small amounts of mono-saccharides. They enhance cell-to-cell communication, modulate the immune system, and increase your body's own stem cell production. They come from plant roots, mushrooms, and other foods, and can be taken as dietary supplements.

Glyconutrients combine with proteins and fats to form a "code" that allows each cell to communicate with other cells. This code is found on the surface of every cell and allows the immune system to distinguish between self and non-self. If you are deficient in glyconutrients, there will be a breakdown in your internal communication system among cells.

People with MS appear to have abnormal galactose molecules, which may be affecting the ability of their cells to communicate with one another. Some MS patients who take supplemental glyconutrients no longer have visible signs and symptoms of MS, and their MRI scans show that their neurological lesions have diminished or even disappeared. This may be because the glyconutrients have helped to restore normal cell-to-cell communication. Welsh doctor Bob Lawrence, who has MS, believes that glyconutrient therapy can be effective in reducing disability and the size and number of MS brain lesions.

Glyconutrients and Stem Cells

Lawrence believes that glyconutrients increase the body's own production of natural stem cells, and that these go where they are needed to repair and heal. He thinks that taking glyconutrients will also help stem cell treatment work more powerfully. (See Stem Cells in chapter 14, page 212.)

Essential Glyconutrients

There are eight essential glyconutrients, and you need all of them. These are:

- *Glucose*
- *Galactose*
- *Mannose*—prompts anti-inflammatory activity and tissue regeneration and helps correct overactive T cells that cause misguided inflammation. It is also an antibacterial agent and has antiviral, anti-parasitic, and antifungal properties.
- *Fucose*—plays a role in eliminating or reversing autoimmunity, cancer, and inflammation. It is profoundly important for efficient neuron transmission in the brain, and is a powerful brain modulator.
- *Xylose*
- *N-acetyl glucosamine*—in the form of glucosamine sulphate, helps repair cartilage, decreases inflammation, is an immune modulator, and has anti-viral properties.
- *N-acetyl galactosamine*—important for proper cell-to-cell communication
- *N-acetyl neuraminic acid* (sialic acid)—plays an important part in the immune system

Complete Sources of Glyconutrients

The eight essential glyconutrients can be provided by just four common food supplements:

- *Kelp.* Contains the five glyconutrients glucose, mannose, galactose, fucose, and xylose. Take four tablets daily.
- *Aloe vera.* Contains the three glyconutrients glucose, mannose, and xylose. Take 15 mls twice a day.
- *Shark cartilage, glucosamine sulphate, and chondoitrin sulphate.* All contain N-acetyl glucosamine and N-acetyl galactosamine, but the

last two are often derived from cattle cartilage, with the possible problems of beef protein sensitivity. Take 2,000 mg a day.

- *Whey or egg protein.* Both whey and egg protein contain one of the essential glyconutrients, N-acetyl neuraminic acid. However, it may not be possible to use egg or whey in MS, due to sensitivity.

Food Sources of Glyconutrients

Glyconutrients can be found to some extent in the following foods:

- *Glucose.* Nearly all ripe fruits and vegetables. Honey, grapes, bananas, mangoes, cherries, strawberries, cocoa, aloe vera, licorice, sarsaparilla, hawthorn, garlic, echinacea, and kelp.
- *Galactose.* Dairy products, fenugreek, kelp, apple pectin, apples, apricots, bananas, blackberries, cherries, cranberries, currants, dates, grapes, kiwi, mangoes, orange, nectarine, peach, pear, pineapple, plums, prunes, raspberries, rhubarb, strawberries, passionfruit, echinacea, boswellia, chestnuts, broccoli, brussels sprouts, avocado, cabbage, cucumber, carrot, cauliflower, celery, potato, eggplant, peas, pumpkin, and spinach.
- *Mannose.* Aloe vera, kelp, shiitake mushrooms, fenugreek, carob gum, guar gum, black currants, red currants, gooseberries, capsicum (cayenne pepper), cabbage, eggplant, tomatoes, and turnips.
- *Fucose.* Kelp, wakame seaweed, and brewer's yeast.
- *Xylose.* Kelp, ground psyllium seeds, guava, pears, blackberries, loganberries, raspberries, aloe vera, echinacea, boswellia, broccoli, spinach, eggplant, peas, green beans, okra, cabbage, and corn.
- *N-acetyl glucosamine.* Shiitake mushrooms, shark cartilage, beef cartilage, and red algae (*dumontiaceae*).
- *N-acetyl galactosamine.* Beef cartilage, shark cartilage, and red algae.
- *N-acetyl neuraminic acid.* Milk, whey protein concentrate or isolate, chicken, eggs.

Some sources, such as the *Wellness Letter* produced by the University of California at Berkeley, say that you can easily get all these from food, and advise against buying expensive products.[21]

....

Gloria: More Flexibility with Glyconutrients

I started taking glyconutrients in 2004. The best improvement has been getting movement back in my left leg, which used to drag and felt like lead. Now I am lifting my foot forward some five inches, and can lift my knee off the bed about an inch! Within eight weeks of taking the powders I had regained full use of my left hand and could eat properly with a knife and fork. I could move my previously wooden body freely and easily. I can touch the tip of my nose with my finger, with my eyes closed. I have regained full circulation in my legs, and they are no longer blocks of ice.

....

Greens

Terry Wahls, who created the Brain Nutrient Diet, is a great fan of drinkable greens, which she thinks "are incredibly good for us and a great energy boost." After starting on a powdered greens product called Kyogreen, she then started making her own greens. She says: "I decided to use my Vitamix blender to create my own green beverages instead of using the instant greens. I've been on rotation blending cilantro, parsley, or kale with water and ice. It's worked well for me. I have more energy immediately following the glass of greens." She does not include wheat grass, as cereal grasses are likely to contain the same antigens as the grain. If you have food sensitivity to gluten, likely you'll have sensitivity to wheat and other cereal grasses.

Curcumin (Turmeric)

Turmeric, the traditional Asian spice that gives curry its yellow hue, can help MS. Turmeric contains curcumin, a polyphenolic compound isolated from the rhizome of the plant *Curcuma longa,* traditionally used in Asian medicine for pain and wound healing. Studies in mice suggest that curcumin may block the progression of MS.[22] Dr. Chandramohan Natarajan, of Vanderbilt University in Nashville, Tennessee, found that mice injected with curcumin showed little or no disease symptoms, while untreated animals went on to develop severe paralysis.

In their thirty-day study, Natarajan's team administered 50- and

100-mcg doses of curcumin three times a week to a group of mice bred to develop the animal model of MS, experimental autoimmune encephalomyelitis (EAE). They then monitored the mice for signs of MS-like neurological impairment. By day fifteen, those mice that had not received curcumin had a marked progression of EAE with complete paralysis of both hind limbs. In contrast, mice given the 50-mcg dose of the curry compound showed only minor symptoms, such as a temporarily stiff tail. Mice given the 100-mcg dose appeared completely unimpaired throughout the thirty days of the study. MS is very rare in India, where curries are eaten frequently.

Exactly how curcumin might work to halt the progression of demyelination remains unclear, but the Nashville researchers believe it may interrupt the production of IL-12, which plays a key role in signalling immune cells to attack the myelin sheath.

Noni Juice

Tahitian noni juice comes from the *Morinda citrifolia* fruit, found in the South Pacific region, where it has been used by native populations for its health benefits for thousands of years. It is claimed to have anti-inflammatory, antiseptic, and antifungal properties. It is also claimed to be a painkiller and to help balance the immune system. The active ingredients of noni juice include carotenoids, bioflavonoids, and anthraquinones, which have antibacterial properties in the intestinal tract and aid digestion.

Proponents say noni juice mimics the secretion coming from the pineal gland, building it up and allowing it to function normally. Noni juice contains an alkaloid precursor to xeronine (proxeronine) claimed to activate the pineal gland, which stimulates two major nerve hormones—serotonin and melatonin. Xeronine may also help enlarge the pores in the walls of human cells and enable nutrients to enter the cells more easily.

Research at the University of Hawaii's Biomedical Sciences Department showed that extracts of noni contain a naturally occurring component that activates serotonin receptors in the brain and throughout the body. Serotonin is an important neurotransmitter. No specific research has been done on the use of noni in the treatment of MS.

In recent years there have been accusations against some of the companies behind noni juice, saying they made fraudulent claims about its benefits and "miracle" ingredients. The basis of the noni juice fraud claim is that it contains proxeronine, a precursor to xeronine, neither of which is listed among the Recommended Daily Allowance list of nutrients.

Also, some potential dangers of noni juice have come to light: Taken in excessive amounts, it can cause liver damage. The dose should not exceed 2 tablespoons a day. Noni juice is also high in potassium, which could be dangerous to people with kidney conditions.

The U.S. Food and Drug Administration (FDA) has warned some of the companies selling noni juice that they made several unfounded health claims about the purported benefits of noni juice as a medicinal product, putting it into the same category as a drug. Under the Federal Food, Drug, and Cosmetic Act, a substance needs to have gone through clinical trials for safety and efficacy to provide compelling evidence to prove that it works in humans. This has not happened with noni, for which the only evidence is anecdotal. There have been some scientific studies, however, showing that noni increases physical endurance in mice and athletes. The FDA has also stated that there is no scientific evidence for health benefits of some specific phytochemicals found in noni juice, scopoletin and damnacanthal.

I have been taking noni juice for about three years with no ill effects. It is difficult to single out how noni juice may be helping since I take so many other supplements. Anecdotal reports about the benefits of noni juice for MS include those from women with MS who say that noni has improved their sex life, making them more orgasmic. The ingredients of different brands of noni juice vary.

Green Tea

A 2007 study conducted by Dr. Orhan Aktas from the Institute of Neuroimmunology, Berlin, showed that green tea can help MS. Green tea contains a powerful antioxidant—EGCG (epigallocatechin-3-gallate)—a type of flavonoid that can boost immunity and combat inflammation by inhibiting autoreactive T cells. Aktas did studies on the animal form of MS (encephalomyelitis, or EAE) and found that green tea improved the condition.[23]

Reishi and Lion's Mane Mushrooms

Reishi mushroom (also known as *ling zhi* in Chinese) and yamabushitake mushroom, also known as Lion's Mane, can help with fatigue and immune modulation. Reishi is also known to improve circulation and scavenge free radicals, thus supporting detoxification. Among other healing properties, Lion's Mane has anti-inflammatory action and helps combat symptoms of peripheral neurological dysfunction. It stimulates the synthesis of nerve growth factor (NGF) and is able to pass through the blood-brain barrier.

Kombucha

Kombucha is a sweet-sour, fermented tea that has been used in China for centuries. Kombucha is a colony of yeast and bacteria that grows in a blend of black tea and sugar from a pure cellulose mushroom. The resulting liquid is a refreshingly sweet and sour, lightly sparkling beverage with a fruity fragrance, that reputedly has antibiotic properties. The tea contains small, but probably significant, amounts of important nutrients, such as B vitamins and essential amino acids.[24] Some people with MS have used it with good results.

Several other supplements are recommended after the removal of mercury amalgam dental fillings and in detoxification. See chapters 18 and 19.

SPECIFIC RECOMMENDED SUPPLEMENTS FOR VARIOUS PROTOCOLS

It is only through trial and error that you will find the best supplement protocol for you. Once you've been tested for deficiencies, consult with your doctor on a recommended daily program. However, a doctor can only tell you so much. If you start on one of the programs described here, give it *at least* three months to take effect before making further adjustments. Some people expect supplements to work virtually overnight, but they do not. See Resources for additional information on the following protocols.

Dr. Tom Gilhooly's Recommended Supplements

Scottish physician Tom Gilhooly, who runs a clinic in Glasgow and treats many patients with MS, advises taking the following supplements. He has researched and formulated his own products specifically for MS, called Baseline am/pm, which simplifies the process of taking supplements into just two capsules. The ingredients contained include:

- Vitamin D: 2,000 IU
- Calcium: 200 mg
- Magnesium: 70 mg
- Selenium: 35 mcg
- Zinc: 50 mg
- Ginkgo biloba: 120 mg
- Pine bark extract (pycnogenol): 100 mg
- Chromium polynicotinate: 400 mcg
- EPA: omega-3 dose as determined by blood test
- A multivitamin

Dermot O'Connor's Recommended Supplements

Dermot O'Connor, Dip. Ac, MMQ, author of *The Healing Code,* was diagnosed with an aggressive form of MS but totally regained his health by following the five-point recovery plan described in his book.

He is now a qualified holistic practitioner, acupuncturist, psycho-therapist, and NLP practitioner who runs his own clinics in Dublin and London. He thinks that the best way to get vitamins and minerals is by eating an organic diet, but he is also in favor of taking specific supplements scientifically shown to help fight serious illnesses. The daily supplements he recommends are not just for MS and include:

- Spirulina: 6,000 mg. Spirulina is the most nutritious concentrated food known to man and contains many nutrients often lacking in people's diets: beta-carotene—a powerful natural antioxidant—vitamin B_{12}, and the essential fatty acid gamma-linolenic acid, all of which are readily absorbed. Spirulina also has protein with a complete amino acid profile. It is the most digestible form of protein and the amino acids are delivered in their "free form" state for almost instant assimilation. It helps protect the immune system and supports absorption of minerals.

- Vitamin A (contained in spirulina): 15,000 IU (*Note:* Do not take additional vitamin A if you are taking spirulina.)
- Vitamin B complex: 50 mg
- Vitamin C: 2,000–10,000 mg
- Vitamin E: 1,000 mg
- Zinc: 30 mg
- Selenium: 200 mcg
- Coenzyme Q_{10}: 400 mg. Coenzyme Q_{10} is like a spark plug, helping us to get energy from every cell. Without coQ_{10}, there is no energy production. It helps bring about increased energy levels and less fatigue. It is also an antioxidant and is anti-aging. Most people don't get enough dietary coQ_{10}, which is lost during the cooking process.
- MSM: 2,000 mg. You cannot overdose with MSM—the body uses what it needs and flushes out the rest. Take morning and evening.

Terry Wahls's Suggested Nutrients

Terry Wahls has made a study of the particular nutrients needed in order for mitochondria, the powerhouse of all cells, to work properly. However, Wahls places great emphasis on getting nutrients from food. Her recommended nutrients were detailed in chapter 6.

9

Vitamin D

WE ARE DEVOTING an entire chapter to vitamin D, particularly vitamin D_3, as it has now been proven beyond a doubt that it is especially critical to MS. It has long been known that vitamin D can suppress autoimmune reactions and slow relapse and progression in MS. Importantly, it has now been shown that vitamin D is definitely one of the environmental, genetic, and epidemiological factors involved in MS.

Vitamin D supplements are available in two forms: vitamin D_3 (also known as cholecalciferol) and vitamin D_2 (ergocalciferol). D_3 is the natural form and D_2 is the synthetic form. Many supplements are in the D_2 form, but vitamin D_3 is the one that is essential and converts in the body to its active form, 25-dihydroxyvitamin D.

Food sources of vitamin D include oily fish, such as kippers, mackerel, salmon, sardines, tuna, fish liver oil, and eggs. However, vitamin D is found only in small amounts in foods. Skin exposed to sunlight produces the greatest amount of vitamin D, according to Michael Holick, professor of medicine, physiology, and biophysics at Boston University Medical Center and author of the book *The UV Advantage*.[1]

∾ WHAT DOES VITAMIN D DO?

Vitamin D helps to regulate immune function and prevent autoimmune disease through its role in T cell development and differentiation. It suppresses the proliferation of T1 helper cells, which are involved in autoimmune activity in MS. When there are high levels of vitamin D, cells called T2 helper cells keep the T1 helper cells in balance, thus reducing autoimmune activity.[2]

Vitamin D is also a powerful antioxidant. It fights dangerous free radicals and combats oxidative damage to the central nervous system. It plays a part in helping to reduce mercury toxicity in the body by radically increasing the amount of intracellular glutathione. Vitamin D also helps the gut absorb calcium, magnesium, iron, zinc, and other minerals.

～ HOW VITAMIN D HELPS PREVENT AND ALLEVIATE MS

Many scientific papers have shown that vitamin D:

1. Prevents MS
2. Helps contol a gene implicated in MS
3. Reduces symptoms and relapses, and lessens disease activity and progression

Vitamin D Prevents MS

Ashton Embry and others are convinced that MS is a disease of long-latency vitamin D deficiency. For many years Embry has been urging people with MS to take vitamin D and also give it to their families to prevent MS in the next generation. One research study after another, conducted at renowned universities and printed in prestigious medical journals, has concluded that lack of vitamin D is linked to a higher rate of MS and that ensuring sufficient vitamin D levels plays a preventive role.

Since Dr. Reinhold Vieth, Canada's leading researcher in vitamin D nutrition, wrote his watershed paper on vitamin D in 1999, it has become very clear that vitamin D deficiency plays a major role in MS.[3] This was one of the first times that the classic recommendations for vitamin D were challenged.

In 2004, Dr. Kassandra Munger of the Harvard School of Public Health, Boston, published a study of nearly 190,000 women showing that those who took vitamin D supplements were 40 percent less likely to develop MS.[4] She also found that a diet high in vitamin D alone was not enough to provide the same protection as supplements.

In 2006, Munger published another major study that confirmed vitamin D's effectiveness in protecting against MS. Researchers examined whether high blood levels of 25-hydroxyvitamin D are linked with a lower risk of MS, and found that those with the highest levels of vitamin D—particularly before age twenty—had a two-thirds lower risk of getting MS compared to those with the lowest levels of vitamin D. The study included more than seven million U.S. military personnel. Each case was matched to two controls by age, sex, race/ethnicity, and dates of blood collection.

Among caucasians there was a 41 percent decrease in MS risk for every 50-nmol/L (nanomols per liter) increase in 25-hydroxyvitamin D. Among blacks and Hispanics, who had lower 25-hydroxyvitamin D levels than Caucasians, no significant associations between vitamin D and multiple sclerosis risk were found. The researchers called for a trial on the preventative role of vitamin D, saying that, "First-degree relatives of individuals with MS are at a higher risk of developing MS, and a prevention trial among this population would be possible and timely."[5]

Other research has found that people with MS tend to have insufficient levels of vitamin D, that periods of low vitamin D occur before times of high disease activity, and that, conversely, periods of high vitamin D precede times of low disease activity.[6]

Several other studies have shown that vitamin D plays a protective role in MS. A study in Norway by Margitta Kampman looked at the risk of MS and differences in outdoor activities and diet of children and adolescents born and living in northern Norway.[7] They found that increased outdoor activities in early life and cod liver oil supplementation (high in vitamin D) were associated with a lower risk of MS.

In Australia, I. A. van der Mei measured vitamin D levels in Tasmanian people with MS and found that "increasing disability was strongly associated with lower levels of 25(OH)D (circulating vitamin D) and with lower levels of sun exposure."[8]

A key paper published in 2007 by Norwegian T. Holmoy came to the same conclusion—that adequate vitamin D in childhood prevents MS by regulating the immune system in such a way that it does not produce myelin-sensitive immune cells during and after infections with childhood viruses, such as Epstein-Barr.[9]

In 2008 another scientist joined the throng saying that vitamin D protects against MS. Sylvia Christakos, Ph.D., of the New Jersey Medical School, wrote in a paper that the incidence of MS decreases as the amount of available vitamin D increases, either through sunlight or diet.[10] The article states that MS is almost unknown in equatorial regions, and that the prevalence is lower in areas where fish consumption is high. Christakos's report focuses on the immunosuppressive actions of the active form of vitamin D, which may inhibit the induction of MS, and emphasizes the importance of maintaining a sufficient vitamin D level.

"Evidence has shown that the maintenance of an adequate vitamin D level may have a protective effect in individuals predisposed to MS," Christakos reported. "One device of vitamin D action may be to preserve balance in the T-cell reaction and thus avoid autoimmunity."

Vitamin D Helps Control a Gene Implicated in MS

A landmark 2009 study showed that vitamin D controls a gene that greatly raises the odds of getting MS. Researchers at the University of Oxford and University of British Columbia, Canada, looked at a section of the genome on chromosome 6, which had been shown to be the primary indicator of MS risk.[11] The researchers found that proteins activated by vitamin D in the body bind to a particular DNA sequence next to the gene, altering its function.

The significance of this is that while around one in one thousand people in the United Kingdom is likely to develop MS, this number rises to around one in three hundred among those carrying a single copy of the gene variant DRB1*1501. That figure rises to one in one hundred in those carrying two copies of the gene variant. The statistics in this research relate specifically to the United Kingdom, however, they are likely to be similar in other places of the same latitude.

Exactly how the gene–environment interaction alters MS risk is yet to be determined. One explanation could be an effect on the thymus—a part of the immune system that produces T cells to attack bacterial and viral invaders. In people who carry the gene variant, a lack of vitamin D during early life might impair the ability of the thymus to delete rogue T cells, which then go on to attack the body, leading to a loss of myelin on the nerve fibers.

This finding has huge implications for protecting the next generation against MS. The coauthor of this study, Professor George Ebers from the Wellcome Trust Centre for Human Genetics at the University of Oxford, said it had been known for a long time that genes and the environment determine MS risk. He stated: "Here we show that the main environmental risk candidate—vitamin D—and the main gene region are directly linked and interact."

Vitamin D Reduces MS Symptoms and Relapses, and Lessens Disease Activity and Progression

Some studies have shown that increased vitamin D lessens disease progression and resulting disability. In an important study published in 2009, Australian scientists found that vitamin D may actually reduce the symptoms of MS. Professor Bruce Taylor, a principal research fellow at the Menzies Research Institute in Hobart, Australia, studied 145 patients in southern Tasmania and tracked their seasonal susceptibility to the disease. He looked at the relationship between vitamin D levels and the risk of having an attack of MS.

Taylor said: "We found that the higher your vitamin D level, the lower your chance of relapse, and for each ten nanomole [a standard measure of concentration of vitamin D in the blood] increase in vitamin D, you can reduce your risk of having an attack of MS by about 10 percent. Doubling your vitamin D will reduce your risk by up to 50 percent—a major result."[12]

A Canadian study done at the University of Toronto and presented in 2009 to the American Academy of Neurology found that taking high doses of vitamin D dramatically reduces the relapse rate in people with multiple sclerosis.[13]

Most of the people in the study had the relapsing form of MS, characterized by repeated relapses punctuated by periods of recovery, and had suffered from the disease for an average of eight years. People in the high-dose group were given escalating doses of vitamin D concentrate that could be added to juice for six months, to a maximum of 40,000 IU daily. Then doses were gradually lowered over the next six months, averaging out to 14,000 IU daily for the year.

The rest of the participants were allowed to take as much vitamin

D as they and their doctors thought was warranted, but it averaged out to only 1,000 IU a day. Everyone also took 1,200 milligrams of calcium daily. Vitamin D is essential for promoting calcium absorption in the gut, and together with calcium, helps promote bone health.

Sixteen percent of twenty-five people with multiple sclerosis, given a daily average of 14,000 IU of vitamin D for a year, suffered relapses. In contrast, close to 40 percent of twenty-four MS patients who took an average of only 1,000 IU a day—the amount recommended by many MS specialists—relapsed.

Also, people taking high-dose vitamin D suffered 41 percent fewer relapses than the year before the study began. Those taking typical doses suffered 17 percent fewer relapses. People taking high doses of vitamin D did not suffer any significant side effects.

Vitamin D appears to suppress the autoimmune responses thought to cause MS. In MS, haywire T lymphocytes—the cellular "generals" of the immune system—order attacks on the myelin sheaths that surround and protect the brain cells. In people given high-dose vitamin D in the study, T cell activity dropped significantly. That didn't happen in people who took lower doses.

In Finland, M. Soilu-Hanninen demonstrated that for MS patients, there was "an inverse relationship between serum vitamin D levels and MS clinical activity."[14]

In a British study, J. A. Woolmore found that there was an association between skin type and disability in female MS patients. Those with sun-sensitive skin types, which produce vitamin D faster, had lesser disability.[15]

ᔐ VITAMIN D DEFICIENCY

There are many things contributing to the widespread deficiency in vitamin D. These include:

- Too few, or too short, sunny days.
- Covering the skin or applying high SPF sunscreen on sunny days.
- Too much time indoors.
- Not enough oily fish in the diet.
- Malabsorption of dietary fats.

- Human body has less ability to manufacture vitamin D as it ages.
- Vegans living in cold climates don't have enough vitamin D in their diets.
- Dark-skinned people may have a reduced ability to produce vitamin D from sunlight.
- Heavy metals can block the synthesis of active vitamin D in the kidneys.
- Deficiency in pregnant mothers causes deficiency in their offspring.

Sun Exposure and Rate of MS

Epidemiological studies have proven time and again that vitamin D from sunlight has an effect on MS. One example is from Australia: Only eleven people in one hundred thousand had MS in Queensland, the tropical part of Australia; whereas in Tasmania, which has a temperate climate, the figure is seventy-five per one hundred thousand.[16]

A California study on twins found that people who spent more time in the sun as children may have a lower risk of developing multiple sclerosis than people who had less sun exposure during childhood, according to a study published in the July 24, 2007 issue of *Neurology*.[17]

For the study, researchers surveyed seventy-nine pairs of identical twins with the same genetic risk for MS, but in which only one twin had MS. The twins were asked to specify which twin spent more time outdoors on hot days, cold days, and during summer, and which one spent more time sun tanning, going to the beach, and playing team sports as a child. The study found that the twin with MS spent less time in the sun as a child than the twin who did not have MS. Depending on the activity, the twin who spent more hours outdoors had a 25 to 57 percent reduced risk of developing MS. For example, the risk of developing MS was 49 percent lower for twins who spent more time sun tanning than their siblings did.

"Sun exposure appears to have a protective effect against MS," said study authors Talat Islam, Ph.D., and Thomas Mack, M.D., with the Keck School of Medicine of the University of Southern California, Los Angeles. "Exposure to ultraviolet rays may induce protection against

MS by alternative mechanisms, either by altering the cellular immune response, or indirectly, by producing immunoactive vitamin D."

The study also found the protective effect of sun exposure was seen only among female twin pairs, but Mack says this novel finding must be viewed with caution, since only a few male twins were involved in the study.

There is also evidence that populations from Northern Europe have an increased risk of developing MS if they live in areas receiving less sunshine. It has been estimated that two hundred cases of MS a year could be prevented in Scotland alone by giving vitamin D to mothers and children. Professor Ebers thinks there should be government intervention to make this available.

Ebers explains: "Human beings spent much of their evolutionary history in tropical and subtropical regions, where dark skin provides useful protection against intense sun. As they migrated north into Europe thousands of years ago, white skin became a necessary adaptation because it allows for more vitamin D production. The sun is too weak in northern Europe to enable vitamin D to be made for several months of the year, but white skin enables people to make use of thin spring or autumn sunlight."[18]

Other experts in this field agree that our exposure to vitamin D from sunlight is too low in some locations.[19] It used to be thought that latitude was the most important epidemiological factor in MS. However, sunlight and genetics are now considered primary.

DISEASE OF THE NORTH:
MS RATES PER 100,000 OF THE POPULATION*

Canada:	240	Australia:	78
Scotland:	150–200	Spain:	59
Norway:	110	Brazil:	18
England and Wales:	90–110		

*Source: Melanie Reid and Oliver Gillie, "Vitamin D Is Ray of Sunshine for Multiple Sclerosis Patients," *The Times* February 5, 2009.

Symptoms of Vitamin D Deficiency

Although many of the symptoms of vitamin D deficiency cannot be seen in their early stages, some are more apparent and suggest that testing should occur as soon as possible. These may include:

- Constipation
- Muscle weakness
- Lowered immunity
- Irritability

ಌ VITAMIN D₃ BLOOD TESTS

The standard blood test, and the most recommended, evaluates the blood level of 25-hydroxyvitamin D, or 25(OH)D, the major circulating form of vitamin D and the precursor of the active form (1,25-dihydroxy-vitamin D).

Of the two available vitamin D tests—1,25(OH)D, or 1,25-dihy-droxyvitamin D; and 25(OH)D, or 25-hydroxyvitamin D—the 25(OH)D test is a better marker of overall D status and is the marker most strongly associated with overall health. Serum calcium levels should be checked at the same time and retested periodically. If you don't understand the results you get from your physician, ask for an explanation.

For people with MS, Ashton Embry says that circulating 25(OH)D level should be between 125 to 200 nanomols per liter (nmol/l). First-degree relatives of someone with MS should maintain a 25D level of at least 100 nmol/l, and preferably closer to 150 nmol/l.

For healthy individuals, optimal levels of circulating 25-hydroxyvitamin D values are 45–50 ng/ml (nanograms per milliliter); 115–128 nmol/l. Normal 25-hydroxyvitamin D lab values are 20–56 ng/ml; 40–50 nmol/l. Your vitamin D level should never be below 32 ng/ml. Any levels below 20 ng/ml are considered serious deficiency states.

ಌ SUPPLEMENTING WITH VITAMIN D₃

Everyone with MS should take vitamin D supplements, according to Professor Reinhold Vieth from the University of Toronto. Many supplements are in the D₂ form, but vitamin D₃ is the one that is essential and converts in the body to its active form, 25-dihydroxyvitamin D. Some supplements and fortified foods have both D_3 and D_2, but vitamin D_3 has been shown to be four times as effective as D_2, so be careful to choose products that include D_3.

The amount of vitamin D in supplements is usually measured in IU (international units), or mcg (micrograms), sometimes shown as ug. One mcg (microgram) of vitamin D equals 40 IUs. Solgar's Natural Vitamin D, for example, contains 25 ug (that is, micrograms), which is the equivalent of 1,000 IU.

If you choose to get your vitamin D from cod liver oil, which also has vitamin A, use no more than 1,500 IU and get the remainder with a D3 supplement that doesn't contain vitamin A.

How Much D₃ Should You Take?

Although there is unanimity about the need for D_3 supplementation, there is disagreement about the quantity. The amount will be partly determined by the results of your blood test.

Your physician may argue that your blood needs no more than normal levels of circulating 25-hydroxyvitamin D. However, Embry and others who have focused on MS strongly argue that it needs to be higher than this when you have MS.

In order to have a circulating vitamin D-25(OH)D level in the blood in the range of 125 to 200 nanomols per liter (nmol/l), Embry recommends taking 4,000 IU of D_3 in the winter and 2,000 IU in the summer. This is considerably higher than the European Union recommended daily allowance (RDA) of 5 micrograms—equivalent to 200 IUs. RDAs are set to prevent deficiencies and are not therapeutic doses. A day in the sun can generate 10,000 IUs of vitamin D. However, the body is effectively able to rid itself of unnecessary vitamin D from sunlight.

Embry is convinced that 4,000 IU of vitamin D_3 is safe, although there are some who disagree. In his words: "A study by Hathcock, et al., provided clear evidence that an intake of 10,000 IU of vitamin D per day is perfectly safe and that such an amount should be adopted as the safe upper limit for vitamin D intake."[20]

When Does Vitamin D Become Toxic?

A trial done in Toronto on the safety of high doses of vitamin D, sponsored by Embry's organization, Direct-MS, found that a dose of as much as 40,000 IU a day can be taken without adverse side effects. These results were presented to the MS World Congress in 2008. MS patients on high doses of vitamin D did better than controls.[21]

Importance of Combining with Calcium and Magnesium

Vitamin D controls the level of calcium in the blood. If there is not enough calcium in the diet, calcium will be leached from the bone, creating risk for osteoporosis. High levels of vitamin D from the diet and/or from sunshine will actually demineralize bone if there isn't enough calcium. Vitamin D supplements should never be taken without simultaneously taking calcium and magnesium.

Also, absorption of all three improves when they are taken together. Cantorna, et al., demonstrated that calcium levels strongly affect the action of vitamin D for suppressing EAE in mice.[22] Calcium intake should be in the range of 600–900 mg daily, with magnesium intake roughly comparable.

✎ PROTECTING THE NEXT GENERATION

Some researchers believe that vitamin D supplementation in pregnant mothers and in childhood could wipe out 80 percent of cases of multiple sclerosis. Dr. Sreeram Ramagopalan, a scientist involved in the Oxford University/British Columbia study, reported: "Our study implies that taking vitamin D supplements during pregnancy and the early years may reduce the risk of a child developing MS in later life."[23]

Ebers' research has shown that developing fetuses whose mothers are deprived of sunlight have an increased risk of MS.[24] He and his team believe that vitamin D deficiency in mothers, and possibly grandmothers, may lead to altered expression of the gene in succeeding generations, and have concluded that 50 mcg (.05 mg) a day could provide a cheap and safe way of staving off the disease.

Adequate amounts of vitamin D need to be taken from birth and throughout infancy and childhood. In 2008, Canadian scientists measured vitamin D levels in more than one hundred children suffering from what may have been their first attack of MS. They found that the children with the lowest vitamin D levels were far more likely to be diagnosed with MS than children with higher levels of vitamin D. Of those with the lowest levels of the vitamin, 27 percent developed MS, whereas only 6 percent of those with the highest blood levels of vitamin D went on to develop full-blown MS within the next two years.[25] More children today may be developing MS because they spend more time indoors than children did in the past. In the United States, the American Association of Pediatrics says that all children should take vitamin D and now recommends a higher dose of vitamin D for children than previously. The following prescription is for a normal, healthy population, and not for children more at risk of MS by reason of a first-degree relative with the disease.

It is now recommended that all infants and children, including adolescents, have a minimum daily intake of 400 IU of vitamin D beginning soon after birth. The current recommendation replaces the previous recommendation of a minimum daily intake of 200 IU/day of vitamin D supplementation beginning in the first two months after birth and continuing through adolescence. These revised guidelines for vitamin D intake for healthy infants, children, and adolescents are based on evidence from new clinical trials and the historical precedence of safely giving 400 IU of vitamin D per day in the pediatric and adolescent population. New evidence supports a potential role for vitamin D in maintaining innate immunity and preventing diseases such as diabetes and cancer. The new data may eventually refine what constitutes vitamin D sufficiency or deficiency.[26]

Health Canada offers the following vitamin D recommendation for children:

Health Canada recommends that all breastfed, healthy term babies receive a daily vitamin D supplement of 400 IU. Supplementation of the vitamin should begin at birth and continue until an infant's diet includes at least 400 IU of vitamin D from food sources or until the breastfed infant reaches one year of age. This recommendation is to help reduce the risk of rickets, a disease that affects bone growth in children. Infants who are formula fed receive adequate vitamin D from formula. After one year, all children should have a daily intake of 200 IU of vitamin D, which is the amount found in two cups of milk or fortified soy beverage.[27]

Health Canada believes this is needed because of Canada's northern geographical latitude, minimized sun exposure to prevent skin damage, prevalence of vitamin D deficiency, the history of safe use of supplementation, and vitamin D's associations with conditions other than rickets. They also say that a population health approach to vitamin D supplementation is warranted because it is neither practical nor cost-effective to screen all mothers and infants for vitamin D deficiency.

There has been a campaign in Scotland to make vitamin D supplements available to all infants and children. Glasgow physician Tom Gilhooly tests the children of some of his MS patients to see if they are low in vitamin D, and most of the children tested have shown a deficiency. He hopes that giving them supplements now will reduce their later risk of getting MS.

Gilhooly said: "Children and first degree relatives of those with MS face a twenty to forty times greater risk of developing the disease. This group numbers around 500,000 people in the United Kingdom, so it makes sense to do everything possible to prevent them from getting MS. We owe it to our families to protect them as much as possible. We can take positive steps to help protect the next generation from MS."

Children who have close relatives with MS need higher doses than those officially recommended for the general population. Andrew Watson, who has MS and runs the Best Bet Diet Group in the United Kingdom, has made sure that his seven-year-old granddaughter Kirsten has received 2,000 IU vitamin D a day from a young age.

10

Fats and Oils and Their Role in MS

WHEN YOU'VE GOT MS, it's important to cut down on saturated fat and consume essential fatty acids in both foods and supplements. This chapter explains fats and oils in more detail.

ཤ TYPES OF FATS

We generally think of fat as something we need to avoid. In fact, there are different types of fat, and some are absolutely essential for healthy body functioning.

Saturated Fats

Saturated fats, which are bad in general and worse when you have MS, are usually solid at room temperature. Examples include butter, hard cheeses, and the visible fat on meat. More subtle examples of saturated fat are in such foods as instant dinners and baked goods. Saturated fat supplies energy, but it is not needed for any essential structures or functions of the body.

Unsaturated and Polyunsaturated Fats

Generally speaking, unsaturated fats are liquid or soft at room temperature. This group includes vegetable, seed, and fish oils. Less easy to identify are the unsaturated fats hidden in foods you would not normally associate with fats at all. This list includes fish, dark green leafy vegetables, organ meats (liver, heart, kidneys, and brains), lean meat, shellfish, and sprouting seeds.

FATTY ACIDS AND ESSENTIAL FATTY ACIDS

Fat is made from smaller components called fatty acids. The body can make some of the fatty acids it needs for growth, but is incapable of making the essential fatty acids. They are called "essential" because your body cannot make them on its own. "Fat" is a rather misleading word when talking about essential fatty acids. These vital nutrients are more like proteins or vitamins; you must consume them to stay healthy. Essential fatty acids are present in every cell in your body and are vital for metabolism. These are the fats that make up a major proportion of the brain and nervous system. This type of fat is an essential part of nutrition.

ESSENTIAL FATTY ACIDS AND MS

Essential fatty acids are required for the growth, repair, and maintenance of nervous tissue. This is particularly important in MS, a disease that attacks the nervous system. If the body lacks these nutrients, any repair of damaged tissue is more difficult. You need both main types of essential fatty acids—linoleic and alpha-linolenic acid, also known as omega-6 and omega-3. (See the following section, Essential Fatty Acid Families.)

People with MS can show an unusual pattern of fatty acids in their blood. With a diet rich in essential fatty acids (EFAs), this can return to normal in nine months to one year.[1]

Some research has shown that the white matter in the brains of people with MS is low in EFAs.[2] In people with MS, the myelin sheath, the red and white blood cells, the platelets, and the blood plasma are also deficient in EFAs, particularly linoleic acid.

EFAs play a fundamental role in all cell membranes of the body. The fluidity and flexibility of cell membranes depends on the EFA level in the cells. The activity of lymphocytes (white blood cells) may be dependent on the state of the cell membrane. They will behave differently according to whether a cell membrane is fluid (plenty of EFAs) or rigid (not enough EFAs.) This influences the ability of certain lymphocytes to react immunologically.

✌ ESSENTIAL FATTY ACID FAMILIES

There are two families of essential fatty acids. Both families are very important to the dietary management of MS. The first family is headed by linoleic acid, which biochemists call omega-6. The other family is headed by alpha-linolenic acid and is known as omega-3.

When foods containing these two families of essential fatty acids are eaten, the body makes them into longer chain unsaturated fatty acids that are more biologically active. It is only these longer-chain fatty acids that are used by the brain. The derivatives of linoleic acid and alpha-linolenic acid are more important for the brain and nervous system than the parent fatty acids. This means that gamma-linolenic and arachidonic acids are more important than linoleic acid, and that eicosapentaenoic and docosahexaenoic acids are more important than alpha-linolenic acid.

HOW LONGER CHAIN FATTY ACIDS ARE MADE IN THE BODY

FAMILY 1: The omega-6 family	FAMILY 2: The omega-3 family
Linoleic acid	**Alpha-linolenic acid**
Found in sunflower seeds, safflower seeds, seed oils, vegetable oils, legumes	Found in green leafy vegetables, such as spinach and kale, broccoli, and certain legumes
↓ *Addition of double bonds*	
Gamma-linolenic acid (GLA)	
Found in evening primrose oil, borage oil, oats, black currant oil, breast milk	
↓ *Chain elongation*	**Eicosapentaenoic acid**
Dihomo-gamma-linolenic acid	Found in oily fish and fish oil
↓ *Addition of double bonds*	↓
Arachidonic acid	**Docosahexaenoic acid**
Found directly in organ meats, such as liver, brains, and kidneys	Found in cold-water oily fish, fish oil, and seaweed
Used in the nervous system	*Used in the nervous system*

∾ DERIVATIVES OF ESSENTIAL FATTY ACIDS

It is fine to eat the parent foods, but only a small amount of the derivatives are actually produced in this way. In any case, it is thought that people with MS may not be as efficient as healthier people in converting the parent essential fatty acids to their derivatives.

In the abnormal EFA blood profile of people with MS, it is better to eat directly the foods containing gamma-linolenic acid, arachidonic acid, eicosapentaenoic acid, and docosahexaenoic acids.

Gamma-linolenic Acid

Gamma-linolenic acid (GLA) is 50 percent more unsaturated than linoleic acid. It is not present in any of the commercially produced vegetable oils; in fact, it is quite rare. From GLA it is easy for the body to make some beneficial prostaglandins, which are vital for good health. The easiest way to take it is in capsules of evening primrose oil, which contain about 9 percent GLA, or capsules made with borage oil or black currant seed oil. It is also found in oats.

VARIOUS WAYS IN WHICH EFAs MAY WORK IN THE TREATMENT OF MS

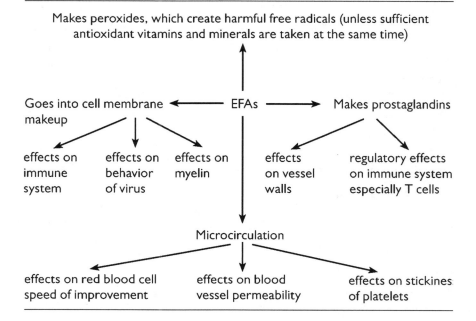

Prostaglandins

Prostaglandins, manufactured from dihomo-gamma-linolenic acid and from arachidonic acid, act as regulatory substances and messengers. Prostaglandins have two particularly important functions related to MS: platelet regulation and immune system regulation.

Platelets are very small particles in the blood that play a role in blood clotting, and there is some evidence of abnormal clumping together of platelets in MS. Using modern testing techniques, it is now possible to show that several months of a diet high in EFAs normalizes platelet behavior in the blood. It is thought that the prostaglandins, which are metabolized from certain EFAs, play a vital role in this process.

The kind of prostaglandins that regulate the immune system may be in short supply in people with MS. A shortage of series 1 prostaglandins may possibly lead to defective lymphocytes, thus increasing the body's susceptibility to autoimmune damage (producing antibodies that act against its own tissues). Series 1 prostaglandins may be of critical importance in regulating the function of some particular white blood cells involved in defending the body—the T lymphocytes. One type of T lymphocyte, the T suppressor cells, prevents the body from attacking itself.

Research has shown that levels of T suppressor cells are very low in MS patients during a relapse.[3] It is known that prostaglandins have the effect of dampening down lymphocytes that are capable of attacking the central nervous system. In short, EFAs help strengthen the immune system.

✥ GOOD AND BAD FATS AND OILS

Good oils to use in cooking are seed oils—sunflower, safflower, sesame, cottonseed; and olive and corn oils. Make sure you buy only pure oils, preferably cold pressed, which are the purest. Whichever oil you use, do not heat it to the point of smoking. Do not use oil more than once; throw it away after one use. Overheating and exposure to oxygen damage the EFA activity. After you have opened the bottle, keep it in the fridge. The best way to eat these oils is unheated, for example, in salad dressing.

Be wary of palm and coconut oils. These two oils give the impression of being unsaturated but are, in fact, saturated. Avoid them! They sometimes are hidden in nondairy products, such as frozen desserts and margarine. It is easy to buy spreads that are high in polyunsaturates, and these usually state their contents very clearly on the lid. Always use a spread that is high in polyunsaturates, but be careful that the product doesn't contain buttermilk, a cultured milk product.

"Cis" Fatty Acids

You may have seen the word *cis* on the label of some margarine tubs. The only type of linoleic acid that can convert into biologically useful substances is cis-linoleic acid, which is found in the oil in its natural, unadulterated state. Only cis-linoleic acid has any real value. Once linoleic acid is processed and hydrogenated, it turns into a biologically different form and behaves like saturated fat. Hydrogenation turns biologically active essential fatty acids into biologically inactive trans-fatty acids.

"Trans"-Fatty Acids

Trans-fatty acids are false friends lurking in our everyday food. On the face of it, they look perfectly innocent: ordinary bottles of cooking oil, cartons of margarine, and a whole range of other things like instant meals, chips, and pastries. But beware! Trans-fatty acids behave like saturated fat. And far from being essential fatty acids, they actually produce essential fatty acid deficiency states and compete with genuine essential fatty acids for your body's time and attention. They elbow the real essential fatty acids out of the action. Trans-fatty acids make their way into tissues like the brain, heart, and lungs, and some scientists are sure that they change the properties of these tissues for the worse.

It is only since the 1920s that significant amounts of trans-fatty acids have been added to the diet (though they always existed in small amounts in dairy products). Some food manufacturers are now taking steps to reduce or eliminate trans fats from their products, and some regulations are now being passed requiring restaurants to list trans and saturated fat content on their menus. Even so, there is still a huge amount of trans fats on the market.

◈ RESEARCH ON FATS AND MS

The first study was done by the late Professor Roy Swank of the Oregon Health & Science University in Portland; the second was done by the ARMS Unit at the Central Middlesex Hospital, London, in the 1980s. Both studies came to the same broad conclusion: people with MS who stick steadfastly to a low-fat diet lower their chances of getting worse, whereas people who do not stick to it *do* get worse.[4]

The Swank Research

Roy Swank was very strict with the amount of saturated fat that he allowed per day—15 grams total. He noticed that if patients exceeded this allowance by even a small amount of fat, they slowly got worse. This even happened to patients who had been stable on the low-fat diet, and Swank observed that once someone slipped or cheated on the low-fat diet, that person was unlikely to return to a stable condition. He said:

> The addition of 8 grams (1.5 teaspoons) of fat often may appear to allow stabilization of the disease, but this lasts for no longer than seven years. Then the disease becomes rapidly progressive, from which there is no recovery. . . . The chance that you can tolerate more than 15 grams of fat daily is no more, and probably less, than 4 percent. Ninety-six percent of patients who have exceeded their saturated fat by 10 grams or more have ended up deteriorating rapidly and suffered a high death rate. There is a sharp increase in disability and deaths upon the addition of 8 grams or more [of] fat to the diet.[5]

Professor Swank noted that a saturated fat intake of 20 to 25 grams will not usually produce any apparent increased disability in a short period. A slow, silent deterioration occurs, and in a few years increased activity of the disease surfaces. To exceed this level repeatedly, he believed, would result in the inability to lead an active life.

Swank did research on a low-fat diet far longer than anyone else. He first started his research in Montreal in 1951. Although his research does not adhere to strict scientific methods, it would be foolish to ignore his very impressive results.

Starting in 1951, Swank followed 150 patients with MS. He looked at the relationship of their fat intake to the progress of disability and the number of deaths. He plotted a graph of those patients who ate fewer than twenty grams of fat a day, those eating twenty to thirty grams of fat a day, and those eating more than thirty grams of fat daily. By the end of the study, 21 percent of the patients eating less than twenty grams of fat a day had died, but Swank concluded that a slight increase of no more than an average of eight grams of fat per day more than doubled the death rate to 54 percent. The patients in his study who ate the most saturated fat deteriorated the most and had the highest death rates.

For those who stuck faithfully to Swank's low-fat diet, the success has been remarkable. Swank reported that 90 to 95 percent of patients who began his diet in the early stages of MS, with little or no evident disability, did not get worse during thirty-five years on the diet.

Patients who started the diet later in the course of the disease, with definite disability, did get worse, but at a much slower rate than would have been expected. In a few cases, the condition stabilized.

Swank observed that his diet prolonged active, productive life. Patients got stronger and remained energetic, stable, and attack-free. Old signs and symptoms may still have been there, but new ones rarely developed.

In the 1970s and '80s, Swank assimilated the research on essential fatty acids and MS and revised his advice: In addition to eating a low-fat diet, people with MS should also take supplements of omega-3 and omega-6.

Patients who started the diet after becoming disabled noted an increased feeling of well-being. Most patients had fewer colds and stomach upsets, and noted an increase in energy. There was a 95 percent reduction in the frequency of attacks, and the attacks that did occur were mild, infrequent, and brief.

Swank found that patients on the low-fat diet were able to work and walk longer. About 50 percent of MS patients on no specific diet who were able to work and walk at the beginning could not do so at the end of ten years, whereas only 25 percent of Swank's patients, all on the low-fat diet, were unable to work or walk after ten years. Death rates were lower, too. By Swank's figures, the average death rate among people with MS on the low-fat diet was two-thirds to three-quarters the normal death rate for MS sufferers.

FINDING THE RIGHT RATIO BETWEEN OMEGA-3 AND OMEGA-6 EFAs

The balance between omega-3 and omega-6 is critical, as imbalance results in the body's inability to successfully monitor the inflammatory/anti-inflammatory response. There is balance when omega-3 and omega-6 work in proper ratio to each other.

Experts differ on the correct ratio between omega-3 and omega-6. Some say the ratio should be 3:1—three times more omega-6 fatty acids than omega-3 fatty acids. (The typical North American diet tends to contain from eleven to thirty times more omega-6.) Others say the ratio should be in favor of omega-3, with a 2:1 ratio of omega-3 to omega-6. Still others endorse a 1:1 ratio.

According to Ashton Embry:

> Experts think that man evolved on a diet which would have had roughly one to two times more omega-6 than omega-3, though there is a school of thought which argues for a 1:1 ratio. Currently, average U.K. intakes are in a ratio of around 8:1 in favor of the omega-6s, while in the U.S. it is around 10:1, and in Australia nearer [to] 12:1. Many individuals within those populations will have an even greater omega-6 to omega-3 imbalance. Because the omega-3s and omega-6s compete on the same metabolic pathway, and the omega-6s may block conversion of omega-3 alpha-linolenic acid to the more useful omega-3 EPA and DHA, (eicosapentaenoic acid and dihomohexaenoic acid) non-fish eaters must be extra vigilant in cutting down on omega-6 intake. Because of their wide-ranging roles, virtually every area of the human body is susceptible to problems if the balance of the two polyunsaturates becomes out of kilter.[6]

Professor Loren Cordain, author of *The Paleo Diet,* says: "The ratio of omega-6 to omega-3 fats in Paleolithic diets was about 2 to 1. You should try to achieve an overall balance of dietary fats from all foods, in which the omega-6 to omega-3 fat ratio is less than about 3 to 1, preferably closer to 2 to 1."[7]

Udo Erasmus, who makes Udo's Oil, thinks the ratio should be in favor of taking more omega-3 to omega-6. He says: "Our practical experience working with people shows that the ratio that gives the best results consistently comes from oils blended to be richer in omega-3 than omega-6. Some people suggest that the traditional perfect balance is 1:1. But traditional ratios have varied widely. The Inuit ratio was 2.5:1. It did not produce omega-6 deficiency. The ratio in Mediterranean diets was about 1:6 and did not produce omega-3 deficiency. The brain of both traditions contains a balance of 1:1, which tells us that the brain takes what it needs from what the body gets, provided that enough of both EFAs are present. In practice, oils richer in omega-3s (but not too rich) consistently produce the best health support and improvement."[8] Udo's Oil is twice richer in omega-3 but contains enough omega-6 to prevent deficiency.

Do We Need Omega-6 Supplements?

Some say there is plenty of omega-6 in the Western diet so we don't need any additional, because omega-6 can be inflammatory. Others argue that omega-6 is beneficial, and its metabolites are vital in tackling an autoimmune and inflammatory disease. They say that although there may be enough omega-6 in the diet, it's mostly as linoleic acid and not sufficiently bioavailable, compared to the more biologically active gamma-linolenic acid.

Dr. Laurence Harbige, a neuroscientist whose specialty is fats and health, thinks that omega-6 taken as GLA (for example, evening primrose or borage oil) is important in MS. One of his experiments found that giving gamma-linolenic acid to mice stopped them from exhibiting the clinical signs of EAE—the animal model of MS.[9] It also protected them against disease relapse, showing that omega-6 fatty acids can alter the progression of an established and ongoing disease. He says: "Omega-6 fatty acid supplementation in MS could therefore have a physiological and/or pharmacological basis. We are currently undertaking phase I/II clinical trials in MS with specific omega-6 fatty acids and investigating further how these fatty acids may exert effects on the immune response in EAE and MS."

The opposing viewpoint is represented by Dr. Artemis Simopoulos from the Center for Genetics, Nutrition, and Health in Washington, D.C., who says:

> Western diets are deficient in omega-3 fatty acids and have excessive amounts of omega-6 fatty acids compared with the diet on which

human beings evolved and their genetic patterns were established. Excessive amounts of omega-6 polyunsaturated fatty acids (PUFAs) and a very high omega-6/omega-3 ratio, as is found in today's Western diets, promote the pathogenesis of many diseases, including inflammatory and autoimmune diseases; whereas increased levels of omega-3 PUFAs (a lower omega-6/omega-3 ratio) exert suppressive effects. A lower ratio of omega-6/omega-3 fatty acids is more desirable in reducing the risk of many of the chronic diseases of high prevalence in Western societies, as well as in developing countries.[10]

My regimen has included evening primrose oil or borage supplements, high in GLA (gamma-linolenic acid), from the start of my MS, and I've never missed a day. I also take good quality high-dose fish oils every day. My ratio is around 1:1. Personally, I agree with the rationale for taking GLA supplements put forward by Dr. Harbige, who has made the subject of polyunsaturates his life's work.

PART THREE

Physical and Complementary Therapies

11

Exercise and Exercise Machines

KEEP MOVING! It doesn't matter what exercise you do, the important thing is to exercise. If you don't, your muscles will lose tone and begin to atrophy, leading to your becoming more disabled than you need be.

✎ EXERCISE IS CRUCIAL

Virtually all the research indicates that exercise is important for maintaining health and vitality, but for those who have MS it is particularly critical. Some of its functions are:

- Improves the circulation of blood and lymph, thus helping with internal cleansing
- Improves all functions in the body
- Increases the amount of oxygen in the blood
- Keeps muscles strong and strengthens weak ones
- Keeps joints mobile and prevents stiffness
- Helps reduce spasticity
- Helps with coordination and balance
- Helps maintain maximum independence
- Lifts depression
- Eases stress

- Engenders a feeling of well-being by toning up the whole system and releasing feel-good endorphins
- Prevents muscles from atrophying
- Helps you do everyday things better
- Gives you more energy
- Helps you look your best
- Helps allay disabilities that are not part of the MS disease process
- Helps stave off cardiovascular disease and diabetes
- Helps prevent pressure sores

USE IT OR LOSE IT

It's really true that "If you don't use it, you lose it." Many of the complications of MS arise from disuse. Contractures, deformities, and reduced mobility are often attributed to being part of having MS, but they are not necessarily part of the disease process at all. They come about because of misuse and disuse. Inactivity can lead to complications. On the other hand, activity can prevent complications, or at least delay them.

Regular exercise can make the difference between being able to stand and walk—or becoming wheelchair-bound.[1]

FATIGUE

You may think—and feel—that you haven't got the energy to do any sort of exercise and fear that it would make you feel drained. The ironic thing about exercise, however, is that it actually energizes you. Of course, you shouldn't exert yourself so much that you're exhausted, but no exercise at all will leave you more fatigued than gentle exercise. Building up stamina also helps you fatigue less easily.

WHAT EXERCISE?

You can do any kind of exercise you like. Obviously, what exercise you do depends on your abilities. Some people who have MS can go skiing or take part in marathons. Others are grateful to be able to touch their toes while sitting in a wheelchair. By exercising and doing other things described in this book, such as changes in diet and taking supplements, some people with MS have regained their ability to cycle, run, or do the sports they used to do.

If you still have normal or nearly normal movement, there is no reason why you shouldn't join an ordinary gym—or any other exercise class—in your local area. Tell the instructor that you have MS so you will not feel compelled to do things beyond your ability or stamina, and so that you don't overexert yourself and can rest when you feel like it.

Any form of exercise will do you good. It does not have to be a formal class. If you have self-discipline, you can exercise at home. Whatever exercise you choose, do it regularly, ideally every day. It will make a real, noticeable difference to your energy, strength, and stamina. If you can, include some aerobic exercise.

Whatever exercise you choose, don't overdo it; overexertion can trigger a relapse.

- Always stop exercising before you get tired.
- Never allow yourself to get fatigued.
- Don't exercise on a full stomach.
- It's fine to stretch your comfort zone, but don't hurt yourself.
- Keep cool. Have the air conditioning or a fan on and a bottle of cold water handy.
- Rest afterward, if you need to.

EXERCISES PARTICULARLY GOOD FOR MS
Pilates, yoga, t'ai chi, and qigong are particularly good for MS.

Pilates
Many of the Pilates exercises are done lying down, and you can choose your own level. Pilates increases core stability, strength, fitness, and stamina.

I have been doing weekly Pilates for the last three years and the benefits are very visible. I have good core strength, which means my pelvic floor and stomach muscles are strong and able to support my body, which helps with walking and balance.

I started out with one-on-one private classes with Pilates teacher Fran Michelman but now go to a Pilates studio in north London (Belsize Studio) where I take a class with other people—men and women. The studio has the full range of equipment, so I am able to work on all mus-

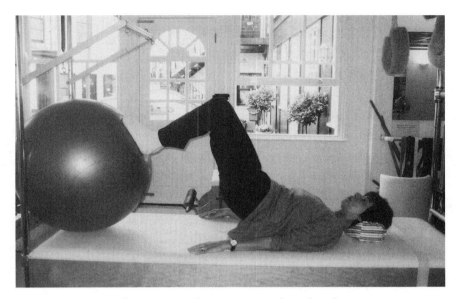

Judy increasing her core strength with Pilates

cle groups—thighs, hamstrings, calves, feet and ankles, abdominals, glutes (bottom), back, shoulders, upper arms, and lower arms. If I don't do Pilates every week for any reason, such as the Christmas break, I always get stiff. Everyone I know with MS who does Pilates raves about it.

Using equipment or doing floor exercises on a mat are both effective. It depends on the level you are working at and what you have available to you. There are easy exercises you can do on equipment and hard exercises you can do on a mat, and vice-versa. There are also props you can use easily at home, such as Swiss balls, which help with balance and core strength; wobble boards, which help improve balance; and rings to exercise your inner thighs and other muscle groups.

....

Judy: How I Got Started on Pilates

It all started at my hairdresser's. Every time I went, my hairdresser Stacey would drop broad hints that I should take up Pilates. "Look what it's done for my slouch!" he announced, showing off his straight back and upright neck. "I don't stoop any longer."

It was true. Pilates had transformed the stooped Stacey into an upright figure, and he looked great. Perhaps it could work wonders for me, too.

After a year or so of Stacey's gentle persuasion, I decided to give it a go. He put me on to his Pilates teacher, Fran, whose praises he rang to high heaven.

The first striking thing about a Pilates studio is the equipment: large exercise contraptions are rigged up with all sorts of springs, pulleys, and bars. It's very different from standard gym equipment.

Each piece of equipment is cleverly designed to work a particular set of muscles. After a warm-up on the exercise bike, Fran starts with my legs. I lie back on an exercise bed and put my feet up on a bar. Then I slide the contraption backward and forward, breathing in and out as she directs.

It's not quite as simple as it sounds. Fran makes sure your whole body is properly aligned. The movement can't be right if you're mis-aligned, as I was. It's all too easy to get a movement horribly wrong, which is worse than useless; so you need to have a trained teacher at hand even if you don't have one-on-one training. If a hip, shoulder, or neck is even a smidgen out of alignment, Fran notices and helps get it where it should be. If I lose concentration for a moment, my body is soon out of whack again.

Using slightly different equipment, an exercise bed called a reformer is used to work your hamstrings, calf muscles, and abdominals. With Pilates, you isolate each muscle group and become aware of those muscles working. Pilates is excellent for stability, muscle control, and being grounded.

Did you know you had muscles up each side of your torso? I didn't, but it turns out that these muscles, which in my case had forgotten they existed, are essential for core stability—a common term in Pilates. There are all sorts of maneuvers to awaken these slumbering muscles: exercises for upper arms, lower arms, shoulders, upper back, lower back, inner thighs, outer thighs, everywhere. There are other ones for stretching every last part of you. It increases muscle tone and flexibility, and helps with balance, coordination, posture, and alignment.

"Engage pelvic floor and breathe in!" commands Fran, several times each session. Encouraging me in my hopeful pursuit of growing tall and straight, she tells me to imagine a line going up from my pelvic floor, through the center of my body, up through my neck, out the top of my head, and up to the ceiling. I try, but haven't quite found it yet.

A one-hour session always ends with the large Swiss ball, or balance ball. The first time Fran asked me to sit on it, I wobbled all over the place and had to grab on to something to stop myself from falling over. Now that I'm more grounded and better aligned, I can sit and bounce sedately in almost perfect balance.

For homework, I bounce a bit on the Swiss ball while watching TV, exercise my hamstrings with some stretchy gadgets, and roll my feet on a tennis ball.

Now I have better core stability, much improved balance and coordination, stronger muscles everywhere, and I do look a bit more upright.

"Isn't Pilates wonderful!" exclaimed Stacey at my last visit to the hairdresser's. I had to agree that indeed, it is.

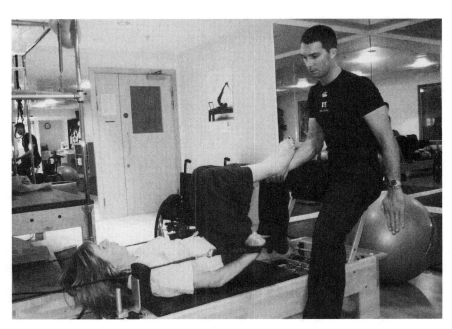

Charlotte using Pilates equipment with assistance from instructor Brett Moreman (Photo by Paul Southall)

Charlotte: Pilates Helped Balance and Bladder

When my physio invited me to join a Pilates class I didn't need much persuading, as my friend Christine, who also has MS, is convinced that doing Pilates has kept her walking. I've been hooked on Pilates ever since.

That class was for people with MS, male and female, who were in wheelchairs. I realized this was well within my abilities and not as difficult as I had feared. When it ended I discovered there were many Pilates classes, and I chose one in Edinburgh that had an accessible loo.

The place I go to is fully equipped with Pilates equipment, but also offers group Pilates mat classes, and I started taking weekly one-on-one Pilates lessons.

More than two years after starting Pilates, I'm astonished at the difference it has made to my fitness, balance, posture, and bladder control. Pelvic floor exercises have had a striking effect on my bladder control and have also helped me sit up straight after years of being in a wheelchair.

I'd become so used to things gradually getting more difficult with MS that I wasn't expecting my overall health and strength to get so much better. It has also improved my mood.

Yoga

Yoga is more than just a simple set of postures or keep-fit exercises, it is a total philosophy that also encompasses the way you breathe, how you nourish yourself, and your whole attitude toward life. However, there is much benefit to be gained simply by doing the poses. Yoga has been widely practiced by people with MS with many reported benefits.

Yoga represents unity of the mental and the physical. Hatha yoga, which is a broad term describing most of the yoga practiced in the West, concentrates on the whole being, so in addition to developing physical health, it also promotes mental health and emotional balance. It involves stretching and holding your body in various poses (*asanas,* in Sanskrit) while simultaneously controlling your breathing and quieting your mind. Done properly, it is both calming and energizing.

The word *yoga* comes from the Sanskrit and means "join" or "union." Hatha yoga is about reaching a balance between the positive and negative within oneself: *Ha* refers to the sun (positive, masculine energy); *tha* refers to the moon (negative, feminine energy).

Yoga and Multiple Sclerosis

The yogic philosophy is that good health is the natural state for human beings. Good health is when the body and mind are in a state of equilibrium. Illness, or disease, is when the body and mind are out of balance.

There is a natural life force within us all that is trying its best to keep us healthy. Even if you have been leading the unhealthy lifestyle of Western civilization, the body's healing powers are still there, just waiting to be given a fair chance.

Yoga has many advantages for someone with MS. Yoga:

- Can help the body's own self-healing mechanism, and may slow or even halt the disease process.
- Stills the mind.
- Lifts the mood and counteracts depression.
- Stimulates functioning of endocrine glands and circulatory and respiratory systems, and improves well-being.
- Does not require any special equipment and can be practiced daily at home.
- Increases energy and counteracts fatigue. A study of sixty-nine MS patients who did six months of yoga or aerobic exercise showed significant improvement in fatigue, compared to controls.[2]

The Yogic Breath

Correct breathing is one of the most important aspects of yoga. You may think that breathing is something that everyone does naturally. In fact, 99 percent of the population breathes incorrectly, with correspondingly ill effects on their bodies.

Breathing is the most important biological function of the body, and closely linked with every other activity of the body. To realize just how important breathing is, remember that you could live for weeks without food, days without water, but only a few minutes without air. Breathing is of primary importance to one's state of health, emotional outlook, and length of life.

Most people in the West take short, rapid, shallow breaths, but it is deep, rhythmic breathing that brings health and energy. Any shock makes people constrict their breath still further. Notice how you breathe out with a sigh of relief when some ordeal is over. When people are anxious, their breathing tends to become shallow, with insufficient exhalation. "I held my breath" is a common expression for being excited or nervous about something. If you hold your breath often enough, or take only shallow breaths, your body can't get the oxygen it needs for energy.

If the energy is not flowing properly, it will affect both your body and your brain. You will fatigue easily, and feel run down and depressed. If you are breathing deeply and rhythmically, you will find it difficult to be tense at the same time. Breath is a source of energy.

All forms of mental unease or physical disease reveal themselves in the way you breathe. Someone with MS may well be breathing incorrectly because of the mental and physical difficulties brought on by the disease. This creates a vicious cycle, because the breathing difficulties themselves only make those problems worse. The way to stop the vicious cycle is

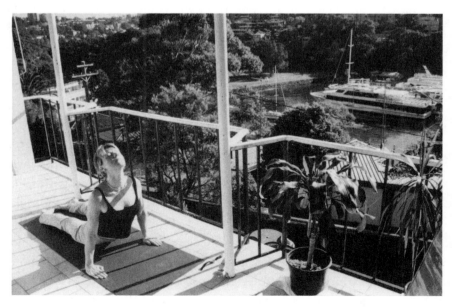

Alison releasing stress and tension with yoga in the sunshine

to exercise control over your breathing. Fortunately, your breath can be under your voluntary control.

Yoga involves deep abdominal breathing. Breath is brought fully into the diaphragm and abdomen, rather than going no further than the chest. An introductory yoga class teaches the essentials of breathing and the differences between a relaxing breath and an energizing breath. Correct breathing is the foundation on which the other aspects of yoga are based. The best place to learn correct breathing is under the supervision of a good yoga teacher.

Release of Stress and Tension

One intrinsic hazard of MS is that stress and tension probably play some part in bringing on an attack of MS. Perversely, the MS itself creates stress and tension, both physically and mentally.

The tension created by having MS can seize up the solar plexus (the network of nerves behind the stomach). This interferes with the movement of the diaphragm, blocking the body's energy flow. Yoga relaxes the body, opens the diaphragm, and frees the energy flow.

Problems with balance and movement will make your body try to compensate by using other muscles. This can create unnatural muscle tension, which will lead over time to spasticity, and also affect the functioning of the area around the tense muscles. Once your postural abnormalities have been corrected and you have learned how to relax through correct deep breathing, your body will be able to move more fluidly. One of the causes of tension in MS is a profound feeling of self-consciousness about your disabled body. Once you lose this disabling self-consciousness, you will be surprised at how much the condition improves. Spasms, spasticity, and clumsiness are worse when you are anxious and self-conscious. If you don't think about it and can relax, these symptoms are far less pronounced. The practice of yoga can help alleviate both physical and mental stress and tension.

....

Sylvia: Invigorated by Yoga

I've just returned from five wonderful days of yoga, relaxation, yoga teaching, sunshine, breathing, gorgeous vegetarian food, fun, and loads of laughter. Where have I been? On a yoga for MS course.

There is such an amazing spirit in this place: invigorating, refreshing, inspiring, motivating, and enlightening. It's a place where you can really unwind and forget about all those things that you think are important.

Everyone is encouraged to participate as much as possible. You simply do what feels right for you. The focus is always on what you can achieve without pushing you beyond your limits.

A Peaceful Mind

Most people's minds are forever buzzing with trivial things. One of the most difficult things to do is to clear your mind. Rubbish piles up and races through your head; yoga aims to clear the debris. "Yoga is controlling the activities of the mind," said Patanjali, one of the great yogis of ancient times.

With a still mind, you can concentrate on what it is you want to achieve and become single-minded. Single-mindedness is the best way to achieve your goals. With a still mind you will have inner calm and peace instead of inner turmoil and hostility.

The body's healing process works better when you are in a positive state of mind, and yoga helps you get into a positive state of mind. If your mind is at peace, your body can be used to the best of its ability. This is an important element of the asanas.

One way to achieve a calm, still mind is meditation. Simply put, you clear your mind of daily trivia by concentrating on just one thing. This one thing could be the breath; a mantra, or chant; or a flower. Practicing meditation every day will help you feel calm and refreshed. (See also Meditation and Guided Imagery in chapter 13.)

Yoga Exercises for MS

Unlike physical therapy exercises, yoga asanas should not be thought of on their own. The correct yoga breathing and the right mental approach are as important as the movements of your body. The late Howard Kent, who founded Yoga for Health, called this the three Bs—brain, breath, and body. He said, "By the correct use of breathing and mental relaxation I have seen people move legs, with control, which have not moved in years; I have seen people get up from the floor unaided for the first time in years. Once the inhibitions are removed, the body's real powers can reveal themselves."[3]

Any book on yoga will show you that there is a vast range of yoga asanas. None are harmful to people with MS. To what extent they can be practiced depends on the individual and the degree of disability.

When people with MS first start yoga, they often find it difficult to do a particular movement or hold a position. With practice, however, many people with MS find that they can make dramatic progress, and they discover quite quickly that they can do some exercises they never thought possible.

If you have never done yoga before, it may be difficult to learn from a book. Try to find a yoga class near where you live, and tell the teacher you have MS. You may find that you cannot do some of the balance exercises at first, such as standing on one leg with your hands in a prayer position, but neither can most healthy people! With a bit of practice you'll be amazed at what you'll be able to do.

Once you've learned some basic exercises in a class, you can do them at home on your own. You may want to purchase a yoga DVD for visual reminders or positions and breath (see Resources). Ideally, to get the best out of it, you should practice yoga every day for at least fifteen minutes.

Remember that yoga asanas tone the neuromuscular system and keep it in full working order, develop and control the respiratory system, and increase oxygen flow and vitality. The internal organs work better, the spine is kept strong and supple, and you enjoy a sense of real well-being.

Bob: My Wife Went from Wheelchair to Walking

When we arrived at the residential yoga course, my wife was in a wheelchair; but when we left she was able to walk out! Yoga really helped a lot.

T'ai Chi

The gentle exercises of t'ai chi are also ideal, improving body awareness, balance, coordination, and strength. In 2003 the National Institute for Clinical Excellence in the United Kingdom issued guidelines stating that t'ai chi may be helpful for people with MS in terms of a general sense of well-being.

In a study published in the journal *General Hospital Psychiatry,* eight people with secondary progressive MS were given individual one-on-one t'ai chi sessions, as well as audio and video tapes. A control group, also of eight people with MS, was not given t'ai chi but asked to continue with their current care. The t'ai chi group was then compared with the control group. The t'ai chi group reported improvement over a broad range of symptoms, including balance and symptom management. These were verified by relatives' independent ratings. The control group showed no improvement. The paper's authors concluded that through practicing "mindfulness of movement" the t'ai chi group had received a self-help method of symptom management that "can maximize physical and psychological functioning."[4]

Qigong

Qigong is a simple form of t'ai chi that uses postures and gentle movements to encourage energy flow and health. The movements have poetic names, such as "The Marriage of Heaven and Earth" and "Cloud Hands," and are designed to help develop a greater sense of connection from each part of the body to the whole body, and between one's body and the earth, sky, and universe.

In a study on t'ai chi/qigong, eight people with MS were assessed by an independent researcher before and after six therapy sessions. Seven of the eight who did the t'ai chi/qigong showed statistically significant specific objective improvements in balance and depression compared with a control group. Participants were also asked for their subjective feedback. Some of the responses included:[5]

> "Qigong has given me an awareness of my body movements, which had been uncoordinated, even clumsy, and are now smoother and more relaxed."
> "I feel I have improved because of finding a form of exercise that does not cause pain or fatigue, and finding myself at peace within myself."
> "I have developed a confidence in getting to know my body in a different way."

"I have an increased awareness of where each part is in relation to each other."

"I used to have problems with balance and bladder control, but six sessions of qigong and craniosacral therapy made a big difference to both my balance and bladder control and increased a sense of vitality."

....

Cathy: T'ai Chi Brings Balance

As a result of doing t'ai chi, I definitely feel more stability and I'm much less likely to lose my balance. My walking is steadier and stronger—I don't wobble like a supermarket trolley so much! It's helped me to feel more confident when I'm out and less reliant on other people.

Most of my class consists of exercises to strengthen and improve balance. Over the past months we covered a small selection of simple exercises, but now that our balance has improved, we are just getting into the first few movements of 'The Form'—set t'ai chi moves.

I try to do these exercises regularly at home, as well as in the t'ai chi class. We do simple t'ai chi walking (sometimes known as 'walking through the forest')—slowly walking from one end of the room to the other in the t'ai chi style, focusing on being stable and grounded.

Other exercises are:
- *The Rainbow Circle.* This involves bending down and reaching up, and improves my balance and feeling of being grounded.
- *Leg swings.* We swing each leg while holding on to the back of a chair for support. This exercise helps me loosen up any stiffness.
- *Leg circles.* We gently circle each leg, which is a great exercise for strengthening leg muscles and improving balance.
- *Hip Circles.* These further improve leg strength and make me feel more flexible.

....

Other Ways to Exercise

No exercise is excluded if you are up to it. I know people with MS who love to go skiing. Gentler exercises include:

- Walking, jogging, riding, rowing, or playing golf in a beautiful, natural outdoors setting such as a forest, mountain, river, seaside, or lakeside
- The martial arts of karate, judo, kung fu, aikido, uechi, budokai, and taekwondo
- Dancing
- Aerobics
- Gymnastics
- Stretching
- Swimming, ideally in non-chlorinated water

✎ EXERCISE EQUIPMENT

While there is plenty of exercise to be had without any special equipment, some of these old standards and recent innovations can be quite useful for managing MS.

Weightlifting

Weightlifting isn't just for the Jack LaLanne types. Used properly, weights can help with balance and strengthening. If you haven't used weights before, it's best to get professional assistance.

. . . .

Donald: Training with Weights

I have had secondary progressive MS and have exercised vigorously, including pumping iron, for the last twenty years. My MS has hardly progressed in all that time. I always feel in fine form for days after a heavy workout. I find training with heavy weights much more beneficial than training with light weights. I've lost count of the number of research bulletins I have read reporting the benefits of exercise for MS.

. . . .

Rebounder

A rebounder, which looks like a mini-trampoline but is designed with individual springs, is very good for building up strength in your leg muscles and for stamina. You will be amazed at how quickly your jumping ability increases, just by using the rebounder for a couple of minutes every day.[6]

✎ PASSIVE EXERCISE MACHINES

There are many electrical exercise machines on the market, known as passive exercisers, which will exercise your legs and arms with minimal effort from you. They are very effective in helping people with MS to buld and maintain muscle strength.

Vibration Trainer

A vibration training machine is reasonably inexpensive and can be used at home or at a gym or MS therapy center. Many anecdotal reports from people with MS say vibration training—also known as whole body vibration training, or WBVT—improves strength, walking ability, muscle tone, and balance. It is also said to increase bone density, improve flexibility, aid circulation, and improve balance by increasing core stability.

The machine has a vibrating platform, and when you stand on it, it sends vibrations through your limbs, "exercising" them for you. Different positions—some standing, some sitting or lying down—on the vibration trainer work different muscles. As little time as thirty seconds in each position, done regularly, can make a real difference. Vibration trainers are particularly good for MS as it is a nonaerobic form of exercise, so it does not make you breathless or lead to overexertion; there is also a grab rail to hold on to.

There are many different vibration trainers on the market, some more suitable for home use. One type of platform is known as a linear, or piston trainer, and moves in a simple up and down motion. With this type of vibration trainer the platform works in one plane—up and down. The more powerful the machine, the more vibrations are generated.

The second type of vibration trainer has an oscillating platform that rocks from side to side, as well as vibrating up and down. Oscillating platforms are said to be much gentler (and quieter) than the traditional up and down linear or piston trainers, and provide the same benefits.

With oscillation you can do more exercise at a gentler pace, making it easier to use without supervision or while training in the home. The key difference between oscillation vibration and piston vibration is that with piston vibration, both legs are simultaneously moving upward or downward, but with oscillation vibration, one leg is moving up while the other is moving downward.

A 2005 study showed that vibration training "may positively influence the postural control and mobility in multiple sclerosis patients."[7]

A small pilot study in Glasgow, Scotland, supported by the MS Trust in the United Kingdom and published in 2009, involved twelve people with MS who carried out a set of exercises with and without vibrations for a fixed number of sessions over a three-month period.[8] Several different measures were used to evaluate and compare the benefits of the two exercise regimens. For most of the measures there was a wide variation within the group, reflecting the range of disabilities of the participants. In general, the results demonstrated small improvements following both exercise alone and exercise combined with whole body vibration (WBV), but there

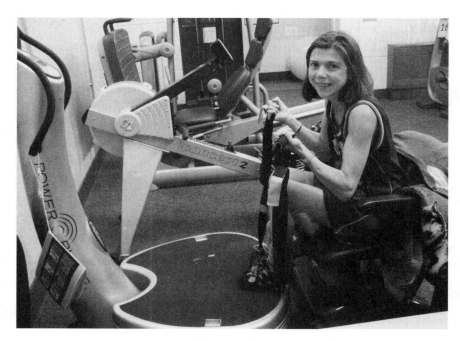

Sylvie using a Power Plate vibration trainer

was no indication that the addition of WBV provided any added benefit over exercise alone. However, although WBV did not lead to a statistically significant improvement in the measures, comments from the participants were generally positive. Participants reported fewer spasms at night, better sleep, improved ability to climb stairs, and better sensation in their feet.

Although this small-scale pilot study showed no significant benefit to using WBV, it's important to note that there were also few adverse reactions, and those that did occur were, with one exception where the vibration caused a flare up of a pre-existing knee condition, not due to the vibration itself.

Vibration training machines are widely available at gyms, as well as at some MS Therapy Centers in the United Kingdom and some U.S. chapters of the National MS Society. The program at the Multiple Sclerosis Center at Vanderbilt University School of Medicine in Nashville, Tennessee, adds whole body vibration to progressive strength training in hopes of hastening the rehabilitation of MS patients beyond what traditional physical and occupational therapies generally accomplish.

....

Vivian: The Vibration Trainer Keeps Me out of My Wheelchair

I can't exercise myself as I can't even walk in a straight line, but the vibration trainer is exercising me rather than my having to exercise myself. Although it hasn't led to any improvements in my MS, I believe the oscillating vibration trainer has stopped me from getting any worse. Family members have remarked that I have hardly used my wheelchair since starting to use the vibration trainer.

....

Anne: Regaining Leg Strength through Vibrations

After talking with MS nurses and physiotherapists, I recognized the importance of exercise for my MS, but realized I needed to find a different way of doing things. Then I read about Power Plate in a magazine and started to use it. The machine contracts and relaxes my muscles through vibrations, or pulses, and within a month I noticed a difference. Mentally I felt more positive and I was simply amazed

at the beneficial effect the machine had on my body and fatigue levels. My balance improved and my legs became stronger; I felt they
started to belong to me again. After several weeks I could stand on
my toes again and stopped falling down in the street.

Neuromuscular Electrical Stimulation

Neuromuscular electrical stimulation, also known as neuro-stim, or
NMES, has been used successfully by Dr. Terry Wahls, who combined
this method with other exercise and a brain-nutrient diet to regain her
health, strength, and mobility.

The electrical stimulation device is placed over the motor nerve of a
particular muscle to induce a muscular contraction. Typically the patient
adds a voluntary muscle contraction to that of the electrical contraction; contracting your muscles while you use the machine is four times as
effective as using the machine by itself, producing gains in muscle mass,
strength, and endurance.

Wahls says she owes much of her improvement to using a neuromuscular electrical stimulation machine on her muscles. During her research
into all the things that might help MS, she came upon some papers about
neuromuscular stimulation that was being used to build muscle mass in
athletes and to help stroke victims recover more quickly. She deduced it
was likely to have the same effect on MS.

Although neuro-stim was not "approved" for MS, a physical therapist
at her university agreed to let Dr. Wahls have a test session on a portable
device—the Empi30—which has two channels, enabling it to work two
muscle groups simultaneously. After a month of neuromuscular stimulation, Wahls found that sitting became less tiring and she could stand in
the kitchen to prepare supper.

Initially Wahls used the Empi at home. The unit is small, light, portable, and runs on rechargeable batteries. The electrodes can be applied
and removed independently if hand coordination remains good. The
manufacturer recommends forty-five minutes every day to strengthen
muscles, and fifteen minutes to maintain muscles. Their website is
www.empi.com.

After six months with the Empi, Wahls acquired a TDR68 from

Tone-A-Matic (www.toneamatic.com) with eight channels. She switched to using the TDR68 for the morning workout and continued with the Empi 300 PV throughout the day, spending a total of four or more hours on the machines daily.

Wahls emphasizes that when using neuro-stim, it's important to work with a physical therapist who will help you design a program, fix electrodes if needed, and make sure it is used safely. She cautions that a trial needs to be done for neuro-stim and multiple sclerosis, adding that on its own, neuro-stim is not enough to bring about recovery.

Resistance Chairs

Resistance chairs enable the user to have a full body workout while seated, which helps in maintaining balance and stability. By pulling on weighted resistance cables, you are able to exercise all muscle groups—abdomen, arms, chest, shoulders, back, and legs. An entire home gym in one piece of equipment, the exercise chair is designed to help with muscle tone, strength, flexibility, and mobility. Resistance chairs are often used in rehabilitation for disabled and elderly people, and are safe and easy to use.

....

Lydia: New Strength with a Resistance Chair

Just when I was about to accept death by flab, I discovered the resistance chair. At last I found something affordable and effective that would fit in my tiny dwelling. It even folds for storage. I ordered mine from Promolife, a U.S.-based company.

My chair arrived unassembled, but with written instructions and an assembly CD. I had a friend help me put it together, and it wasn't difficult. However, the tools they provide aren't the best, so I recommend the person helping you bring along basic tools, such as Allen and socket wrenches.

What an incredibly compact home gym! I can perform a multitude of exercises while sitting down. It's based on elastic resistance cables that use pulleys. The handles on the cables are attached to a large chair, so it's difficult to drop anything. If I do, it doesn't cause any damage. At last I can exercise my arms, shoulders, chest, abdomen, and back without fear of falling over.

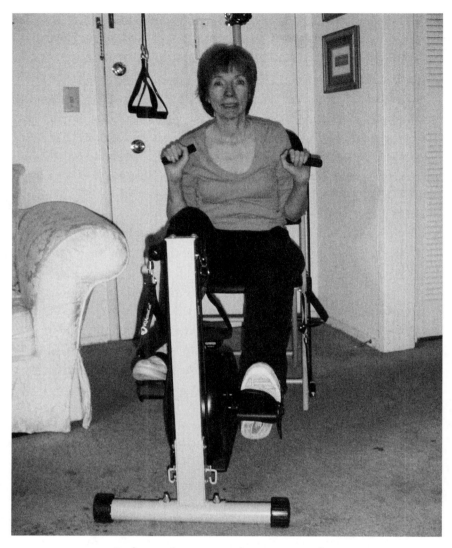

Lydia working out on her resistance chair

My resistance chair came with a set of cables, but as I get stronger I can order heavier ones to tailor the resistance level. I also ordered the Freedom Flex, a pulley system designed to improve shoulder flexibility and range of motion; and a Smooth Rider Mini-Bike, so that my legs can be exercised and I'll get a cardio workout.

My resistance chair came with an exercise DVD that is not strenuous and includes a section on stretching. I'm really grateful for the DVD. If left to my own devices, I'd do one or two exercises and that's it. Did I mention I'm lazy?

The chair is sturdy for sitting, but can tip if I grab it for balance. It comes with a posture attachment to ensure I do the exercises correctly.

I've noticed that my spasms and tremors are less with consistent exercise. I'm getting so strong that I don't have to wait by the building's front door for someone with muscles to open it; I now have muscles of my own. I actually look forward to exercising, a first for me. I'm even considering putting racing stripes on my resistance chair. How's that for a shift in attitude?

⮞ RESEARCH INTO EXERCISE AND MS

Exercise was formerly discouraged for someone with MS, but in recent years attitudes have completely changed.

- Researchers from Alberta, Canada, now say that exercise helps alleviate some of the symptoms of MS, especially fatigue, stiffness, numbness, and pain. It also helps increase flexibility, balance, and coordination; elevates mood; improves bladder and bowel function; and helps maintain independence.[9]
- Researchers from the University of Illinois found that exercise can have "an overriding positive effect on walking ability," and that it improves the quality of life in people with MS. Exercise also improved their self-efficacy and confidence.[10]
- A study was done in Iceland to determine the effect of aerobic and strength exercise on physical fitness and quality of life in sixteen patients, ages eighteen to fifty, who had mild MS. These were divided into two groups, half of whom were put in an exercise group that exercised three times a week for five weeks, and half of whom were put in a control group and did not change their habits regarding exercise. In the exercise group, there was a tendency toward improved quality of life, but no change in disability. The study confirmed that brief, moderate, aerobic exercise improves physical

fitness in individuals with mild MS. No evidence was found for worsening of MS symptoms from exercising.[11]

- An American study found that similar to their non-MS counterparts, people with mild to moderate MS are capable of improving their aerobic fitness levels. In addition, those individuals with MS who exercised regularly reduced their risk of cardiovascular disease and diabetes. The researchers found that aerobic fitness improved by 10 percent in the MS subjects.[12]

12

Physical Therapy, Physiotherapy, and Rehabilitation

THERE IS NO DOUBT that physical therapy (also called physiotherapy) is of significant benefit to anyone with MS, and there is a great deal of research to back this up. Physical therapy is now accepted as an integral part of any MS management program.

It's best to see a physical therapist as soon as possible, so you can maintain your present abilities or even improve on them, and avoid secondary handicap. Physical therapy improves movement, strength, balance and coordination, helping people with MS to achieve more normal and easier movement, and enjoy a more active life. It also prevents secondary disability arising from disuse and has beneficial effects on specific MS symptoms, such as fatigue, tremor, and spasticity.

Physical therapy teaches the correct way to stand and walk, get up from a sitting or lying position, and coordinate movements. A physical therapist will help you be aware of your posture, your movements, and your sensory perception. The aim is to bring your body back into balance so you can move more normally and freely and enjoy an active life as much as possible.

A physical therapist—ideally one who is neurologically trained—

works out a set of exercises based on the particular needs and circumstances of an individual with MS. This program is adjusted as necessary. The physical therapist also assigns exercises to be done between appointments, ideally every day.

In the United Kingdom, the National Institute for Clinical Excellence (NICE) states that people with MS should have access to physiotherapy as, and when, it is required. All types of physical therapy are beneficial to people with MS, whether done in a hospital, rehabilitation, or respite care setting, or elsewhere. Individual chapters of the National Multiple Sclerosis Society in the United States will have information about local physical therapy options.

In a good partnership between a patient and a physical therapist, the patient is not just passively on the receiving end of treatment, but is actively involved and responsible. This means seeing the management of multiple sclerosis as a way of life, rather than just a series of therapies. It also means understanding the benefits of rest, as well as the benefits of activity. It means being proactive and doing the exercises designed for you.

⤳ POSTURE, SECONDARY HANDICAP, AND STRETCHING

Poor posture may be the first sign of muscle imbalance. It may be difficult to stand properly because of damage to neural mechanisms. It is very important to take steps to correct bad posture because it can have a domino effect: apart from throwing the body out of balance, it also has a deleterious effect on breathing and on the internal organs, which will make constipation and incontinence worse than need be. Slouching can also cause pain in the neck and shoulders, depression, and flabby muscles. In time, postural abnormalities will have an effect on movement. All of these are examples of secondary handicap, which can be avoided.

The best way to prevent postural abnormalities from becoming fixed is a daily stretching routine. A physical therapist will give you simple stretching exercises to do every day at home. These stretching exercises will stimulate good posture and good balance. Yoga is also very good for correcting postural faults, as is Pilates (see chapter 11).

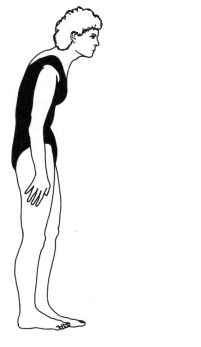
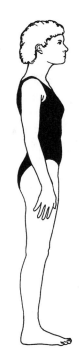

Poor posture   *Correct posture*

✎ BALANCE

The loss of balance typical of MS may be due to abnormalities in the
inner ear caused by the disease itself. However, walking as if you're falling off a tightrope could also be because of poor posture. You are literally
thrown off balance because your body is out of alignment and your center
of gravity falls outside the base of support. To get you centered again, the
physical therapist will suggest activities and exercises that promote balance. Yoga and Pilates are also very effective.

✎ MUSCLE TONE

One of the things a physical therapist will identify is abnormalities in
muscle tone, which can create problems with movement. As with bad
balance, poor muscle tone can be a secondary effect of poor posture. In
people suffering from MS, muscles can be flaccid (no tone), spastic (too
much tone), or atrophied from disuse.

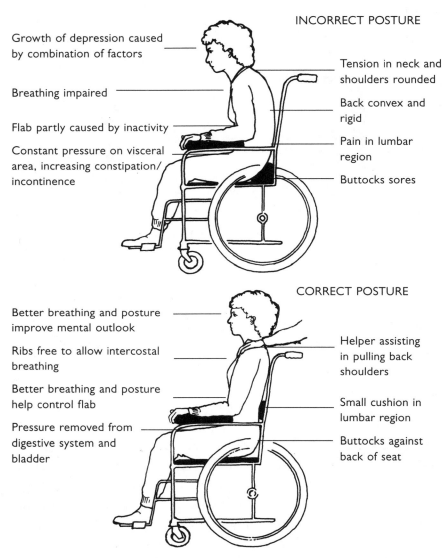

INCORRECT POSTURE

Growth of depression caused by combination of factors

Breathing impaired

Flab partly caused by inactivity

Constant pressure on visceral area, increasing constipation/incontinence

Tension in neck and shoulders rounded

Back convex and rigid

Pain in lumbar region

Buttocks sores

CORRECT POSTURE

Better breathing and posture improve mental outlook

Ribs free to allow intercostal breathing

Better breathing and posture help control flab

Pressure removed from digestive system and bladder

Helper assisting in pulling back shoulders

Small cushion in lumbar region

Buttocks against back of seat

Correct and incorrect posture in a wheelchair

In the rehabilitation process, it's important to be alert for associated reactions—things that occur on their own in response to something you do. For example, one part of your body may be compensating for another part: the more you use your right hand, the weaker your left hand gets; the more you use your arms, the weaker your legs get. Concentrate on the weak areas to help bring your body back into balance.

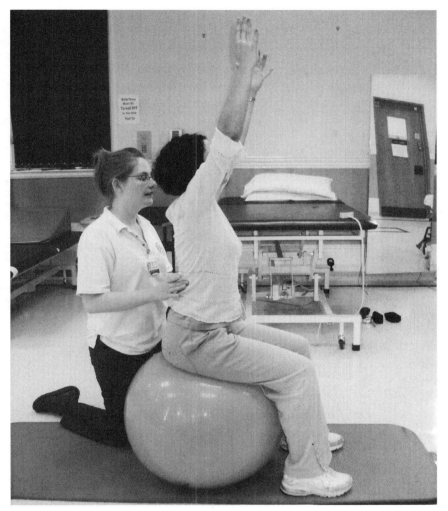

Joanne doing a balance exercise with assistance from a rehabilitation therapist

It is not helpful is to increase the strength of muscles that are already strong. If you only build up the strong muscles, the weak ones stand no chance, and the more out of balance you will be. If, for example, you are strong from the waist up but weak from the waist down, there is the temptation to use your arms and trunk a lot, rather than your legs and lower half. This is why you should be careful not to put your weight on your hands when you sit down or get up from an armchair. Use your legs as much as you can.

A physical therapist will design a set of exercises tailor-made to your particular needs and disability. Gentle stretching exercises are likely to be part of this. Such exercises will be designed to make the most of what you've got, correct any postural faults, get you back on balance, and rectify abnormal muscle tone.

If the muscles are spastic, the physical therapist will design a program that avoids positions and activities that increase tone or reinforce abnormal ways of moving. The program will include daily walking or standing, carrying weights, and regular stretching. The therapist will also advise ways to avoid pressure sores, constipation, and bladder infections.

REHABILITATION

Checking into a neurological rehab unit for one, two, or more weeks can bring about big functional improvements. Much of the therapy is physiotherapy based, but you also work with a multidisciplinary team that can help you with problems such as bowels, bladder, and eyesight. In the United States, ask your local chapter of the National Multiple Sclerosis Society or the National Rehabilitation Information Center about the options available in your area (see Resources).

Liz: Physical Therapy Was Surprisingly Helpful

At my assessment, I talked to a nurse and doctor and was examined by a physiotherapist. They offered me two weeks in the community rehab unit as they thought I could be helped. And how right they were! I didn't know quite what to expect beyond the physiotherapy, which was the main treatment they thought could help me.

When I first went there, I was using my walking frame, or walker, very badly, standing too far away and stooping. But by the end of my two-week stay, the physios had helped me exercise the right muscles and given me the confidence to be able to walk unaided indoors— something I hadn't done for years.

In addition to helping me in many practical ways, the rehab unit was a good respite and a great morale booster. It's not surprising that I left better than when I arrived, but the challenge is to keep yourself motivated, so they also provide excellent follow-up visits.

ꙮ PROVEN BENEFITS OF PHYSICAL THERAPY

Results of a study in the *Journal of Neurology, Neurosurgery & Psychiatry* suggest that an individualized rehabilitation program is effective in reducing disability in MS patients. Researchers in Australia conducted a study with 101 patients who were randomly assigned to an individualized program or standard care. Patients in the treatment group received comprehensive multidisciplinary rehabilitation over twelve months, which included intensive treatment aimed at patient education, health promotion, bladder retraining, and mobilization. Compared with patients who received standard care, those given individualized rehab showed greater overall functional independence as well as specific improvements in walking and self care. Their disability was significantly reduced. Overall, 70.8 percent of patients in the treatment group improved, compared with 13 percent of those in the standard care group. More patients in the standard care group also deteriorated over the study period.[1]

At Cardiff University, Wales, a study done in 2000 on the effects of mobility in chronic MS found a statistically high beneficial effect of exercise over no exercise. Those who had physiotherapy had improved mobility, walked better, and felt a greater sense of well-being and mood compared to those who did no exercise.[2]

Treadmill training has also proven effective. A study published in February 2009 found that exercise training is associated with a small improvement in walking mobility among individuals with multiple sclerosis. Several patients who took part in a study on improving gait in MS showed significant improvements after doing repetitive, robot-assisted, body weight-supported treadmill training.[3]

Several years ago the charity ARMS (Action and Research for Multiple Sclerosis), the predecessor of the Multiple Sclerosis Resource Centre in the United Kingdom, carried out research into the effects of exercise and physiotherapy on MS. It found they had a vital role to play in learning to control and coordinate movements, reduce spasticity, encourage more normal movements, and regain functional abilities. Physiotherapy and rehabilitation are also firmly endorsed by the National Multiple Sclerosis Society in the United States.

13

Complementary
Therapies

MANY THERAPIES that come under the broad heading of holistic, complementary, or alternative medicine can be very helpful in MS. These include such well-established schools as naturopathy and osteopathy; familiar therapies, such as acupuncture and homeopathy; and less well-known therapies, such as reflexology, aromatherapy, applied kinesiology, and electromagnetic crystal therapy, that are often quite effective.

Many of the holistic therapies emphasize some of the concepts of the ancient Eastern systems of medicine, in which balance is synonymous with good health. Good health is harmony: a balance between opposing forces, between yin and yang, or between acid and alkaline.

Harmony goes beyond biochemical balance. As in the traditional Eastern forms of medicine, it also means right life, wisdom and love, right fellowship, meditation, healthy eating, and exercise.

Complementary therapy is holistic in its approach. Unlike the orthodox doctor, a complementary therapist or integrative medicine doctor will treat you as a whole person—mind, body, and spirit—and not just treat the diseased part. The whole approach of alternative therapies is radically different from that of orthodox medicine.

By and large, complementary practitioners are not very interested in disease labels, such as multiple sclerosis or arthritis. They generally speak more of a loss of balance in the body, imbalanced lifestyle and thought patterns, and blocked energy, or *chi*. Their goal is to help you bring your body back into balance so that good health can be regained.

Orthodox medicine diagnoses symptoms and tries to find ways of suppressing those symptoms, usually through drugs. By contrast, holistic therapists aim not to suppress symptoms, but to get to the root cause or causes of the symptoms and treat those root causes instead. The general starting point with complementary medicine is the conviction that the body has innate powers to heal itself given the right conditions. The task of any complementary therapist is to help bring about the right conditions so the body can get on with the business of healing itself.

The therapy itself is likely to be only one part of a holistic treatment program that may involve quite dramatic changes in diet, lifestyle, exercise, and thought patterns. The whole attitude of holistic medicine transforms your way of thinking and makes you think seriously about how you came to have MS, and how you might be inadvertently making it worse. You may well, with the help of the therapist, discover aspects of your old lifestyle that must be changed if you want your health to improve.

Some already-disabled people may experience increased well-being as a result of seeing a holistic practitioner, and some with only mild MS symptoms may find that their symptoms become even milder or go away. Everyone, no matter how healthy or ill, should experience a greater sense of well-being as a result of treatment in the chosen therapy, if accompanied by the recommended lifestyle changes.

Although few would claim to "cure" MS, many complementary therapists say the condition can be stabilized and the downward spiral can be stopped or reversed. You're no longer classified as someone with an incurable illness. Instead, you are someone who is making profound changes to help regain health.

One mistake some patients make is to view a particular alternative therapy as just a technique. This is a very conventional, passive view of medicine. If you want any kind of holistic therapy to be helpful, you have to be an active participant in the healing process and not just a passive recipient having something done to you. Before you see any holistic practitioner (including integrative medicine M.D.s), you should be psychologically prepared to fundamentally change many aspects of your life.

I have had good personal experiences with several complementary therapies, and they may have played a part in helping me stay as well as I am. I've explored nutritional medicine, acupuncture, shiatsu, osteopathy, cranial osteopathy, conductive education, homeopathy, hydrotherapy, herbalism, naturopathy, applied kinesiology, massage, magnet therapy, reflexology, Alexander Technique, and electromagnetic crystal therapy.

If I did all of these all of the time I wouldn't have time to do anything else and would also be broke. Right now I have weekly shiatsu, and when I'm in pain I have osteopathy or acupuncture. Nutritional medicine is a way of life.

Nearly all of the complementary therapies you'll find here have been used to treat patients with multiple sclerosis.

ACUPUNCTURE AND ACUPRESSURE

Acupuncturists believe illness is an imbalance in the body's energy. The aim of acupuncture is to restore this balance. In traditional Chinese medicine, it balances the yin and yang. Fine needles are inserted into the skin at particular points along invisible energy channels called "meridians," which are named after the organs they represent. The needles help unblock *chi,* or life force energy. By stimulating these points, blockages are released and energy flow is restored. Heat or electrical stimulation can sometimes be applied at acupuncture points. The needles may be uncomfortable at first if you are far out of balance.

Acupressure is similar to acupuncture. Instead of inserting needles, however, acupuncture points are pressed with fingertips or a massage tool. Acupressure is used to relieve pain and tension. Acupuncture and acupressure can help alleviate pain, spasticity, eye problems, and bladder urgency.[1]

They can also improve movement, increase energy, relieve fatigue, give a boost to the immune system, and improve quality of life.[2]

One study that looked at acupuncture as a treatment for spasticity in MS found the results "encouraging enough to invite further investigation."[3]

In another study that explored acupuncture for bladder dysfunction, forty-one people with MS were divided into four groups, receiving no intervention, conventional treatment, acupuncture, or conventional treatment plus acupuncture. Those receiving either conventional treatment plus acupuncture or acupuncture alone benefited most.[4]

ᴂ ALEXANDER TECHNIQUE

Alexander Technique is particularly good for correcting poor posture that results from using your body incorrectly. An Alexander Technique teacher helps you to unlearn bad habits and perform all movements correctly, whether walking, standing, sitting, or lying down. Correctly implemented, the technique can improve balance, posture, and coordination; correct rounded shoulders and a slouched back; and help you to stand taller. This usually involves addressing and correcting tension held in the neck and shoulders, which affects the whole body and causes chronic tightening of the muscles. Doing the Alexander Technique properly makes all your movements more fluid, which helps in everyday life and improves quality of life.

Alexander Technique has been used with a great deal of success in multiple sclerosis. You can learn it in a one-on-one lesson with a teacher or be part of a group or workshop; in either case, you practice at home between sessions. It is widely available in the United States, Canada, Australia, and New Zealand. In the United Kingdom, some multiple sclerosis therapy centers offer sessions in Alexander Technique. The following testimonial is from an MS therapy center.

....

Kevin: Taller, More Stable, and Out to the Market

I will admit that I was a little sceptical at first and only went to lessons sporadically. However, I came to realize that it was doing more than I thought when one day someone said to me, "You look taller!" After that I began to take weekly lessons and started to markedly improve. In the beginning, I didn't really understand what was going on during a lesson. The teacher's touch is very light but the impact is quite dramatic. As each session progresses I feel myself getting taller and my stability improving. My right leg, which is weaker and less stable than the left, becomes steadier and I get more feeling from my back down into my legs and out through my toes (which usually feel clawed). During the part of the lesson when I'm lying down, although the touch is subtle, I feel as if I've been really stretched. During the session it also becomes easier and more natural to move in and out of the chair with less effort. A session makes me feel better and I really like the positive approach. The next day I always feel that I can cope better and feel happier in myself.

The Alexander Technique has had a big impact on my life. A year ago I had to lean on the sink to brush my teeth, and now I can stand unsupported. I used to sit in a slumped, unhealthy way, and now I can sit upright, unsupported, and comfortable for longer periods of time. Six months ago I had to do my shopping on the Internet, and now I physically go to the local supermarket. It's made me more aware of how I do things, but the changes also feel natural so I don't have to think about them. The Alexander Technique has improved me, without a doubt, mentally and physically. I'm managing to help myself, making the conscious effort to make my life a little bit better.

ANTHROPOSOPHIC MEDICINE

Rudolf Steiner, an early twentieth-century Austrian scientist and philosopher, stressed that good health has a spiritual as well as a physical dimension. Steiner believed that many illnesses—including MS—can be caused by a sickness of the spirit, life, and soul.

In anthroposophic medicine it is believed that a patient's health and vitality are chiefly influenced by an inherent "life force"—or chi—that shapes the person's ability to recover from illness, and which maintains good health. This life force regulates a healthy immune system and keeps the body running at optimum levels, balancing physical performance with a healthy mind and positive spirit, and enabling you to feel energized rather than drained, and optimistic rather than depressed.

Therapies offered by anthroposophic practitioners aim to invigorate the life force, and in the case of MS, to rebalance it. Medicines are conventional, herbal, and homeopathic, as well as anthroposophic. One of the most common remedies used to treat MS patients is derived from the parasitic plant mistletoe and is usually given by injection. Mistletoe preparations are said to stimulate T cell development and have immune-modulatory effects.[5]

In addition to natural medicines, complementary therapies may be offered that help MS symptoms of stiffness, weakness, and pain. These include massage, hydrotherapy, art therapy (painting or sculpture), and eurythmy, a kind of movement therapy that can help build a sense of well-being and lead to improvements in coordination, control, and mobility.

Medical and biographical counseling from trained professionals are often an integral part of an anthroposophic treatment program.

In the United States, the Rudolf Steiner Health Center (RSHC) provides anthroposophic medical care in combination with traditional Western medicine in one facility. A true integrative medicine center, it houses all the therapies that anthroposophic medicine encompasses. Their website is www.steinerhealth.org. (See also Resources for more complete information.)

Until recently, there was an inpatient anthroposophic medical facility in the United Kingdom called Park Attwood, but this has now sadly closed. Two of their practitioners continue their work with outpatients at the Raphael Medical Centre, Hildenborough, near Tonbridge, Kent. Other U.K. facilities that offer this type of medicine include the Camphill Medical Practice in Aberdeen, Scotland, and other clinics in Maidstone, Kent, and Bristol. (See Resources for more information.)

....

Vicci: Healing through Art

Park Attwood is a good reminder of the fact that you are not the MS. At Park Attwood, you are an individual where the focus is not all about the MS condition. The emphasis is all on healing. It's the full program of therapies, medication, emotional support and even the place itself, that all works together. It works on nurturing your own strengths so that you are not overwhelmed by the disease. Of the various therapies at Park Attwood, I found the painting and sculpture therapies the most energizing. Even though on a recent visit to Park Attwood I was only able to work with one hand, I did some relief sculpture and was amazed at what could be achieved despite the limitations. But if you're feeling low, massage therapy might be the therapy of choice.

....

APPLIED KINESIOLOGY

Applied kinesiology uses muscle testing to identify food and environmental sensitivities, nutritional deficiencies, and health problems. This technique is based on the belief that weakness in certain muscles relates to specific disease states or imbalances in the body. Kinesiologists may use this modality to diagnose organ dysfunction or energy blockage. Applied kinesiology may include specific joint manipulation or mobilization, myofascial (muscle tissue) therapies, cranial techniques, meridian therapy, good nutrition, dietary management, and various reflex procedures. In MS, applied kinesiology is most often used to help identify food sensitivities.[6]

ᔓ AROMATHERAPY

Aromatherapy uses volatile, essential plant oils that have a beneficial effect on mind and body. Essential oils are extracted from herbs, flowers, shrubs, or trees. The most widely accepted theory of how aromatherapy works suggests that our olfactory senses chemically convert the fragrance and relay information to the brain. However, there is some evidence that pure essential oils are able to penetrate the skin and enter the bloodstream.

Each essential oil is different, with its own fragrance and therapeutic use, often in conjunction with massage. Some essential oils have anti-inflammatory properties, others bring about a feeling of relaxation, and still others are stimulating. Many are known to have such potent effects on the mind that they can alter your mood in minutes. To get the full health benefits of aromatherapy, it is best to consult a professional aromatherapist.[7]

If you are purchasing essential oils, be sure the label specifies "essential oils," rather than "natural ingredients," and doesn't include any chemicals. When using, be careful to always dilute oils in water or a carrier oil. Undiluted, they should not be applied directly on the skin. You can add a few drops of essential oils to a bath or to a room vaporizer. A bowl of warm water works equally well but cools quickly.

In treating MS, juniper stimulates the urinary system and rosemary is a neuromuscular relaxant. Neroli oil can also be very useful, especially if there are neuromuscular problems. Hypericum (St. John's wort) is an antidepressant. For constipation, a gentle oil such as black pepper may help. Disturbed sleep patterns can be helped with Roman chamomile; low spirits with grapefruit oil.

ᔓ AUTOGENIC TRAINING

This is a relaxation and body awareness technique that involves visualization. In daily sessions, specific visualizations are repeated almost like a meditation mantra, training your body to respond to your words. It is said to restore balance between the sympathetic and parasympathetic functions of the nervous system, and to be helpful in reducing stress and improving positive outlook.

A study done on relaxation and quality of life in people with MS found that those who did autogenic training had more energy and vigor than those who did not.[8]

AYURVEDIC MEDICINE

Ayurveda, Sanskrit for "science of life," is an ancient system of traditional medicine and philosophy native to India. It is a holistic lifestyle approach that treats mind, body, and spirit in multiple ways, including food, herbs, massage, yoga, and meditation. An ayurvedic doctor will expect you to take responsibility for your own health in order to be well and live in harmony with the environment.

Ayurveda evaluates each person as a specific body-mind type, or *dosha: vata, pitta,* or *kapha.* You are treated according to your dosha or combination of doshas. For example, you may be pitta-vata or kapha-pitta.

Vatas tend to be visionary, imaginative, and full of creative energy, but when they are out of balance they can be forgetful, spaced out, anxious, and uptight. Typical vata problems are erratic digestion, bloating, anxiety, or joint disorders. Pittas are confident, passionate leaders, organized, and perfectionists, but excess pitta can make them fiery, snappy, and irritable. Pitta people have a tendency to suffer from skin irritations, overheating, heartburn, and ulcers. Kaphas are loyal, kindhearted, calm, and full of love, but a kapha overload can make them lethargic and overindulgent. Kaphas are prone to congestion, excess weight, and sluggish digestion.

At your first consultation, your ayurvedic practitioner will ask many questions to determine your likes, dislikes, and tendencies. The doctor will analyze your pulse to help determine your body type and any imbalances. Three fingers are placed on the left wrist if you're a woman, on the right wrist if you're a man, while the doctor tunes in to what's going on in your body through your pulse. It may take up to several minutes as different impulses are detected. From the pulse diagnosis, the doctor can tell you your dosha balance and may suggest an herbal remedy, dietary or behavioral change, or an in-house treatment.

....

Cathy: Fantastic Results with Ayurveda

Over the years, I have had lengthy ayurvedic treatments with fantastic results, not just with my MS symptoms, but also with my general health and happiness.

When I was first diagnosed with MS, I had become pretty disabled almost overnight, needing a wheelchair or strong arm to hang onto to move around, then two walking sticks. The neurologist was astonishingly discouraging, telling me there was nothing I could do but rest and come back and see him again in three months. When I asked him what he thought of alternative approaches, he said, "Save your money and buy a crate of champagne."

Luckily, I didn't take his advice. I consulted an ayurvedic doctor who was uplifting, helpful, encouraging, and caring, making me feel listened to and that I mattered—a great start to my healing process.

The standard ayurveda treatment begins with a preparation process that involves drinking melted ghee (clarified butter) in increasing amounts over several days to loosen toxins and start the cleaning process.

The hands-on treatment begins with Indian head massage, then a full body massage, or *abhyanga* (loving hands), which is always given by two therapists (female for women, male for men), who work in synchrony, using warm herbalized oil. This is performed in silence, allowing for even deeper relaxation and inner awareness. It is followed by *shiro dhara,* in which a steady stream of warm oil is drizzled over the forehead for half an hour. This is so profoundly relaxing that patients usually fall asleep.

Then comes an herbalized steam bath and finally an internal cleansing (a gentle oil enema) that removes loosened toxins. This treatment left me feeling extremely settled, contented, and wonderfully clear mentally.

I have been to India twice for treatment, each time for three weeks at an ayurvedic clinic. The most effective treatment for my MS was *navara kizhi.* Two therapists massaged my body briskly with coarse linen bags filled with hot rice cooked in milk and herbs. The milky, starchy rice seeped through the linen bags, covering me in a sticky mess! The combination of heat, friction, and the milky residue was instantly healing for my stiff, numb limbs, and after several days of this I began to notice I was more flexible, walked better, and had better balance.

Another very effective treatment for me was called *pizichil* and involved being massaged with a constant flow of warm herbalized oil. I also had *nasya,* which treats the sinus and nasal passages, leaving my head feeling clear and unfogged. *Netra tarpan* treated my eyes by bathing them in ghee (clarified butter), which had the effect of soothing my sore eyes and clearing my sight.

Every afternoon my chakras were balanced with *kati vasti, griva vasti, hriday vasti,* and *chakra varti vasti,* which I nicknamed "the doughnut treatment." Large, doughnut-shaped circles made from a paste of chickpea flour and water were placed on a chakra area (heart, stomach, lower and upper back) and filled with warm herbalized oil, and then I had to lie still for twenty minutes.

Since coming back from India, I have gradually become aware of the main improvements in my MS: energy and walking ability. A couple of months after I got home I was able to walk downhill without a walking stick. That felt like a big breakthrough for me, and I use my walking stick less and less.

There are many ayurvedic clinics throughout the world, which can be found easily on the Internet. For specific listings, see Resources.

BIORESONANCE

Bioresonance is an energy therapy based on the principle that every material structure in the universe vibrates, or oscillates, in a unique energy signature, or frequency. It was first developed in the 1970s in the early days of microelectronics, which perceived the human body as a complex electronic circuitry made up of conductors, capacitors, and inductors. The assumption made by the originators of bioresonance was that if the body is mainly electrical circuitry, disease (malfunction) must be found in the distortion of electrical signals as they travel through this circuitry. Bioresonance practitioners say they can use this therapy to treat disease by stimulating a change of bioresonance in the cells, reversing the disruption caused by the disease.

One modern form of bioresonance is a device called the Bicom that claims to strengthen the natural electromagnetic oscillations of the body and/or cancel pathological oscillations, thus enabling the body to regain healthy function. Practitioners say they are able to use the Bicom to pinpoint the real, underlying causes of chronic and degenerative diseases, which they believe is the accumulation of toxins in the space between cells in the tissues of the body. These toxins are thought to block the cells' ability to receive oxygen and nutrients and to eliminate metabolic wastes. The toxins eventually enter the cells and produce symptoms of chronic illness. The Bicom machine uses biofeedback to test the body's electrical reaction to specific substances that might be toxic. Skin resistance measurements at specific locations reveal how the body reacts to things like chemical toxins, drugs, heavy metals, fungi, parasites, viruses, and allergies. The bioresonance device then sends the body an inverse oscillation pattern of the energy of the toxin to neutralize its electromagnetic charge. This allows the immune system to easily remove the remains of the toxin from the body. This program can also identify chemical imbalances, vitamin/mineral imbalances, yeast, candida, mercury toxicity, and food imbalances.

The Bicom program claims to be able to neutralize the frequency of any toxin present in the body. More than just removing toxins, it actually "rewires" the body by enhancing healthy frequencies using bioresonance technology.[9]

BOTANICAL MEDICINE

Botanical medicine, or herbalism, uses plant extracts, tinctures, tablets, and teas. Herbs can be powerful and have side effects, so it is wise to consult a medical herbalist or practitioner trained in traditional Chinese medicine or ayurvedic medicine.

Herbs can strengthen the immune and nervous systems and also ease certain MS symptoms, such as muscle spasms, fatigue, paralysis, and urinary problems. The particular herbs used to treat MS include antimony, gotu kola, ginkgo biloba, and cannabis, which is addressed in chapter 14.

Ayurvedic remedies include food concentrates high in antioxidants and ashwaganda, another Indian herb useful for loss of muscular energy and paralysis. Perhaps the most commonly used herb in MS is evening primrose oil. Other herbs, such as barberry, are used for specific problems.

Barberry is a very powerful anti-candida herb that supports the helpful bacteria in the gut and prevents the growth of candida after antibiotic use. It cleanses and regulates the liver, helps the stomach, and balances the action of the gallbladder and bowels, combining well with other herbs.

Chamomile is a nerve relaxant that calms the mind and body and aids sleep. It is also anti-fungal. Cramp bark is good for muscular cramp. Echinacea helps the immune system, elderflower helps with elimination, and ginger is useful for circulation and digestion. Ginseng (Siberian, Korean, or American) is a tonic that boosts the immune system and supports the adrenal glands, which, in turn, assist the nervous system.

Gotu kola is said to be one of the most important rejuvenative herbs in ayurvedic medicine and the main revitalizing herb for nerves and brain cells. Hawthorn berry is rich in vitamin C and flavone glycosides, good for stress. *Huo ma ren* is a cannabis extract from China that qualified and registered herbalists can legally prescribe. It helps to relax the muscles but is not mind altering. Licorice is anti-inflammatory, providing natural steroids.

Milk thistle (silymarin) cleanses, purifies, and counterbalances the effects of eating rich, junk foods. It is a powerful liver detoxifier and helps to protect and regenerate liver cells. It also increases secretion of bile from the gallbladder. Myrrh is anti-inflammatory. Oat seed and straw feed the nerves. Sage is anti-spasmodic and aids digestion. Schizandra berries work like Siberian ginseng. Skullcap works as a nerve tonic to feed and strengthen the nervous system and is also anti-inflammatory. Slippery elm nourishes and heals the digestive tract. Rhodiola is high in antioxidants.

Stevia rebaudiana is an herb that grows in the rain forests of Brazil and has been used as a natural sweetener in South America for centuries. It is calorie-free and does not feed candida. A leaf or a pinch of leaf powder can be added to drinks, and powdered Stevia can be added to food or used in baking. A liquid extract is also available, which is said to be three-hundred-times sweeter than sugar. It has no calories and only a negligible effect on blood sugar. Woodbetony nourishes the nervous system. Other herbs sometimes used for MS are lemongrass, yucca, burdock root, red clover, dandelion root and leaf, peppermint, bee pollen, bilberry leaf, and astralagus.

Certain plants used in herbal medicine are foods. Examples are sesame seeds, flaxseeds and flaxseed oil, oats, pumpkin seeds, onion, garlic, almonds, sea kelp, hemp oil, watercress, lettuce, asparagus, and lemon.

Medicinal herbs used in cooking include ginger, coriander, saffron, turmeric, cumin, cardamom, nutmeg, cinnamon, anise, oregano, rosemary, basil, parsley, sage, and thyme.

Herb teas are delicious alternatives to black tea, and some of these are rooibos, pau d'arco, green tea, chamomile, fennel, mint, sage, borage, and lime tree flowers.

A mixture of herbs based on a traditional Tibetan herbal formula, called Padma Basic (Padma 28 in Europe) is sometimes used in MS. In a small study Padma Basic was given to one hundred people with MS. After taking two pills, three times per day for one year, 44 percent experienced increased muscle strength and overall improvement.[10] (See also chapter 8, page 79.)

Another herb frequently taken in MS is ginkgo biloba, which helps boost circulation to the extremities. It is also taken to boost brainpower. When intravenous injections of a constituent of ginkgo biloba, known as ginkgolide B, were given to people with MS for five days, 80 percent of them reportedly improved.[11] This specialized treatment is experimental, and it is not known whether oral use of ginkgo extracts would have a similar effect. (See also chapter 8, page 68.)

☙ BOWEN TECHNIQUE

The Bowen Technique addresses the whole body, because ailments of one body area are frequently due to problems somewhere else in the body. It can help in cases of MS, though it is not a cure. It is frequently used as a form of stress management and to help boost energy; improve balance, bladder, and movement; and help restore sensation to the limbs.

The Bowen Technique is gentle and involves fingers and thumbs moving in a series of light rolling moves over muscles, fascia, and ligaments. There is no cracking and crunching, friction or rubbing. It is not a massage and no oils are used. No heavy pressure is needed and the light moves can be made through clothing.

When the body goes out of balance, the Bowen Technique can help with realignment. The gentle moves send powerful neurological impulses to the brain, improving communication between body and brain, and increasing blood and lymph flow. Sometimes patients may feel warmth on an area recently touched, or claim the sensation of a hand still on them. It is believed the technique encourages the body's own power of healing to do whatever is necessary. The moves used in Bowen Technique trigger the parasympathetic nervous system and put the body into a state of deep relaxation, making it ideal for stress relief. To achieve the full benefit of these moves, there can be breaks that may last from two to five minutes to allow the body to integrate the stimulus received. Bowen treatments last typically forty-five minutes to an hour.

For more information about Bowen Technique, see Resources.

CHIROPRACTIC

Chiropractic focuses on the diagnosis, treatment, and prevention of mechanical disorders of the musculoskeletal system, especially the spine. These disorders are thought to affect general health via the nervous system. The main treatment involves manual therapy, including manipulation of the spine, joints, and soft tissue. Treatment also includes exercises and health and lifestyle counseling. Traditionally, chiropractic assumes that spinal joint dysfunction—subluxations—interfere with the body's innate intelligence and ability to function properly.

A recent journal study revealed that correction of upper neck injuries might help improve or even reverse the progression of MS.[12] The study evaluated the data from forty-four MS patients, of whom 91 percent showed improvement over five years of treatment. These findings led researchers to believe the correction of neck injuries could activate a reversal of MS. Head and neck injuries have long been thought to be contributing factors to the development of MS. These results are the first to confirm the relationship between the two.

COGNITIVE BEHAVIORAL THERAPY

Cognitive behavioral therapy (CBT) is a form of psychotherapy that emphasizes the important role of our thoughts in how we feel and what we do. It aims to help a client think more positively—and has been the subject of trials for depression and fatigue in MS.

In a study done in northern California published in 2001, individual cognitive behavioral therapy sessions brought about significant reductions in depression, and produced the same results as the antidepressant sertraline and supportive expressive group therapy.[13]

Another Californian study, which examined the efficacy of an eight-week telephone-administered cognitive behavioral therapy for the treatment of depression in MS patients, found that depression decreased significantly in the group treated with CBT.[14] In the telephone sessions, patients were counseled on how to cope with MS.

A study done in 1984 came to the conclusion that the results "clearly support the use of cognitive behavioral treatments in patients with MS."[15]

Cognitive behavioral therapy is being used successfully at the University of Southampton in England to help treat adjustment to MS and fatigue. A study coordinated by Southampton University and the University of Auckland, New Zealand, tested cognitive behavioral therapy and relaxation therapies for fatigue in MS, and found that both groups showed a significant decrease in fatigue.[16]

The goal of CBT is to help people to adjust to having MS and to create a better quality of life. Clients are encouraged to fully engage in life to the best of their abilities while accepting that they have the condition. A CBT psychotherapist will help the client address common problems, such as avoidance and denial.

When there is good psychological adjustment, the person acknowledges negative emotions surrounding MS, yet has the flexibility to alter or adapt life goals or values. A poor adjustment to MS is characterized by high levels of stress and distress, with MS having an unhealthy negative impact on quality of life.

According to Rona Moss-Morris, professor of health psychology at the University of Southampton, several psychological factors have been shown to be important in successfully adjusting to MS. These include seeking social support, accepting the illness but not giving up, seeing difficult experiences in a realistic rather than negative light, and having a sense of control over the illness. Being able to reinterpret upsetting or difficult experiences in a more positive light is an important part of cognitive behavioral therapy. Another example would be going through a difficult relationship break-up but later being able to say that in some ways the experience was very helpful, because you learned a lot about yourself and are now better able to deal with relationships.

Good adjustment to MS also involves looking after yourself with a healthy diet, regular exercise, a good sleep/wake pattern, and avoidance of harmful things, such as smoking.

Moss-Morris has been conducting a randomized controlled trial of CBT in MS. At the time of writing, the clinical part of the trial was complete (ninety-four patients randomized) but they were still collecting follow-up data and are unable to determine as yet whether or not this is an effective treatment approach. Data will be analyzed during 2010.

COLONIC IRRIGATION

This therapy involves gently filling the colon with warm filtered water through a small sterile tube. You lie on your side and a tube is inserted into your anal orifice, through which the warm water will gradually irrigate your intestines. The water is flushed in and when it flushes out, carries with it any material that has accumulated in the intestine, including water, waste matter, toxins, and trapped gases. The entire process is completely contained so if you don't want to see what is being flushed out of your body through the semi-transparent tube, you can look the other way. However, it can be illuminating to see what has been trapped in your body.

The process does not cause pain or discomfort, though there can be a full feeling. During the session the therapist presses gently on parts of the lower abdomen to encourage the release of blockages. The final part of the therapy involves replenishing the colon with friendly bacteria, which is done by squirting a probiotic liquid up the back passage.

Sylvia: Lighter after Colon Hydrotherapy

During the actual session, which lasted about an hour, I had approximately fifteen gallons of warm water gently flushed through my colon, and I lost more than five pounds of waste matter! Some people may experience a healing crisis as toxins are eliminated from the body (and so feel worse before feeling better). The next day I felt as good as new and somewhat more buoyant. Since that time I have had daily bowel movements, which is most unusual for me. It makes sense to me that if you are constipated due to a sluggish digestive system, it's a good idea to give the colon a good cleaning occasionally. The muscles of the colon get a workout as well.

I believe this therapy is proving beneficial to my overall health and that it could be helpful to people with a variety of medical conditions, such as irritable bowel syndrome, constipation, recurrent urinary tract infections, candida (yeast overgrowth), and fatigue, among many others. I have been feeling less bloated, more energetic, and somewhat lighter and clearer generally, though I would hesitate to give all the credit for this to this therapy.

◈ CONDUCTIVE EDUCATION

Conductive education teaches people with motor disorders how to use their bodies more effectively. This gives them greater confidence and more control over their lives. The teaching is very verbal and can be hard work, but is often fun and a great boost to self-esteem. It was initially developed as a system of rehabilitation by the Hungarian physician Andras Peto in Budapest, Hungary, for the needs of children with cerebral palsy, and later used for those with neurological conditions, including MS.[17] Professor Peto theorized that in MS, new neuronal pathways could be built to do the work of damaged nerve cells.

Conductive education helps you regain lost skills and improve new skills through active learning and repetition. Clients work with motivating teachers, or "conductors," who help them become active learners.

During a typical conductive education session, time is spent on improving movement, balance, and the fluency and rhythm of walking; and also on reducing muscle spasm, fatigue, and tremor. The exercises also help with speech, circulation, and general well-being.

The National Institute for Conductive Education in the United Kingdom says: "Conductive education is an educational approach to multiple sclerosis that helps individuals develop the skills and motivation they need to overcome problems of movement and bodily control they encounter in everyday living."

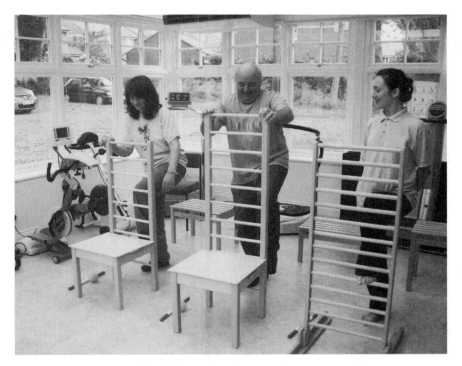

Louise (far left) at a conductive education session

Louise: Loves the Feeling of Wind in Her Face

I attended my first session of conductive education at the beginning of June, 2009. It was tiring but also exciting, as I was told I'd be walking without a stick within a couple of months. I'm pleased to say that after just three weeks I tentatively abandoned my stick and began to walk unaided.

I can't claim to walk well but I can certainly walk short distances without a stick. Some days I have a pronounced limp but I'm standing straighter and the discomfort in my neck and shoulders is gone. Many people have commented that I seem more upright. I am able to enjoy and take part in normal family life, where I had previously felt excluded.

Conductive education has also helped me to realize which parts of my body don't function properly, which can help me to concentrate my efforts when things start to malfunction. It has also increased my self-confidence and improved my feelings about MS and what the future holds. Lately I have rented an adult trike and pedalled it along the canal path. I can really get that wind-in-my-face feeling, and it's wonderful!

Kelly: Developing a "Can Do" Attitude

With conductive education the approach is: "You can do this." They enable you to do things you thought you couldn't do any longer. I learned how to maneuver myself out of bed when my legs stiffened, enabling me to overcome the frustrating situation of having to shout for my husband or children. Now I can roll on to my side, bring my legs up, and use my body as a lever to throw myself up. You learn how to work with your body rather than it working against you. In some ways it is very simple and practical, but no one had told me how to do it before.

Much of what I learned can easily be integrated into everyday life, such as maintaining control as you sit down, rather than flopping into a chair. I'll be in the kitchen making a cup of coffee and I'll hear the conductor's voice in my head. If I'm not having a good day, I can imagine her encouraging me: "You can do this."

Find out more about conductive education in Resources at the back of this book.

CRANIAL OSTEOPATHY

Cranial osteopathy, a very gentle osteopathic treatment, focuses on relieving stress and tension in the body.[18] Stresses and tensions disrupt the body's natural cranial rhythm; though gentle, cranial osteopathy can be powerful in its effects. Cranial osteopaths feel and interpret a very delicate, rhythmic shape change that exists in all body tissues. This motion, known as cranial rhythm, is due to the movement of cerebrospinal fluid bathing the spinal cord and the pull of the soft tissue connections to the cranial bones. This involves a rhythmic elongation and narrowing, followed by a shortening and widening, a cycle that repeats approximately every ten seconds.

Treatment involves observing and correcting disruptions in the cranial rhythm, which can be due to events that have happened recently or past physical or emotional experiences.

You may experience a feeling of slight pressure as the therapist cradles your head. Most people find this treatment deeply relaxing and energizing. You may feel tired after a treatment as stress is released and your body and mind adjust to new patterns.

ᐸᔑ CRANIOSACRAL THERAPY (CST)

Craniosacral therapy helps to bring awareness into the body and helps develop your ability to switch off and unwind so you are not constantly in a state of fight or flight, or red alert. In craniosacral therapy, the practitioner makes gentle contact usually on the head, feet, or spine, and tunes in to where the energy flow of the body is constricted or interrupted. He or she then works to release areas of constriction. Sometimes this may involve pressure at points inside the mouth, which can be a bit uncomfortable. After a session clients generally feel more alive and clearer. Sensations of a "tide-like" movement flowing up and down the body are very common.

In MS, craniosacral therapy is sometimes used successfully to relieve temporomandibular joint pain (TMJ). It has also been found to be an effective means of treating lower urinary tract symptoms—such as inability to empty the bladder completely, which can lead to incontinence—and improving the quality of life in MS patients.[19]

ᐸᔑ CRYSTAL THERAPY

Crystals use electromagnetic energy to help balance the body's energy. Crystals have an atomic structure very much like our own, but different chemical composition. Particular crystals have particular properties, and when placed on specific chakras—centers of energy in the body, according to Eastern medicine—they create a constant energy flow. There are chakras on the front and back of the body from the groin to the top of the head.

Some crystals—amethyst, angelite, and lepidolite—have a generally balancing effect and help to steady the immune system and correct emotional imbalances. Others have particular characteristics: yellow citrine is uplifting, rose quartz may help to ease heartache, amethyst may calm a busy mind and help you sleep, and ruby is good for energy.

At least five crystals help MS in a more direct way: amazonite supports the nervous system, aquamarine boosts the immune system and balances the thymus chakra, hematite reduces inflammation, iolite activates the nervous and endocrine systems, and pyrite is claimed to increase the oxygen supply in the blood.

Pearl: Energized by Crystals

After the first session, and within minutes of the end of the session, my bladder was communicating with me for the first time in two years. Further sessions gave me renewed energy and soon I was walking unaided.

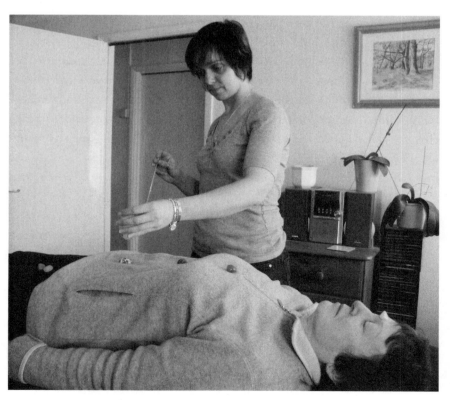

Pearl receiving crystal therapy

I have found crystal therapy to be such a help for the pain and fatigue I was suffering. The fatigue has gradually lessened and my quality of life has improved so much in just a few months. Crystal healing is ideal if you suffer from fatigue, as it gives you energy while you simply relax. You don't even have to believe in it for it to be of benefit, but I'm certainly convinced now that I am benefiting by having more energy and bladder control. All that is required in my sessions is to lie fully clothed on a couch. There is no massage and the only time there is any contact is when the crystals are placed on the chakra points on my back or wherever needed.

The approach was always professional but friendly, with notes being taken to build a profile; anything I mentioned or asked was always noted and explained. I have become so interested in this therapy that I am now doing a foundation course online. I have had so many people comment on how much better I am moving and how well I look.

The main crystals used in my therapy were male quartz, which energizes; female quartz, which helps remove negative energy from the body; the mangano calcite wand, which aligns the subtle bodies; the vogel crystal, which removes emotional wounds; and the quartz wand, which magnifies the energy of the other crystals.

EMOTIONAL FREEDOM TECHNIQUE

Unhappy feelings and memories, and unresolved emotional issues, can cause blockages in body energy, bringing disease. The aim of Emotional Freedom Technique (EFT) is to free these blockages. Using EFT, people revisit the unhappy event(s) in question and balance the disturbed meridians, resolving both the anguish and the physical symptoms. Based on acupuncture, EFT uses a tapping technique on meridian points on the head, torso, and hands.

Jules: Facing the Truth about Secondary Benefits

For me, EFT was astonishing. I have used it on everything from headaches, anxiety, numb fingers, and claustrophobia, to symptoms of IBS (irritable bowel syndrome). The essence of EFT is that you repeat affirmations of acceptance of yourself regarding a particular issue in your life, while rubbing on the "sore spot" or "karate chop" point on your body. I use a shortened version of the tapping procedure that has evolved from the basic, longer form of EFT.

The first time I used EFT for my MS, I really faced some of my demons. One demon was my thoughts surrounding secondary gain, something that I regard as a big issue. Secondary gain is what psychologists refer to as "unconscious psychological motivators" for symptoms/diseases. With MS, an example of secondary gain might be the release from the pressure of having to work in a stressful job and it being okay to be at home; undivided attention or care from a loved one that might not otherwise be available; the benefits, if you like, of having the disease. This is not to say the disease is not real or apparent, just that there may be unconscious benefits.

Nothing prepared me for the moment when I was asked to stand up, leaving my stick beside the chair. I find it quite hard to explain the emotions I felt as I proceeded, with unusual ease, to walk back and forth in front of so many people. Amazingly, I felt as if I was strolling, rather than struggling. Here I was, facing the reality of the fact that I could obviously get up and do the walking without aid. Why hadn't I been able to until now? What had stopped me? I was elated, confused, and horrified all at once! This extraordinary event made me realize that my feelings about my disability (and possibly a substantial amount of my disability itself) are inextricably bound up with a plethora of painful emotions and fear. The most wonderful thing is that feelings are entirely able to be dealt with, and now I know how.

Find more information about EFT at www.emofree.com.

✥ FELDENKRAIS METHOD

This body work method helps people to reconnect with their natural abilities to move, think, and feel. It also helps make people with MS aware of ways the body accrues tension. Gentle Feldenkrais lessons can improve all these and increase flexibility, convey a sense of overall well-being, and make daily life easier due to being able to move with less effort. Some evidence suggests that balance and confidence with daily movements, depression, anxiety, self-esteem, and overall quality of life may improve in patients with multiple sclerosis who use Feldenkrais body work.[20]

✺ HOMEOPATHY

Homeopathy is based on the theory that like cures like. It uses highly diluted substances, usually in the form of tablets or drops.

There is no universal homeopathic treatment for MS and individual homeopaths may use different remedies. A homeopath looks at the whole person, including personality, temperament, state of mind, and lifestyle, before prescribing the appropriate remedies. Emotions and state of mind are as important as physical factors.

In MS, homeopathy can sometimes help lessen fatigue, increase energy, warm cold extremities, get rid of vertigo, and detoxify the body. It can also help with bladder and bowel problems, spasms, and double vision. One author lists fifty-six homeopathic remedies that could be used in the treatment of MS.

Specific remedies for particular symptoms:

- Bladder symptoms, including incontinence and retention, can often be helped by Causticum in a 6c or 30c potency. (Causticum is also used for paralysis.) In cases where people use intermittent self-catheterization, Staphysagria can help void urine from the bladder.
- Remedies for constipation and bowel problems include Opium, Alumina, Silica, Nux vomica, and Sulphur.
- For eye problems in MS, Phosphorus 30c every day can help optic nerve inflammation. Gelsemium can help double vision. Gelsemium is also used for dizziness and trembling, bladder problems, and other eye problems, such as blurred vision.
- For cramps and spasms, a common remedy is Cuprum metallicum, 30c every night.
- For sensory symptoms, Secale can be useful.
- For pain, pins and needles, and numbness, Oxalic acid is sometimes used.

Depending on the homeopath, you could be treated with either classical homeopathy, which involves taking one remedy at a time; or complex homeopathy, which involves taking several remedies in combination. Certain substances work better when they're combined with other substances, and since MS is such a complex illness, complex homeopathy may be more appropriate.

The practitioner may use a special machine, called a Biological Functions Diagnosis (BFD) machine, to find out what is going wrong in your body, and where. It is similar to a Vega machine (described on page 36), but used in a different way. It works by a galvanic skin response through the acupuncture points, or meridians, which correspond to different parts of the body. During diagnosis, you hold a metal tube in one hand. This is attached to the machine, and the practitioner uses a small metal rod, also attached to the machine, to contact different meridian or energy points on your hands and feet. If there is a problem in any part of the body, a gauge on the machine may indicate this.

Small vials containing different substances in homeopathic potencies are then placed on the machine to gauge your response—this way the cause of illness may be found, as well as the correct remedy. The process is painless and noninvasive, and is thought to be highly accurate, although this has been called into question in some scientific circles. It is used in many German hospitals, and by doctors who are general practitioners in the Netherlands.

During diagnosis, your whole body is also checked for bacterial infection, viruses, and parasites, which can be anywhere in the body, including the brain and spinal cord. For treatment you are given bottles of homeopathic tinctures, or tablets. You will be prescribed a daily dose of a specific number of drops in water or juice, or a specific number of tablets.

Flushing out toxins is also part of homeopathic treatment. You are given tinctures that help remove debris from your body. These toxins accumulate as the harmful organisms and poisons are eliminated.

There is no hard evidence to show that homeopathy can prevent the progression of MS, but homeopath Dr. Thomas E. Whitmarsh of Glasgow Homoepathic Hospital in Scotland says: "there is a feeling amongst those of us who treat a lot of people with the condition that the frequency of relapse is sometimes cut down. As a complementary treatment in addition to conventional drugs, homoeopathy is particularly good at helping some of the complications of the condition."[21] Whitmarsh finds homeopathy "of particular benefit in MS . . . because of its whole-person approach, which allows for complete individualization of treatment, taking account of the minutiae of someone's life."[22]

ᥐ HYDROTHERAPY

Hydrotherapy may include exercises done in water, hot tubs, or hot and cold pools. It works primarily by increasing oxygenation in the blood. In addition, hydrotherapy increases the white blood cell count, which aids healing and promotes repair of damaged tissues.[23]

Hydrotherapy treatments are especially suited to people with MS because water supports the weight of your body and there's no risk of falling. Also, it keeps you from getting overheated while exercising. In hydrotherapy pools designed specifically for people with MS, the water is kept at a comfortable temperature, not too hot. Usually the exercises are devised by a physical therapist. They can improve walking and alleviate muscle stiffness, and confer other benefits similar to those seen in conventional exercises.

Several chapters of the National MS Society in the United States offer hydrotherapy, as well as some private centers, such as the Rocky Mountain Multiple Sclerosis Center in Colorado. In the United Kingdom, a few MS therapy centers have hydrotherapy pools.

Also beneficial is thalassotherapy, based on the healing properties of seawater and climate. When the water is heated, trace minerals are absorbed by the human body. Circulation is increased and toxins are released, bringing relaxation and a sense of well-being. It is widely used in European spas.

· ·

Judy: Taking Great Pleasure in Taking the Cure

A big thing in France is to "take the cure." What this means is going to some stylish seaside spa and getting a liberal dose of water therapy— what the French call thalassotherapy. In thalasso clinics, they find half a dozen ways to blast you with seawater.

The essential ingredients of thalassotherapy are seawater, sunshine, sea air (climate), and seaweed. That's why most French thalasso clinics are right by the sea, so they can pump seawater straight into the place, you can prostrate yourself to the sun and sea air, and they can gather seaweed to pour green gloop into your bathwater. It's a very curative combination.

I've been to two thalasso clinics in France, one in St. Malo and one in Le Touquet, and began to feel a wonderful sense of well-being within a day or two each time. Before I went, I was a bit put off by ads that show lithe young beauties frolicking on the sand next to the clinic. But when I actually got there, the reality was a bit different. Far from being nubile and beauteous, most clients are in various stages of dodderiness, shuffling around in white bathrobes between one appointment and the next. Many are ill, some are old, and a few—unusual for French women—are reassuringly fat.

Taking the cure doesn't actually mean you get cured of anything. It just means having a bit of an overhaul using water therapy. Until very recently, the French government actually paid for (French) people to take the cure (that's my idea of a national health service!).

Some old spoilsport put an end to that, but going to a thalasso clinic still doesn't need to cost the earth. The expensive part can be the hotel accommodation. But in Le Touquet, for example, you can stay in a beachfront two-star hotel quite cheaply, and just pay for whatever thalassotherapy appointments you have.

I stayed in the three-star Novotel, which was right on the sandy beach and had a lovely gourmet restaurant. The location was perfect, and less than one hour's easy drive on the new highway direct from the port at Calais. The thalassotherapy clinic in St. Malo is a bit grander, but again, very easy to find.

Thalasso clinics dot the coastline of France, with some in Spain and Italy, too. My idea of a blissful holiday is to go to a different one each time. For future trips, I have earmarked those in Carnac, Dinard, Corsica, and Sardinia.

So what about the lingo? Well, it certainly helps to know the difference between *froid* (cold) and *chaud* (hot) when it comes to water temperature. In aquarobics classes you could get by just watching what all the other people are doing, then doing the same thing half a second later. Other than that, you wouldn't come to much harm by just letting the therapists do their stuff while shouting at you in incomprehensible French. Just lie back and enjoy it.

Therapy sessions are scheduled either just in the morning or just in the afternoon, so you have half of every day to relax and soak up the sea air and sunshine, or do some sightseeing. To the French, taking the cure also means eating the most delectable food. At thalasso clinics you can choose between the mouth-watering *menu gastronomique*, or the more spartan *menu dietetique*, which is lighter on the calories but nonetheless delicious.

Either way, a week of thalassotherapy and I guarantee you will come back very clean, with some new French vocab and revived *joie de vivre*. Oh, and remember to bring back a bottle of seaweed gloop for your bath.

HYPNOTHERAPY

Hypnotherapy helps to release stress and visualize goals. People with MS use hypnotherapy for a range of problems, including pain control, chronic worry, and fear for the future.[24]

First, clients are taken through a series of relaxation exercises, which entrains them in switching off and allowing the unconscious mind to be accessed. Then they are helped with a series of visualizations that show them overcoming their particular problem. For example, if someone is lacking in confidence, a visualization will help them to see themselves in a very positive way in a social situation. It's quicker and easier to get results by working with a hypnotherapist, but anyone can learn basic self-hypnosis, which includes relaxation and visualization.

INDIAN HEAD MASSAGE

The aim of Indian head massage, also practiced in ayurvedic medicine, is to release stress that has built up in the tissues, muscles, and joints of the head, face, neck, and shoulders. The subject stays fully clothed, seated in a chair. The therapist uses kneading and compression movements over the neck, shoulder, and scalp areas, and also gently stimulates and strokes pressure points on the face. Indian head massage is especially good for relieving stress, tension, fatigue, insomnia, headaches, migraine, and sinusitis. It is also very relaxing and deeply calming.

⌘ LAUGHTER

Although laughter is not a complementary therapy as such, it is included here because it is so beneficial for health. Laughter strengthens the immune system, boosts energy, lessens pain, and is a powerful antidote to stress.[25]

Laughter relaxes the whole body and triggers the release of feel-good endorphins. Laughter also binds people together and increases happiness, joy, and intimacy, and helps you surmount problems.

Watch some humorous films and TV shows; see the funny side of life. Have a belly laugh every day; it gives an inner massage. And take a look at Squiffy's House of Fun—Laughter for MS, on the www.msrc.co.uk website. Squiffy, alter ego of John Habkirk, says: "Jokes and humor, that's what this site is all about! I hope through the laughter contained on my site to lighten the load of those with MS and entertain those without the disease." One of many excellent entries on this site is:

Clown Prayer
Dear Lord, help me to create more laughter than tears,
dispense more happiness than gloom, spread more cheer
than despair. Never let me grow so big that I fail to see
the wonder in the eyes of a child.

⌘ MAGNETIC THERAPY

Electromagnetic stimulation (EMS), also known as electromagnetic field therapy (EMF), is a natural, noninvasive, drug-free treatment. It's well established in mainstream European health care and has been particularly used to treat acute and chronic pain, but it is also claimed to help MS. This therapy is administered either by lying on a special mattress or blanket, by a small device that fits into the palm of your hand, or by being connected to a small magnetic field machine.

For every cell in your body to work properly, you need a constant supply of energy. This comes from what we eat and drink, from oxygen, and from Earth's electromagnetic energy. EMS produces electromagnetic energy at the same strength as our planet's natural magnetic field. This is delivered in slow-induction magnetic wave frequencies directly to the cells, increasing circulation and, by working with the body's natural frequencies, speeding up the healing process. EMS improves blood supply and oxygen to cells, which allows them to detoxify, regenerate, and reproduce. When your body cells are in good condition, all your bodily systems start to work as well as they possibly can.

Since the early 1990s, Professor Reuven Sandyk has found that electromagnetic stimulation therapy has helped reverse MS symptoms in many patients he has treated. Sandyk theorizes that in MS there may be a dysfunction of the pineal gland, which produces hormones such as melatonin.[26] Melatonin regulates the neurotransmitter serotonin. Serotonin works to prevent fatigue, sleep disorders, spasticity, poor bladder function, cognitive defects, and depression—all common symptoms of MS.

Research done at the University of Washington, Seattle, and published in the *Journal of Alternative and Complementary Medicine* found that the pineal gland is very sensitive to EMF and can be treated using low intensity pulsed electromagnetic fields, which "energize" the pineal gland.[27] The studies showed that EMF treatment was successful in creating a marked improvement in 60–70 percent of the patients in the study, and mild to moderate improvement in the rest. The treatment was most effective at the early stages of the disease. EMF had previously been shown to boost the release of melatonin, and following from that, serotonin. EMF increases the feel-good hormones—endorphins. The majority of MS patients who received magnetic therapy showed symptom improvement in bladder problems, cognition, double vision, and clarity of speech. The machine used was an Enermed (see page 178).

One 1998 American research study that reviewed electromagnetic applications for multiple sclerosis found that "it is possible that EM fields could be developed into a reproducible therapy for both symptom management and long-term care for MS."[28]

Electromagnetic field therapy can be delivered by a mattress, blanket, or machine. One U.K. mattress model, the Viofor JPS System magnetic bed, has been clinically demonstrated to help reduce fatigue, alleviate pain and spasticity, increase mobility, improve bladder control, increase energy levels, oxygenate the body, aid restful sleep, and improve mood in MS patients.

It is being used in MS therapy centers such as the Mercia MS Therapy Centre in Coventry, England. Matthew Ally, an osteomyologist who works at the center and operates the professional model of the Viofor machine, says: "I've been here ten years and no therapy works as well as this. Normally the best we can hope for with MS is to keep people stabilized. One of the studies on the Viofor electromagnetic bed showed how it reversed the long-term clinical course of patients with MS."

MS patients treated at this center undergo a six-week intensive course of treatment, with twenty-five-minute Viofor treatments twice a week in two cycles. The first cycle is for the whole body and the second cycle concentrates on a particular area, such as the lower back, or where pain is felt. Patients lie on the bed fully clothed. The treatment is totally noninvasive, but some mild tingling might be felt.

Molly: Electromagnetic Therapy Loosens Both Feet and Tongue

After having electromagnetic stimulation therapy, I felt normal again. My chronic symptoms are loss of balance, fatigue, depression, heaviness around the middle, numbness in both feet, and speech problems. After treatment my cognitive behavior and balance improved so much that I felt like skipping through fields and doing cartwheels, like I did as a youngster. My friends couldn't stop me from talking, and told me I was a different person.

In Canada, the Enermed machine is perhaps the most widely used device for delivering EMF. This is an extremely low frequency, pulsed, electromagnetic field generator. It is battery operated and around the size of a man's wristwatch. Each device is programmed for the needs of each particular client. At the time of writing, this particular product was not approved for sale in the United States. Other delivery methods include a small box from which attachments are placed on the patient's head. There are also magnetic bracelets available, such as those by Bioflow, which some people with MS claim give them more energy and relieve pain.

In the United States and other countries, some companies adver-

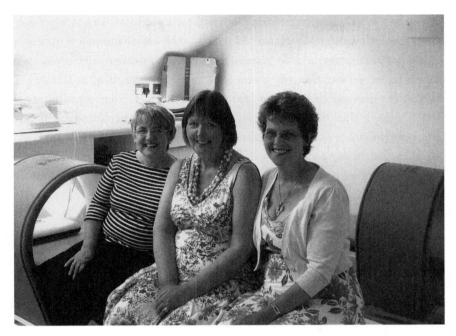

Pauline, Janice, and Janice with the Viofor electromagnetic therapy machine, which is used at the Trafford MS Therapy Centre in Manchester, England

tise magnetic mattress pads for home use by people with MS. These are easy to find with an Internet search. Although magnet therapy and EMF products are available, they are not yet (as of 2010) approved as treatments for MS in the United States and are not covered by medical insurance.

For further information, see Resources.

☙ MASSAGE

Various types of massage are useful for MS, including traditional Swedish, Thai, acupressure (see page 150), aromatherapy (see page 154), manual lymphatic drainage, and shiatsu (see page 188). Massage helps with many MS conditions, especially pain, mood, sluggish circulation of blood and lymph, and flagging energy. It also reduces stress and helps people relax. Stomach massage is also used to relieve constipation.

It has been estimated that 23.3 percent of MS patients in the United States have used massage therapy.[29]

In one small American study, twenty-four adults with MS were randomly assigned to either massage therapy for forty-five minute massages twice a week, or standard medical treatment. The massage group was found to have lower anxiety and a less depressed mood immediately following the massage sessions. By the end of the study they had improved self-esteem, better body image, and enhanced social functioning status. They also had a more positive attitude about having MS.[30]

Another small study found that a slow stroking massage (that uses the flat of the hand) over the spine was associated with improvement in anxiety and muscle stiffness.[31]

An article in *Massage Today* quoted several practitioners as to how and when they would perform massage therapy on MS patients. Some prefer not to do anything during a flare-up, but to wait for a remission.[32]

In the United Kingdom, massage is available at many of the multiple sclerosis therapy centers around the country.

꩜ MEDITATION AND GUIDED IMAGERY
(See also Visualization on page 190, and Yoga in chapter 11.)

Meditation involves relaxing deeply, focusing awareness inward, stilling the mind, and blocking out the outside world. It works well as a stress management technique. Meditation has been shown to strengthen the immune system and aid positive thinking. Scientists found that volunteers who meditated for a short time every week showed lower anxiety levels than those who did not.

The American study found that meditation produced lasting results both in the brain and the function of the immune system. Researchers used "mindfulness meditation" as an antidote to the stress and pain of chronic disease.[33] Mindfulness meditation is designed to focus one's attention intensely on the moment, noting thoughts and feelings as they occur but refraining from judging or acting on them.

....

Anne: Frantic to Peaceful through Meditation

If you'd said to me a couple of years ago that very soon I'd be spending a large part of every afternoon doing nothing and enjoying it, I wouldn't have believed you. That I would discover my best friend is me, and like her? Absolutely not. That I would turn down the extraneous volume in my life and find peace in silence? No.

When I was diagnosed with MS I was rapidly forced to change my lifestyle—from a frenetic rollercoaster ride of canned laughter and flashes-before-your-eyes to a more thoughtful existence that gave me time to calm down and reassess my life.

It's amazing how you change when you have to, what different things you are forced to learn, and finding out how close you were to self-destruction. In other words, MS was a blessing for me, though of course I didn't appreciate it at the time.

....

Transcendental Meditation

Transcendental Meditation (TM) is a simple meditation technique introduced to the West in 1958 by Maharishi Mahesh Yogi. It involves sitting and "practicing" TM for twenty minutes each day, focusing on a particular mantra that you repeat over and over. It has met with excellent results in individual cases of MS. Used for deep relaxation and revitalization, it allows the mind and body to gain a unique state of very deep rest; your mind achieves inner calm while remaining alert. The intention of TM is to reach the quietest level of the mind, known as trascendental consciousness, and in the process dissolve deeply rooted stress and tension, and relieve fatigue. This supports energy, clearheadedness, creativity, and efficiency.

During meditation, the brain switches to an alpha (resting) or theta (relaxing) brain wave state. In these states, the brain's rhythm slows and endorphins—feel-good hormones—are released. Metabolism is lowered, the heart rate and breathing are slowed, and blood pressure drops. This induces relaxation, which counteracts stress and fatigue. There has not been any specific scientific research on TM and MS. However, MS is one of the conditions that practitioners of TM claim they can successfully treat.

Some people with MS have found Transcendental Meditation to be their most helpful therapy.

....

Frank: Free Meditation Therapy Keeps Him in High Spirits

With MS we have many physical symptoms, but our state of mind also plays a big role in how we are feeling at the end of the day. We still have a choice in that if we choose to allow ourselves to feel miserable, we will end up feeling a lot worse than if we choose a sunny outlook. There are many ways to help us to keep a bright attitude.

The one I find most effective is Transcendental Meditation. There is a lot of talk about it, as if there's a veil of mystique or magic about it, but that's a load of old cobblers, as it is quite easy, simple, and safe to practice. All you really need is to want to do it. Find yourself a quiet room where you will not be disturbed. Just sit down quietly and breathe in and out from the diaphragm.

Next, make sure that you are deeply and properly relaxed. Then start breathing in and out really deeply, listening to the natural rhythm of the breath. When I breathe in I like to use the mantra (which is a word or short phrase) "raising" (as my tummy rises up). And when I breath out, "falling" (as the diaphragm relaxes back). I try not to think of anything else, but if my mind wanders, I simply note the thought (or chain of thoughts) without getting involved with them, and then simply bring my focus back to my breath.

It will probably take you between five and ten cycles until you set your mind free, but don't worry too much if you cannot quiet the "mind chatter" straight away. This will happen in its own time. Whatever level you are at, you will still benefit from this daily practice.

When you successfully meditate, you feel as if you are millions of miles away, although you obviously haven't physically moved at all. I practice it every day and it keeps me in very high spirits. Give it a go and see how well you feel. It costs nothing and will make you feel great.

....

Dynamic Meditation

American psychologist Aretoula Fullam, a research fellow at Harvard Medical School, found that dynamic meditation can gradually improve the symptoms of patients with MS. After reading about the disease,

Fullam discovered that the one common element is stress. By learning how to relax, people with MS can deal with stress, anxiety, depression, and memory problems. The brain cannot tell the difference between what is real and what is imagined. This is how improvements occur. Fullam describes an "amazing result" with one MS patient who was able to stop using a scooter and eventually went back to using a walker.

In dynamic meditation you gradually clear your stress by expressing contained feelings physically and verbally. You begin by standing with your eyes closed, breathing rapidly through your nose, and moving or swaying so that you start to pump more oxygen into your body. Gradually you move into letting go and expressing physically and verbally whatever you are feeling. From here you move into jumping up and down and yelling, "Hoo, hoo," loudly enough that the vibration of your voice pushes your energy upward. The final stage is quiet and relaxed, as you surrender to the universe.

Guided Imagery

In guided imagery, a practitioner or CD guides you through visual images, such as of a beautiful beach or mountain where you feel relaxed. Using your imagination, you use the senses of sight, sound, smell, and touch to achieve a tranquil state. Once there, you are guided to imagine things like the myelin sheath being repaired or your immune system being healed.

While you are relaxed and in a happy, delightful place, the brain cannot discern whether you are on a real or imagined beach; it simply sends out messages via the nervous system to the muscles, glands, and organs to relax. Once this has occurred, there are beneficial effects on all of the body systems—immune system, nervous system, and digestive system.

It isn't difficult to learn guided imagery, although it may seem so when you first try. To help, there are several scripts available on CD. The technique is to find a comfortable place, close your eyes, take deep breaths, and allow the body and mind to slow down. Now you imagine yourself in a beautiful place of your choice, using all of your senses. Imagine warm sunlight on your body, perhaps the sound of lapping water, the scent of frangipani, and so on. Continue with this image for fifteen minutes before gently bringing yourself back into the present.

One study on guided imagery and MS followed thirty-three patients with MS and trained half of them in relaxation sessions involving the use of imagery, focusing on imagining the repair of damaged myelin and positive immune system responses.[34] The control group followed their normal medical treatment. After a six-week course of treatment, the imagery group had a significant decrease in anxiety, but there were no changes in other psychological variables or in MS symptoms. The authors comment that this is a simple, cost-effective approach that can significantly reduce anxiety in people with MS.

Miriam Franco, Ph.D., has designed guided imagery scripts for multiple sclerosis on CD (www.imagerywork.com). She has found this effective in reducing anxiety, muscle tension, spasticity, fatigue, headache, and sleep problems associated with multiple sclerosis. Guided imagery can also help patients with anxiety about medication injections. Franco conducted a patient education study in 2008, using guided imagery, and it was found to be efficient and effective in lowering general anxiety and for injection anxiety in 97 percent of MS patients, even several weeks post-workshop.[35]

⬥ NATUROPATHY

This natural and holistic approach to health care embraces a wide array of noninvasive techniques and therapies, including, potentially, everything described in this chapter. It is particularly suited to chronic conditions.[36] Among the basic principles of naturopathy are the healing power of nature and the body's inherent ability to heal itself. The aim of the naturopathic treatment is to harness the body's own healing ability.

Another basic principle is that mental, physical, spiritual, and environmental factors all play a part in ill health and must be addressed in treatment. Naturopaths try to get to the root causes of illness, rather than just deal with symptoms. They also teach patients how to take responsibility for their own health, which may involve nutritional, emotional, dietary, and other lifestyle changes. For naturopathy resources, consult the Resources section at the back of this book.

⬥ NUTRITIONAL MEDICINE

One of the main thrusts of this book is nutritional medicine, which uses food and diet to help the body's own healing ability to maintain good health and to prevent or alleviate illness.[37] Practitioners look for nutritional deficiencies, allergies, or intolerances to food, or for factors that can cause poor digestion or absorption in the stomach or intestine. Treatment involves dietary change and may include the use of nutritional supplements, such as vitamins and minerals. If you see a doctor trained in nutritional medicine, you'll get a program tailored to your individual needs, rather than a "one size fits all."

I began seeing doctors trained in nutritional medicine when I first became aware of my MS. Every four to six months I have had a very detailed biochemical examination, based on blood and urine (and sometimes sweat and hair analysis). A computer printout reveals any abnormalities, and the doctor prescribes accordingly. This is an expensive option, but highly specific and personalized.

ᢒᢧᢧ OSTEOPATHY

Osteopathy is a drug-free, noninvasive type of medicine based on the body's musculoskeletal system—bones, joints, muscles, and ligaments. It is designed to have a positive impact on the body's nervous, circulatory, and lymphatic systems.

Osteopaths use their hands to diagnose and treat any problems found. Techniques include manipulating muscles, sometimes using short, sharp movements; gentle massage; and rhythmic joint movements. One small, short-term study found that a combination of osteopathic manipulation and a specific exercise program led to improved strength and walking ability in people with MS.[38]

ᢒᢧᢧ REFLEXOLOGY

Archaeological evidence points to the use of reflexology since ancient times. Reported benefits of reflexology for MS include improvements in movement, bladder and bowel problems, balance, lymphatic drainage, eye problems, and circulation; increased sensation in feet and legs; and reduction of swelling.

Reflexology is based on the principle that every part of the body is represented, or "reflected," in the feet. Reflexologists apply gentle hand pressure to specific areas of the feet (or hands), pressing what they call reflex points, or "reflexes." By working on the parts of the feet that correspond to the head and the neck, they stimulate healing in the referral area. Some parts of the body, such as the lungs, are mapped on both feet while other organs—such as gallbladder and spleen—are represented on one foot only. Reflexology foot charts show in detail where the different parts of the body are represented on the feet.

Reflexologists usually think of health problems as occurring because of a blockage of life force, or chi, at various points in the body. Massaging, squeezing, or pushing on the appropriate parts of the feet helps to restore the flow of energy through channels, or meridians, that have been blocked or disrupted by illness. It also relieves tension and improves circulation.

Specific health problems with internal organs can sometimes be felt during reflexology work. The texture of the feet in these referring areas may feel slightly lumpy, or "grainy," and can be painful. The color and temperature of the feet may be indicators as well. Reflexologists are also "foot readers" on the lookout for areas of the feet that look or feel different. They believe that waste products such as calcium and uric acid accumulate around the nerve endings, of which there are seven thousand in each foot. By feeling these deposits, a therapist is said to be able to identify a problem in a corresponding area of the body. Massaging these points may crush the deposits and stimulate the body to eliminate them, thus healing and revitalizing the problem area while restoring balance and harmony to the whole person.

In the United Kingdom, the 2003 NICE (National Institute for Health and Clinical Excellence) published guidelines on MS report some evidence that reflexology may be helpful for people with MS in terms of their general sense of well-being.[39] Many multiple sclerosis therapy centers in the United Kingdom offer reflexology.

A 2003 Israeli study of twenty-seven people with MS who received reflexology showed some improvements in bladder problems and in relieving spasticity and improving muscle strength. Physiotherapists' assessments backed up this observation. In this trial, seventy-one MS patients were studied. Half received the active reflexology treatment for eleven weeks. The treatment included manual pressure on specific points in the feet, and massage of the calf area. The control group received nonspecific massage of the calf. Both groups were tested for numbness, bladder problems, muscle strength, and spasticity. The results showed a significant improvement in the group given reflexology.[40]

Cynthia: From Bleak to Hopeful after Reflexology

This has been the best year since I have been chair bound—regaining movement I thought was gone forever. This has given me more independence and hope for the future, which looked very bleak and depressing with no hope of improvement. I didn't think my legs would ever work like this again. When people meet me these days they tell me I'm moving better and don't seem so stiff. From lying in bed unable to move a muscle to being able to move and stretch is incredible.

Beth: Reflexology Eases Swelling and Fears

My weekly reflexology sessions that began last year have worked wonders for me. My feet are no longer blue, the swelling has reduced quite a lot, and my leg tremors are not so frequent. Now my arm and fingers are very supple. Reflexology has put my mind at ease about the fear of losing my legs.

REIKI

Reiki healing originated with Mikao Usui in Japan in the early part of the twentieth century. The word *reiki* means "universal life energy" in Japanese. A Reiki practitioner uses this energy, which is passed to the receiver through the practitioner's hands, to encourage the body to heal itself.

A limited test of thirteen volunteers, treated for six to ten sessions in 2002 at the Reiki Research Foundation, showed positive results, with 90 percent experiencing reduction in pain, but only 42 percent experiencing a reduction in symptoms in their arms.[41] For more information, see www.reikiresearchfoundation.org.

Therapeutic Touch (TT), developed by nurses Dora Kunz and Dolores Krieger, uses similar methodology.

ᕍ RELAXATION BOOSTERS

Relaxation techniques can reduce stress and boost the immune system.[42] They can easily be learned and benefits gained from just five minutes a day (see Meditation on page 180 and Visualization on page 190). One excellent relaxation booster is lying flat on your back in the buoyancy of a flotation tank, which takes all stress off joints and spastic muscles.

Jacuzzis and hot tubs can also be very relaxing and reduce stress and pain. The combination of heat and water buoyancy loosens muscle tension, increases circulation, and encourages release of endorphins.

ᕍ SHIATSU

Shiatsu, which originated in Japan, uses a combination of pressure and assisted-stretching techniques, some of which are common to other therapies, such as physiotherapy, acupressure, and osteopathy. Shiatsu works on the flow of energy (chi) that circulates through our bodies in specific meridians. The actual treatment approach and philosophy is similar to acupuncture in its usage of the meridians and pressure points, as well as diagnostic methods, but without the use of needles. Unlike most other forms of bodywork, in shiatsu the receiver usually remains clothed for the treatment and no oil is used.

Shiatsu is a variant of acupressure, as it involves the stimulation of the acupoints with pressure. Pressure may be applied precisely over acupoints using fingers and thumbs, or over a wider area, using palms, elbows, knees, and feet.

In addition to the pressure itself, shiatsu involves gentle stretch and manipulation. Shiatsu practitioners apply rhythmic and gradual pressure to the meridians and *tsubos,* or stress points. Sometimes very light "holding" techniques may be used, usually with the palm. Stretching exercises and other corrective techniques create flexibility and balance in the body, both physically and energetically. In shiatsu, the physical touch is used to assess the distribution of chi throughout the body and to try to correct any imbalances accordingly.

Shiatsu treatment stimulates the circulation and flow of lymphatic fluid, releases toxins and deep-seated muscle tension, stimulates the hormonal and immune systems, and acts on the autonomic nervous system. In MS, shiatsu is used to treat pain, spasm, postural abnormalities, and to help patients relax.

❧ TRADITIONAL CHINESE MEDICINE

Traditional Chinese medicine (TCM) takes a holistic view of MS, teaching that emotional and spiritual factors are important in the disease, which is thought to be triggered by an infectious illness.[43] Emotions such as fear, anxiety, and depression are considered to be major causes of MS, taking priority over biologic or genetic factors. Doctors who practice TCM view MS as the loss of a vital fluid essence (*jing*). The aim of treatment is to replenish this essence and normalize organ function. This is done by changing the diet and prescribing particular herbs. Acupuncture can also be used to help reestablish harmony. Underlying emotional and spiritual issues can be addressed with psychotherapy or counseling as well as herbs.

TCM diagnostic protocol includes examining the tongue and taking the pulse on the wrist. (In TCM, pulse diagnosis is used to reveal far more than in Western allopathic medicine.) Depending on what the practitioner finds, a combination of herbs based on the patient's unique needs is generally prescribed. These are often in the form of dried herbs that need to be brewed at home.

There is no one formula to treat every MS patient; herbs have to be formulated for each individual. TCM practitioners claim that symptoms of MS can be controlled as long as the herbal prescription is correct, the dosage is appropriate, and the treatment is carried out consistently and for a sufficient period of time (which can be anywhere from a couple of months to several years, if relapses are to be prevented). If relapse occurs after the patient stops taking the herbs, starting them again can often alleviate symptoms. Although treatment may take several years in some cases, in other instances it is possible to see improvements within the first two months.

In a Chinese study involving thirty-five MS patients, four different complex combinations of herbs were developed and given to those patients most suited to each particular formula.[44] The herbs were prepared by boiling them for about 45 minutes; once cool, the decoction was consumed. Patients who were in an active phase of the disease were also given anti-inflammatory drugs. All patients who completed the study (three discontinued treatment within the first ten days) experienced some improvement from taking the Chinese herbs. Of these, two individuals were considered to be cured (after taking forty-five and sixty-eight doses), fifteen significantly improved, and another fifteen somewhat improved (most taking from twenty to forty doses).

In another study by the same researchers, thirty MS patients were given a formula of seventeen herbs, called Ping Fu Tang (also known as Fu Tang Ping or Pacify Relapse Decoction).[45] The goal was to see whether this could prevent exacerbations. Patients took two to three divided doses each day for a period of three to thirteen years. In all this time, there were only two mild exacerbations. However, in the control group of fifteen MS patients, exacerbations occurred between one and four times per year.

Good results with traditional Chinese medicine have also been reported by Dr. Domei Yakazu in Japan.[46] One of his patients was a forty-eight-year-old man who took an herbal formula for two and a half years. Another, a thirty-eight-year-old woman who was considered to be cured after taking herb decoctions for about fifteen weeks followed by herb pills for a year. Other individual cases of MS patients who benefited from TCM can be found in Chinese journals.

It is interesting to note that high dosages of herbs tend to be used in the Chinese clinical studies that have shown good results. It is also important to recognize that side effects such as stomach upsets, nausea, and rash can sometimes occur when taking herbs. These can usually be resolved by adjusting the herbal formula or by taking something to aid digestion, such as ginger tea.

❧ VISUALIZATION
(See also Guided Imagery on page 183.)

Visualization is, quite simply, mentally envisioning things happening, training your mind to see the positive outcome in a particular situation, and getting your mind to accept a particular route. This could be compared to daydreaming, but in a very focused way. When you visualize, it can leave a lasting positive impression. With visualization, it's important to set goals and focus on what you want to achieve. A famous person who extols the virtues of visualization for MS is TV show host Montel Williams.[47]

14

Other Modalities that Can Help MS

THERE ARE A NUMBER of other therapies and products that can also be helpful for MS. I have personally tried some of these, though not all. Those I have not tried have been recommended by others with MS. What works for one person with MS may not necessarily work as well for the next person, so it is a question of trying things and seeing the effects on your condition.

The following is not an exhaustive list and does not include mainstream disease-modifying drugs, such as Avonex, Copaxone, Tysabri, and Campath, which are not the focus of this book. Nor does it include the many suggestions listed in the following part 4, such as eliminating toxic substances (for example, mercury), fasting, and cleansing.

❧ AIMSPRO (GOAT SERUM)

Aimspro has powerful anti-inflammatory properties. It is derived from the blood serum of goats that have been specially vaccinated to generate neutralizing antibodies, and is composed of a set of peptides that stimulate the release and regulation of a molecular cascade that modulates the hypothalamo-pituitary-adrenal (HPA) axis. It is administered by injection under the skin, which patients can learn to do themselves. Some people with MS were able to try Aimspro for free when it was first marketed, and some reported good results, with improved walking and alleviation of other MS symptoms. It is currently available for purchase through certain U.K. doctors, and at the time of writing, Aimspro was undergoing trials for bladder function in secondary progressive MS at a London hospital. Since October 28, 2009, the U.S. Department of Health and Human Services has designated Aimspro as an orphan-drug (one designed specifically to treat a single rare medical condition) for the treatment of amyotrophic lateral sclerosis (ALS), the most prevalent type of motor neuron disease. This compassionate dispensation did not extend to MS, so until all the trials have been done and all the regulatory authorities satisfied, doctors in the United States cannot prescribe Aimspro for MS.

✎ CANNABIS AND SATIVEX

Many people with MS find that cannabis and Sativex (derived from cannabis) help with symptoms of pain, spasticity, and spasm, and also improve their mood. Both remedies reportedly help with some bladder and eyesight problems.

Cannabis

Cannabis can be smoked in a pipe or a hand-rolled cigarette, infused into liquids, or cooked into foods However, strong varieties of cannabis, known as skunk, have been linked to impaired memory and mental function, and psychosis.[1]

....

Clare: Spasm Relief with Cannabis

Over the years I've been given steroids, tranquilizers, painkillers, muscle relaxants, and antidepressants. At best they only helped in the short term, and many have intolerable side effects.

My main problem was that my bladder was in constant spasm, and no prescribed medicines helped me. Then in 1992 I read an article in a U.S. journal about how some doctors had observed cannabis could help people with MS. Before I did anything I talked to different doctors. None of them knew much about it, but they thought it wouldn't do harm.

As I was a middle-class mother of two young children, I had a bit of a problem obtaining cannabis, but eventually I found a woman who helped me.

The physical relief was almost immediate. The tension in my bladder and spine was eased, and I slept well. I was comfortable with my body for the first time in years. Just as important, I felt happy that there was something that could help me.

It took a couple of months to work out how to self-medicate. To begin with, it was easy to take too much or too little. I then established a routine of nine grams of herbal cannabis per week, drinking it in milky drinks during the day and smoking it at night before bed. To make the drink, I simmer the cannabis in milk for a few minutes, sieve the milk to remove the leaves, then drink the milk. However, I've found smoking is the easiest way of regulating the dose.

I don't feel in any way addicted or tempted to take harder drugs. I don't crave it or suffer withdrawal symptoms when travelling abroad. I've been using cannabis for more than ten years. I eat better, sleep better, and feel more positive and motivated.

Medical Research on Cannabinoids

Medical trials have been done on cannabinoids taken in capsule form, and also on Sativex, a commercial product taken as an oral spray.

In noncommercial trials, cannabinoids have been tested for several MS symptoms: spasticity, lack of mobility, bladder problems, cognitive problems, pain, and tremor. Results have been mixed, but in general, patients on the trials have had a more favorable subjective response than the objective results reported by researchers. Results for Sativex have been still better (see Sativex on page 196).

CAMS (Cannabis in MS) Trial

To date, CAMS has been the largest study of cannabis-based medicine for MS. Six hundred participants from many parts of the United Kingdom took part in a randomized, controlled, double-blind trial funded by the Medical Research Council, a government body, with results published in November 2003.[2] Participants were given either capsules containing extract of cannabis plant (Cannador), standardized to contain 2.5 mg delta-tetrahydrocannabinol (THC); dronabinol (Marinol), a synthetic delta-tetrahydrocannabinol (THC); or a placebo. The main aim of the trial was to look at spasticity. The dose was gradually increased over five weeks, treatment continued for a further eight weeks, and then tapered off over two weeks, with regular assessments for spasticity and mobility.

Researchers found that cannabis had no significant effect on spasticity; however, there was some improvement in the time taken to complete a ten-meter walk (about thirty-two feet). Also—in contrast to the scientists' findings—when participants were asked to give their own subjective view, they reported improvements in spasticity, pain, and sleep quality. No significant side effects were experienced and the treatment was considered safe. There was little difference in the effect on symptoms between Cannador and dronabinol, suggesting that the whole plant or synthetic versions of cannabis may be equally effective.

In an extension of this trial, participants were given the option of continuing with the cannabis medicine for another year, which about 80 percent did. Results from this trial suggested that over the longer period of time, cannabis-based medicine had a small effect on muscle spasticity, most notably in the group taking dronabinol, when compared with Cannador and placebo. However, there was some suggestion that dronabinol and Cannador might delay increased disability over a period of time.[3]

Cognitive Performance, Mood, Pain, and Fatigue Trial

For this trial, which started in 2001, 150 participants with MS and spasticity were recruited from two U.K. centers. The main aim was to evaluate whether cannabis-based medicines have any psychological impact and/or any impact on cognitive performance, mood, pain, and fatigue in participants undergoing treatment. The preliminary results, presented in 2003, were that medicinal cannabis had no significant effect on cognition.[4]

Spasm/Tremor Trial

This randomized, placebo-controlled, double-blind crossover study involved fifty-seven people with MS who were hospitalized while undergoing rehabilitation treatment. The active drug was a whole plant cannabis extract containing 2.5mg THC and 0.9mg CBD in a gelatin capsule.

Participants received either active or placebo ingredients for two weeks in the main part of the study. The aim was to investigate whether this helped people who had poorly controlled spasticity. Results showed no statistically significant differences between cannabis-based medicine compared with placebo. However, minor improvements were observed in subjects on cannabis-based medicine for spasm frequency, mobility, and getting to sleep. More side effects were seen in people receiving cannabis-based medicine rather than placebo, although these were manageable. The researchers suggest cannabis-based medicine might be useful for people with MS whose spasticity is not responding to other drugs.[5]

CUPID Study

CUPID (Cannabinoid Use in Progressive Inflammatory Brain Disease) is a long-term follow-up study from the CAMS trial.* It recruited 493 subjects with primary or secondary progressive MS from twenty-five hospitals across the United Kingdom to be followed for three-and-a-half years. Participants' MS had worsened over the year before entering the trial and they were still able to walk twenty meters (about twenty-two yards), with or without a walking aid.

The trial was created to see whether delta-9 tetrahydrocannabinol (THC) can slow the increase in disability in people with progressive MS or relieve spasticity, and also whether it is safe. The cannabis-based medicine used in this trial is different from that used in the CAMS or Sativex trials. This trial is randomized and placebo-controlled, so people receive either the cannabis-based medicine or a placebo. All capsules look identical and neither those receiving it nor the doctor knows which treatment each patient is receiving. The trial finished enrolling in June 2008 but results are not expected for several years.

Other research at the University of London showed that cannabinoids can reduce nerve damage and slow the progression of MS.[6]

---

*Since this trial is still in progress, no articles on it have yet been published. Professor John Zajicek is the study's lead researcher. The main website for CUPID is http://sites .pcmd.ac.uk/cnrg/cupid.php.

Sativex

Sativex is a commercial cannabis-based medicine composed primarily of two cannabinoids: CBD (cannabidiol) and THC (delta 9 tetrahydrocannabinol). It is sprayed under the tongue or in the cheeks, with each dose containing 2.7mg THC and 2.5mg CBD. Cannabinoids are molecules found only in the cannabis plant. Different cannabinoids appear to have varying pharmacological effects, including analgesic, antispasmodic, anticonvulsant, anti-tremor, antipsychotic, anti-inflammatory, antioxidant, antiemetic and appetite-stimulant properties.

The drug is supplied in packs of four vials—on average, six weeks of treatment. Side effects reported in trials have included dizziness, drowsiness, and dry mouth. It is not recommended for pregnant women, anyone less than eighteen years of age, or anyone with a history of psychotic problems. Sativex may impair the mental and/or physical abilities required for certain potentially hazardous activities, such as driving.

In 2005, the Canadian regulatory authority granted approval of Sativex for neuropathic pain. In the United Kingdom and Spain, it is expected to get approval for spasticity during 2010. Until that time, it can be prescribed only on a "named patient basis," meaning that the patient is the direct responsibility of the prescribing doctor. At the time of writing, Sativex had not yet been approved by the FDA in the United States.

Sativex has had trials for overactive bladder, neuropathic pain, and spasticity in MS with promising results.

Trials for Treatment of Bladder Problems

A Savitex trial involving twenty-one MS patients with advanced bladder problems—urinary urgency, frequency, and incontinence—was done at London's National Hospital for Neurology and Neurosurgery.[7] Patients in this trial found the number of Sativex sprays that best suited them, gradually building up the dose (titrating). On the first day, they had a maximum of one spray of Sativex every four hours, up to a maximum of four sprays a day. During the first week or so, doses were spread evenly throughout the day. After that, patients could gradually increase the total number of sprays according to their own personal need and how well they tolerated the drug. All problems improved significantly after treatment with Sativex. Participants also reported subjective improvements in pain, spasticity, and sleep.

In Belgium, a study was carried out at the Leuven/National MS Center on 135 patients with overactive bladder who suffered from urge incontinence. The main aim was to see whether Sativex reduced the number of daily episodes of urge incontinence, but researchers were also looking at night incontinence, overall bladder condition, frequency of needing to go to the toilet, quality of life, and patients' own impression of change.

Results showed that Sativex decreased the number of incontinence episodes per day but was not statistically significant. On the other things being tested, it was statistically significant in favor of the Sativex group. Also, more patients in the Sativex group (83.6 percent) than in the placebo group (58.2 percent) subjectively reported their bladder condition improved. The authors concluded that Sativex improves voiding control in MS-related bladder dysfunction.[8]

Multiple Symptoms Trial

A trial with 160 people in the United Kingdom looked at the effect of Sativex on five MS symptoms: spasticity, spasms, bladder problems, tremor, and pain. There were some statistically significant results for spasticity and quality of sleep improved. Slight, but not statistically significant, improvements were seen on a number of other measures.[9]

Neuropathic Pain Relief Trial

It is estimated that more than 25 percent of MS patients suffer from neuropathic pain. Twenty-eight patients completed a two-year, open-label extension trial at the Walton Centre for Neurology and Neurosurgery in Liverpool, England. Patients required fewer daily doses of Sativex and reported lower median pain scores the longer they took the drug. Authors also reported that the drug's administration was not associated with an increase in patients' use of other analgesics—noting that several of the study's participants reduced or ceased their use of pharmaceutical pain medications while taking Sativex.[10]

Dysesthetic Pain Relief Trial

Another Liverpool trial found that Sativex was effective for people with MS experiencing dysesthetic pain—uncomfortable sensations, such as pins and needles, burning or crawling feelings, numbness or tightness, or painful spasms. Of the sixty-six subjects who received either Sativex or placebo, the treatment group reported an average reduction in pain intensity of 2.7 points, as opposed to 1.4 in the placebo group. The effect on sleep disturbance was also marked, with a reduction of 2.5 points in the treatment group and 0.8 in the placebo group.[11]

Spasticity Trials

A fourteen-month study involving 137 people studied its effect on spasticity and other symptoms. Sativex remained effective in those who had perceived initial benefit.[12]

In March, 2009 there were positive results from a pivotal Phase III double-blind, randomized, placebo-controlled study of Sativex in patients with spasticity due to MS. In this study, 573 MS patients with spasticity who had not been adequately treated by other means were recruited from fifty-two hospitals in five countries. At the end of the trial, there was a statistically significant difference between those taking Sativex and those on placebo. Of the Sativex patients, 74 percent achieved an improvement of greater than 30 percent in their spasticity score, versus 51 percent who achieved improvement on placebo. Statistically significant improvements were also seen in spasm frequency, sleep disturbance, patient impression of change, and physician impression of change.[13]

....

Geoffrey: Spasms Stopped and Happier with Sativex

I have nothing but praise for Sativex. It has helped with sleeping, which I didn't do much of before, and has stopped my spasms by 80 percent. It is very good for urinary problems, meaning I don't have to urinate half as often. One of the biggest things it has alleviated is my depression. Before Sativex, my wife said I was getting unbearable to live with!

....

COLLOIDAL SILVER

Colloidal silver is a powerful, natural, antibacterial, antifungal, antiviral, antiparasite, body-normalizing substance. In MS, colloidal silver is particularly useful in treating urinary tract infections.

Colloidal silver is silver particles suspended in a liquid—usually water. Different products have different quantities of silver held in suspension, varying from less than 10 ppm (parts per million) to 100 ppm. It is odorless and nontoxic.

Silver in its colloidal form has been proven to be useful against many different infectious conditions and is nontoxic in its micro-concentrations. However, according to tests done in March/April 2000 by Mark Farinha, Ph.D., at the Department of Microbiology at the University of North Texas, colloidal silver at just 15 to 30 parts per million is fatal to virtually all species of fungi, bacteria, protozoa, parasites, and viruses.[14] These destructive microorganisms are killed within minutes of contact. Reports of these kill-time test studies confirmed neutralization was achieved in less than six minutes, with most in less than four minutes. The many bacteria tested and neutralized included *Enterococcus faecalis, Salmonella typhimurium, Candida albicans, Staphylococcus aureus, Staphylococcus epidermidis,* and *Pseudomonas aeruginosa.* Other tests have shown it to be effective against *E.coli* and streptococci.

....

Trish: Colloidal Silver Knocked out UTIs

For those of us who battle with constant UTIs (urinary tract infections), I definitely give colloidal silver the thumbs up. I ordered a couple of bottles—which were not expensive—and began taking 10 ml (about one-fourth teaspoon) of colloidal silver morning and night on an empty stomach. The results for me were very effective. UTIs no longer rule my life, thanks to colloidal silver.

....

COLOSTRUM

Colostrum is the first secretion produced by the mammary gland, and precedes milk. During the first one or two days following birth, colostrum provides life-supporting immune and growth factors (IgG and IgF) that help form the building blocks for healthy development. Colostrum has many health benefits for a newborn mammal and without it the immune system can be seriously impaired. Bovine colostrum used in the treatment of MS is claimed by some to enhance the immune system, promote nerve regeneration, help build muscles, and increase energy, mobility, and well-being.

Colostrum contains immunoglobulins, amino acids, and growth factors that help with cell regeneration. It also contains immune-regulatory factors called proline-rich-polypeptides (PRPs) that can help to enhance an underactive immune system and suppress an overactive immune system. Insulin-like growth factor-I (IgF-I), platelet-derived growth factor (PDgF), fibroblast growth factor (FgF), and ciliary neurotrophic factor (CNTF) form a complex of multifunctional growth factors that promote cell proliferation, differentiation, and survival. IgF-I has been shown to "reduce lesion severity and promote myelin regeneration in experimental autoimmune encephalomyelitis (EAE), an animal model of MS."[15]

A particular colostrum product made in New Zealand, called Colostem, is claimed to promote production of the body's own stem cells. Although I cannot personally recommend this product, one New Zealand woman named Shauna McLean claims to have reversed her MS by taking this. She is currently sponsored by the company.

☙ COMBINED ANTIBIOTIC PROTOCOL

Combined antibiotic protocol (CAP) as a treatment for MS began in the United States with Drs. Stratton and Sriram of Vanderbilt University, Nashville, Tennessee.[16] In the course of other research, they discovered that people with MS had colonies of the Cpn (*Chlamydia pneumoniae*) bacterium in their brain and central nervous systems. They then formulated an antibiotic protocol to try to eradicate it.[17] Cpn also affects people who do not have MS.

Cpn is initially a respiratory disease that can cause asthma, sinusitis, and a host of other diseases. Unfortunately for MS patients, the bacteria cross the blood-brain barrier and infect the central nervous system. When first formulated, the treatment was so unpleasant that many people dropped out. Then British doctor David Wheldon, whose wife has MS, suggested some changes that would give people the option of going more slowly, but without inducing possible bacterial resistance to the antibiotic.

One problem in treating Chlamydia pneumoniae with a combined antibiotic protocol is that the dying bugs tend to make people feel worse than they did previously, until the bacteria are substantially reduced. Another problem is that Cpn has three phases to its life cycle. In its first phase it migrates as elementary bodies (EB) to colonize other parts of the body. When it finds suitable cells it infiltrates them, steals their energy, and becomes a parasite, reproducing in vast numbers. If the environment is suitable, the cell will burst open and release these EBs into the bloodstream to colonize more cells. If the environment is not suitable, Cpn will remain dormant within the cell. When Cpn hides like this, it is sometimes difficult to detect. If it is dormant, no one will know it is there, as it may not be apparent in the blood.

Three antibiotics are used to treat Cpn: two to stop Cpn replicating and one to kill Cpn within the cells. Patients usually take these antibiotics for months and years, rather than day and weeks, to ensure that all dormant Cpn is eradicated.

The antibiotics used are:

1. Doxycycline, 200 mg once a day
2. Azithromycin, 250 mg three times a week
3. Metronidazole (Flagyl), 400 mg three times a day

Doxycycline and azithromycin work in synergy to prevent the replication of Cpn; not only are they more effective together at stopping it from replicating, but Cpn cannot find a way around the twin antibiotics to evolve a resistance to them.

Metronidazole is taken in five-day courses every three weeks or so. This antibiotic kills Cpn and causes the dying bacteria to release toxins, which can cause some discomfort. Initial treatment is a minimum of a year, with many patients treated for much longer.

Treating Cpn takes time, patience, and tenacity. These antibiotics cost very little, especially compared to the usual MS drugs, but doctors often feel reluctant to use this as a treatment for MS because of the antibiotic resistance problem. Dr. Wheldon explains that if the antibiotics are taken as recommended, there is little chance of resistance. Additionally, patients take a complex list of daily supplements to support the metabolism and digestive system, listed on the next page.

- B-12: 5,000 mcg sublingually
- Best-quality omega-3 fish oil: 4,000 mg
- Evening primrose oil: 1–5 g
- Vitamin D: 4,000 mcg
- Vitamin B-50 complex with C: 1,000 mg
- Vitamin E: 800 mcg
- Selenium: 100 mcg
- Coenzyme Q_{10}: 200–400 mg
- N-acetyl cystein: 600 mg twice daily
- Combined acetyl L-carnitine: 1,000 mg and alpha-lipoic acid: 300 mg
- Magnesium: 300 mg
- Calcium: 500 mg
- Acidophilus or lactobacillus sporogenes, as required: 200–300 mg
- Melatonin: 0.5–50 mg

Calcium, magnesium, and acidophilus should be taken at least two to three hours after doxycycline.

Ella: Helped by Multiple Antibiotics

When I first started taking the antibiotics, they made me feel sick and depressed. My breathing got worse and I was pretty ill. Because of my initial reactions, Dr. Wheldon cut me back to one antibiotic—doxycycline. It was about two weeks before I was able to tolerate the second antibiotic, azithromycin, and when I started taking it again I only took one a week, gradually increasing to three weekly. I continued taking only these two antibiotics, during which time I gradually recovered some function, became more stable, and experienced fewer fluctuations in my symptoms. I was also looking more healthy, had more energy, lost the brain fog, and was able to start living independently again.

During that time, I received a lot of support from other people on the help site, www.cpnhelp.org, who are following the same protocol. This has been so important because some of the symptoms people with MS experience on this treatment, especially when starting the third antibiotic, appear remarkably like another relapse. For example, when I started taking the metronidazole (the killing antibiotic) six months after starting the other two, I had a marked loss of function in my right arm. I could no longer write or carry anything for about four weeks, and then, slowly, over the course of three to four months and without the benefit of steroids, function returned. I now found my hand to be stronger and more dextrous than it had been previously. The difference between these pseudo relapses and a real MS relapse is that after you recover from it your function is marginally better than before it happened, and as time goes by, improvement continues slowly. Taking the third antibiotic, Flagyl (metronidazole), does precipitate symptoms and this can be scary, but you learn that these are good signs and will lead to healing. Reactions to antibiotics are common and can include nausea, depression, and respiratory symptoms. When first starting the metronidazole, people can experience nausea, brain fog, vertigo, and neurological symptoms, but these reactions show that the antibiotics are doing their work. Reaction to these antibiotics varies from one person with MS to the next. It is important to realize that the CAP is not a magic bullet and won't cure you overnight, but it will give your immune system a helping hand and give your body a chance to heal itself.

COOLING

Heat and humidity can drain the energy of anyone with MS, leaving you feeling like a wet rag. If you lower your core temperature by as little as one degree, these symptoms are likely to subside. There are many practical solutions for cooling, including:

- Air conditioning
- Fans and evaporative air coolers
- Cool suits filled with frozen gel pads, Cool Ties (or Kool Ties) and hats (containing polymer crystals)
- Cool pads you put on your skin
- Cooling pillows, sheets, and special pads to go under your fitted sheet

- Cooling sprays
- Ice cold water and ice in baths
- Cryotherapy—ice cold chambers

Extreme cold is claimed to boost the immune system, heal nerve damage, ease pain, revive tired skin, and be a general pick-me-up. It is anti-inflammatory and can also help with depression, stress, and insomnia. By boosting blood circulation it also increases the delivery of oxygen and nutrients and speeds up the removal of toxins. There are claims that cryotherapy also eases the effects of MS. In the United Kingdom, this therapy is offered at Champneys spa in Tring, Hertfordshire, and the London Kriotherapy Centre in Battersea. Some European spas also offer this treatment, which was first used as a healing modality in Poland in 1983; and it is more widely available in the United States.

Emma: Benefits of Freezing to Life

I went to a hotel in the Austrian alps called the Hotel Alpenmed Lamm. After settling in I was ready to try the cryotherapy chamber. First, I had a health check with Dr. Kettenhuber, who also explained about proper breathing while in the chamber. Isabella, one of the cryotherapy specialists, checked my blood pressure to make sure it was safe for me to go in. Dressed bizzarely in socks and training shoes, gloves, mask, ear muffs, and my swimsuit, I prepared to become literally freezing cold.

A cryotherapy chamber has three areas. You enter the first at minus 15°C to acclimatize to the cold. It was a little like stepping into a freezer—as the door opened, swirls of cold air swept around my feet. Next I went into chamber 2 at minus 60°C, and then into the third chamber—where the treatment really starts, at a staggeringly cold minus 120°C—for up to three minutes.

It took me three attempts over a couple of days to be able to stay up to three minutes, and there is no way of describing it other than it is extremely freezing cold. When I managed to stay for three minutes, I felt a slight stinging feeling on my legs and arms but nothing too uncomfortable.

You can choose the music you want to listen to during the treatment. I was dancing to "Thriller" by Michael Jackson, as you really do need to keep moving around.

Outside the chamber but connected to me by intercom, Isabella talked to me, kept an eye on me through the window, and checked that I was okay. There is also a camera in the chamber. Knowing I was safe helped me to stay calm and not feel claustrophobic.

When I got out I felt fantastic—I had a real rush of energy and the release of endorphins made me feel amazing: really alive, bright, and fresh.

After a treatment, I was guided to the luxurious relaxation area to relax and chill out—literally. It is recommended you stay for half an hour minimum, but I stayed longer just because I was taking advantage of doing nothing for a change.

Not only did I experience a surge in energy and feeling great, my muscular aches and pains also seemed to disappear, along with an old calf injury. I also slept better after that.

Cryotherapy is thought to work by shrinking the molecules in the body so that when you emerge from the cold, the molecules expand and blood flow increases, which helps ease pain and swelling and fight inflammation.

Dr. Kettenhuber said that for many of his MS patients cryotherapy was beneficial for spasms, pain, and sleep. He recommends a stay of two weeks with two cryotherapy sessions per day.

....

Gary: Cold Baths "Chill Out" Symptoms

I have an ice cold bath every night for thirty minutes. I started with just cold water, then gradually added ice cubes over the next couple of weeks. I now add one hundred ice cubes. Since starting the ice cold baths I have seen a great improvement in all my MS symptoms.

I can be really tired, but after an ice cold bath I lie down for five minutes and then feel great, able to go out without any problems. I can walk three times as much I used to, I can walk upstairs without holding onto anything, my balance is better, and I have better bladder control. My sports therapist, Simon, describes the benefits of ice:

"The principle of ice is to reduce all aspects of inflammation, such as swelling, heat, redness, and scar tissue production. The theory behind ice baths is to help break down the scar tissue (scleroses) on the nerves so the myelin sheath can regenerate. The increase in Gary's energy is probably due to reducing his core temperature."

ESPERANZA HOMEOPATHIC NEUROPEPTIDE

Esperanza Homeopathic NeuroPeptide is a homoeopathic substance that contains tiny doses of modified Thai cobra venom. It is being researched by its manufacturer, the Esperanza Research Foundation, but not by independent bodies, and has no peer-reviewed published studies. It is an unlicensed treatment that is claimed to reverse some of the symptoms of MS, regulate the immune system, and work against viruses. It is taken by puffer spray under the tongue. Some people say they have benefited; others not. I tried it and nothing happened. It is available at centers throughout the United Kingdom and in the Bahamas, as well as on the Internet. In some case vitamin D_3 has been added to the product.

HEAT

Just as people with MS are often very sensitive to heat and humidity, it is also common for many to suffer from cold, particularly in the feet and legs, which can feel like blocks of ice even on mild days. Conventional heating methods work well, such as electric heating pads, electric blankets, hot water bottles, warm socks and gloves, and pads and pillows made from various materials that can be warmed in the microwave.

HUMAN GROWTH FACTOR

Human growth factors are made by the body to regulate cell division and cell survival, and can also be produced in a laboratory by genetic engineering.

This therapy is used in some of the more specialized clinics for treatment of MS, including the Baxamed Clinic in Basel, Switzerland (www .baxamed.com). The doctors who run the clinic, Anita Baxas and Sam Baxas, claim very good results. I don't have firsthand knowledge of anyone who has had this treatment.

≈ HYPERBARIC OXYGEN THERAPY

Hyperbaric oxygen therapy (HBOT) administers oxygen at an increased level of pressure. The subject enters an atmospheric pressure chamber where each seat is equipped with an oxygen mask and connected to an oxygen feed. During the treatment (sometimes called a "dive") an oxygen mask over the mouth and nose enables the subject to breathe pure oxygen. This higher concentration of oxygen saturates tissue and blood. For MS, it is most likely to help symptoms of incontinence and fatigue.

Exactly how HBOT works is unclear, but one of the more popular theories is that of Dr. Philip James of Dundee University, a consultant in occupational medicine, who believes MS may result from fatty blockages in tiny blood vessels.[18] The damaged vessels leak toxic substances into the surrounding nerve tissue, damaging the myelin sheath and producing the scattered scars of multiple sclerosis in the central nervous system. If the fatty blockage theory is right, HBOT works because oxygen under pressure dislodges and disperses the fat globules.

Interestingly, divers who get "the bends" when they come up from a deep-sea dive too quickly suffer from symptoms very similar to MS, as a result of air bubbles in the circulation. Dr. James suggests that fat globules in the blood block blood vessels in the nervous system in the same way in multiple sclerosis.

People sometimes ask why they can't just breathe oxygen sitting at home in an armchair. When you breathe oxygen at normal pressure you cannot reach the same oxygen content in the blood as when you breathe it under increased pressure.

From research to date, it seems that maintenance treatments are essential to improvement and stability. Realistically, HBOT can't instantly repair long-term deterioration. Many people do respond in some way once the right pressure and length of treatment have been determined.

Since 1983, hyperbaric oxygen has been widely used in more than sixty self-help therapy centers throughout England, Scotland, Wales, and Ireland. The centers first based their operations on information gleaned in a controlled clinical trial in New York from 1980 to '82, although this has since been updated. The results of this trial indicated both an improvement in symptoms and some protection from deterioration in more than half of those treated.[19] The results of subsequent studies have varied from "no obvious change" to a variety of positive changes.

HBOT is essentially a long-term treatment and may take six months to a year before any significant improvement becomes apparent. The treatment is mainly intended to maintain stability.

Hyperbaric oxygen therapy is widely available at MS therapy centers around the United Kingdom.

LIBERATION TECHNIQUE FOR CCSVI (CHRONIC CEREBROSPINAL VENOUS INSUFFICIENCY)

The Liberation Technique is the name given by Dr. Paolo Zamboni to the treatment of chronic cerebrospinal venous insufficiency. In this condition, veins in the head and neck become narrowed, restricting normal outflow of blood from the brain, causing alterations in the blood flow within the brain and a reflux of blood back into the brain—something that eventually causes injury to brain tissue and degeneration of neurons. Zamboni found that CCSVI almost doubled the risk of developing MS.[20]

The liberation procedure begins by using Doppler ultrasound to get a picture of which veins are affected and where. The affected veins in the neck are then opened and repaired using either balloon angioplasty or, in more serious cases, expandable metal tubes called stents. Surgery is usually done under local anaesthetic—sometimes as an outpatient, other times requiring a short hospital stay. Balloon angioplasty is relatively safe and uncomplicated. However, putting in a stent is more controversial. At Stanford University, one MS patient died when a stent became dislodged. After that, all treatment was halted until more research can be done.

In uncontrolled trials, the liberation procedure has been shown to reduce some MS symptoms, but it is not a cure and may need to be repeated. Improvements can sometimes happen quite quickly—in a day or two—after the procedure. In some spectacular cases, nearly all MS symptoms have disappeared and people have gone back to leading normal lives; but in others, only some symptoms are modestly improved. Individual patients have sometimes reported improvements in bladder function, walking, brain fog, and fatigue. There have also been reports that relapse rates have been greatly reduced. At the time of writing, more research is underway internationally. MS patients who do not want to wait may have to travel to countries such as Poland, Bulgaria, or India for private treatment.

ᕈ LIGHT THERAPY

Exposure to full spectrum light is believed to alter the circadian rhythm and stop the body from discharging melatonin, both of which may cause biochemical changes in the brain. The subject sits or works for specific lengths of time near a light therapy box that gives off specific wavelengths of light and mimics natural outdoor sunlight. Full spectrum lightbulbs are also available for use in the home. Light therapy has been used by some people with MS to help treat depression and seasonal affective disorder (SAD).[21]

ᕈ LOW DOSE NALTREXONE (LDN)

Naltrexone is a class of drug called an opiate antagonist, or opioid receptor, usually used to treat alcohol and drug addiction. At doses of 50–150 mg, it blocks the response to opiate drugs, such as heroin or morphine, and it decreases the craving for alcohol. The idea of using a low dose of naltrexone (LDN) for MS was devised by the late Dr. Bernard Bihari, who was a practicing neurophysician in New York. The way it works is by briefly obstructing the effects of brain endorphins (the brain's natural painkillers). This has an effect of stimulating the increased production of these same endorphins, which in turn stimulate the immune system, thus reducing the activity of MS. In those for whom LDN works, it can help with walking and reducing neuromuscular spasm, fatigue, and bladder problems. It also helps stop attacks. For MS, the recommended dose is from 2.8–4.5 mg either in pill or liquid form, usually taken late each evening. Early research shows that a 3 mg dose of naltrexone is able to increase the level of T cells by 300 percent. This benefit lasts approximately eighteen hours.

Around two-thirds of those who try it have some symptomatic improvement within the first few days. Dr. Bihari, who had more than seventy people with MS in his practice, claimed that as many as 99 percent remain stable once on LDN. This applies to those with both relapsing/remitting and chronic/progressive MS. LDN cannot be used by people on beta interferon, as the two therapies are incompatible. LDN does not work for everyone, and some (including me) cannot tolerate even the lowest dose, because it can cause muscle aches.

Linda: A Magnificent Zero with Naltrexone

In early December 2003, I started taking LDN, and the results were amazing. By Christmas I was functioning again, and my liver tests were back to normal. I felt like myself again—okay, a me with MS, but that didn't matter.

In February 2004, I had to be assessed again on the EDSS disability scale. When I started taking Interferon I was supposed to be monitored for ten years, although by now I had stopped taking it. I scored a magnificent 0 (indicating no symptoms), even though the neurologist wouldn't recognize that it might have something to do with taking low doses of naltrexone (although that was all I was taking). It was confirmed that I had reverted to relapsing and remitting MS and was now officially in remission.

Thanks to LDN and Dr. Bob Lawrence, who prescribed it for me, I have a life again and hope for the future. I can plan things and actually do them. I founded the LDN Research Trust in May of 2004, and it is the most exciting thing I have ever done. I am able to give many hours a week to the Trust, helping people to obtain naltrexone and trying to raise funds for a clinical trial of naltrexone for multiple sclerosis. A successful clinical trial could make LDN an accepted treatment for MS and help others.

My head is clear, energy levels up, and I have greater muscle strength. Balance, vision, hearing, bowels, and bladder are good. In March 2005, I was re-assessed on the EDSS scale and achieved another 0. Throughout the last year I have had no relapse. To sum up, I know I have MS and I haven't been cured. I'm not back to the old me, but if I can remain as I am now (a major improvement in symptoms and no further progression), I will be more than happy.

A study titled "The Effects of Low Dose Naltrexone on Quality of Life as Measured by the Multiple Sclerosis Quality of Life Inventory" was started in 2007 at the University of California, San Francisco, by neurological researcher Bruce Cree, M.D., and colleagues.[22] Some eighty patients with MS were involved in this double-blind, randomized, placebo-controlled, crossover-design study. Each subject received either LDN or a placebo for eight weeks, followed by one week without either, and then a further eight weeks on the other capsule.

Dr. Cree reported the following conclusions to the World Congress on Treatment and Research in Multiple Sclerosis, held in September 2008 in Montreal:

- Eight weeks of treatment with LDN significantly improved quality of life indices for mental health, pain, and self-reported cognitive function of MS patients as measured by the MSQLI (MS Quality of Life Inventory).
- An impact on physical quality of life indices, including fatigue, bowel and bladder control, sexual satisfaction, and visual function, was not observed.
- The benefits of LDN were not affected by disease course, age, treatment order, or treatment with either interferon beta or Copaxone.
- The only treatment-related adverse event reported was vivid dreaming during the first week of the study drug in some patients.
- Potential effects of LDN beyond eight weeks of treatment were not addressed in this study.
- Multicenter randomized clinical trials of LDN in MS are warranted.

More information about LDN with many testimonials can be found at www.lowdosenaltrexone.org and www.ldnresearchtrust.org.

⁕ PROKARIN

Prokarin was devised by Elaine DeLack, an American nurse with MS, based on research first done in the 1940s. Prokarin comes in ready-made patches that you put on your skin, one patch every day. The active ingredients are histamine and caffeine.

DeLack's company, EDMS, funded a double-blind study that showed promising improvements in fatigue among a group of twenty-nine patients.[23] The National MS Society disputed the design of the study, and thus the results. DeLack challenges this. I am not aware of any independent study having been done on Prokarin and MS.

Note: Prokarin includes caffeine, which is prohibited from the Best Bet Diet. These are two very different approaches to treating MS. More information on Prokarin can be found at its website www.edmsllc.com.

✑ REST AND SLEEP

Rest is a great restorative. Ideally, you need to build rest periods into your daily routine to recover from a period of exertion, exercise, or activity. You need to totally switch off and relax, and if you can sleep, so much the better. If you take a rest or nap in the late afternoon, you may find you have enough energy to go out for the evening. If you feel an MS attack approaching, it is sometimes possible to nip it in the bud by lying completely still and resting. Be sure to get plenty of undisturbed sleep at night.

✑ STEM CELLS

Stem cells may hold the most promise as a mainstream treatment for MS. A great deal of scientific research is underway on both sides of the Atlantic and in Australia to make this happen as soon as possible.

There have been some startlingly good accounts of people with MS recovering from MS after stem cell treatment. In December of 2009, scientists in Canberra, Australia reported the case of a twenty-year-old man, Ben Leahy, who made a remarkable recovery after receiving stem cell treatment. Before the treatment he had lost his ability to stand, and was in a wheelchair. After the treatment, he was able to walk again. Doctors first removed stem cells from Leahy's bone marrow and used chemicals to destroy all his immune cells. The stem cells were then transplanted back into his body to replenish the immune system—effectively resetting it. Colin Andrews, a neurologist from Canberra, said that the stem cells may have arrested the disease in this young man. The outstanding results mean that others will now be able to get this treatment. Andrews believes that for some patients there would be a 60–80 percent chance that the progress of the disease could be stopped, and many would have a good chance of symptom reversal.

Before this, American scientists were the first to succeed in reversing some of the damage in early stage MS. Richard Burt, of Northwestern University Feinberg School of Medicine in Chicago, and his colleagues had previously tried using stem cells to reverse this process in patients with advanced stages of the disease, with little success.[24] Burt believes that stem cell treatment needs to be administered *before* neurodegeneration has taken hold.

For the two-year trial, Burt's team recruited twelve women and eleven men in the early relapsing/remitting stage of MS who had not responded to six months of treatment with interferon beta drugs. They removed stem cells from the patients' bone marrow, and then used chemicals to destroy all existing immune cells in the body before re-injecting the stem cells. These then developed into naive immune cells that do not see myelin as alien, and hence do not attack it. At the end of the trial, seven of the patients had improved by at least one point on a standard disability scale, while none of the patients had deteriorated.

Although these results are very good, more research needs to be done before stem cell treatment is approved and is available to MS patients, which is very frustrating for those who want to be treated as soon as possible.

Stem cell treatment is presently (2010) available at clinics in Germany, Ukraine, China, Mexico, Panama, and some other countries, with some people with MS reporting good results and other people not. Evaluations, but not the actual treatment, can be done in the United States, Canada, Australia, United Kingdom, Ireland, and many other European Union countries. Some international clinics, (for example, in Germany and Panama), use autologous (coming from your own body) stem cells taken from your own bone marrow; others (Ukraine) use stem cells from babies' umbilical cords.

Mainstream scientists working in the field of stem cells warn that we have not yet (as of 2010) reached the stage in the science of stem cell treatment when it can be given safely and effectively to MS patients, and believe more research and trials are needed. The U.S. policy on stem cell research recently changed when President Obama came into office, and research has started to move more quickly. "Promising" stem cell treatment research has also been done in the United Kingdom at Bristol University, published in 2010. However, some with MS may not wish to wait through several more years of research before stem cell treatment becomes available, and are ready to chance their luck and money at unofficial clinics. Although we are not promoting this, a Google search brings up several stem cell clinics around the world offering treatment to MS patients. See also www.adultstemcellfoundation.org.

Promoting the Body's Own Stem Cells

A New Zealand company claims that one of its colostrum products, called Colostem, helps the body produce its own natural stem cells from bone marrow. (See Colostrum, this chapter, page 199.)

Another stimulus to self-production of stem cells may be glyconutrients. Dr. Bob Lawrence reports cell counts in the blood of patients taking glyconutrients for only one week have increased exponentially. (See Glyconutrients in chapter 8, page 83.)

◦ WATER

Water flushes out toxins and waste products with the help of the lymphatic system, arteries, veins, liver, and kidneys. Water also enables body cells to take in nutrients and eliminate waste—both of which require water. A loss of just 3 percent of the body's water can cause a 10 percent drop in strength. Fluid retention and excess weight can actually be caused by insufficient fluid intake.

The reason we survive this deficiency is that our food contains so much water. Signs of dehydration are:

- Dry skin. The body robs moisture from the skin if it is needed for vital organs.
- Dark yellow urine—it should be clear and pale. Concentrated urine is also bad for the bladder, as there is a risk of infection.
- Dry mouth.
- Flushed skin.
- Fatigue.

We don't always realize we're thirsty, and can become dehydrated without knowing it.[25] One reason for this may be that the control mechanisms for thirst and hunger are very close together in the brain. They can get mixed up, so you may think you're hungry when in fact you need to drink. By the time you do feel thirsty, you may be very dehydrated, so it's best to rehydrate before you even feel thirsty.

In ayurvedic health care, drinking very cold water is thought to weaken digestive fire—the energy required to digest food. Very cold water is known to be a diuretic, whereas hot (boiled) water is detoxifying and can have a settling effect on the physiology.

Still water is better than carbonated. Carbonated drinks contain phosphoric acid. Too much of this gives you too much phosphorus, a mineral that needs to be carefully balanced with calcium. If you have too much phosphorus and not enough calcium, the body takes calcium from the bones to deal with the excess phosphorus in the blood. Also, if you drink artificially carbonated fluids, the carbonates bind to minerals in the body and remove them.

Remember to drink water regularly—it's easy to forget when you are tired or stressed. Drinking water can also give a mental boost when you are flagging. Drink two glasses of water (or the equivalent) when you get up in the morning, two at midmorning, two in the afternoon, and two in the evening. In other words, a total of eight glasses of water over the course of the day. Don't drink a lot of fluids with meals; it can make you feel bloated and dilute your digestive juices.

15

Hormones and MS

HORMONES PLAY A ROLE in MS, both good and bad. However, increasing research shows that hormones can be useful in the treatment of MS.

Hormones may also help to explain why:

- Almost twice as many women have MS than men.
- Females tend to get MS at an earlier age.
- Some people have more severe symptoms than others.
- Pregnant women with MS often go into remission.
- Bearing children seems to offer some protection against severe disability.
- Breastfeeding has a protective effect against relapses.
- For some women, MS symptoms get worse before menstruation and during menopause.

Hormones first came to the forefront of MS research in 1994. At that time the National MS Society of America set up a special task force to research how estrogens, progesterone, testosterone, prolactin, growth hormone, insulin-like growth factor 1, and other hormones interact with the immune system in men and women with MS.

A later study conducted in Italy found that sex hormones play a role in the inflammation, damage, and repair mechanisms typical of MS.[1]

ᴇᴗ PREGNANCY HORMONES

It has been noted for many years that pregnant women with MS often experience remission, particularly in the third trimester. A landmark clinical study published in 1998 in the *New England Journal of Medicine*, known as the PRIMS study ("Pregnancy in Multiple Sclerosis"), followed 254 women with MS during 269 pregnancies and for up to one year after delivery. The PRIMS study demonstrated that relapse rates were significantly reduced by 71 percent through the third trimester of pregnancy from pre-baseline levels, and that relapse rates then increased by 120 percent during the first three months postpartum before returning to pre-pregnancy rates.[2]

Estrogen

Dr. Rhonda Voskuhl, professor of neurology at the University of California, Los Angeles, has been investigating the specific physiological role estrogen plays in MS. Why pregnant women often go into remission could be explained by the neuro-protective effects of estrogen (and other female sex hormones) during pregnancy. In 2003, a pilot study using estriol (a form of estrogen) in ten women with MS showed decreases in MS severity and an 80 percent reduction in brain lesions.

A larger, two-year, placebo-controlled multi-center trial treating women with relapsing/remitting MS with estriol followed.[3] Given as a pill named Trimesta, estriol provides patients with hormone levels equivalent to six months of pregnancy. One group took Trimesta with Copaxone, an amino acid formulation; the other group took only Copaxone. The goal of the study was to determine if estriol leads to a reduction in relapses, symptoms of fatigue and depression, and brain atrophy. Another aim was to see if estriol leads to better neuro-protection by reducing the ability of immune cells to attack the brain, while at the same time making the brain more resistant to damage. Results indicate that estriol helps modulate the immune system and is also neuroprotective, and more studies are now underway.

Progesterone

Progesterone may have profound neuroprotective effects in addition to helping women with MS combat premenstrual tension and menopause symptoms. Research published in 2010 by American researcher Donald G. Stein, Ph.D., from Emory University in Atlanta, Georgia, showed that progesterone has profound neuroprotective effects that improve outcomes and reduce mortality following brain injuries, and may also help those suffering from central nervous system damage, strokes, spinal cord injuries, and multiple sclerosis.[4]

During pregnancy, progesterone gives powerful neuroprotection to the fetus by suppressing neuronal excitation that might otherwise damage the baby's developing brain tissue. It now appears that progesterone can have a similar effect on injured brain tissue, while also helping it heal. The reason progesterone may help multiple sclerosis is that it may also have protective and regenerative effects on myelin, the protective coating along the nerve fibers. Stein advises that the best delivery method for progesterone is drops of around 1 mg under the tongue, rather than a pill or a cream. This can be prepared by a compounding pharmacist.

In 2007, doctors at the University of Paris found that progesterone promotes the formation of myelin and can have an impact on neurotransmitters, the substances that carry messages from one nerve to another.[5] Progesterone is produced in the human body in Schwann cells, which are a collection of nerves that branch off from the central nervous system.

Prolactin

Another pregnancy hormone is prolactin. In a Canadian study, researchers from the University of Calgary showed that prolactin was directly responsible for the formation of new myelin in the brains and spinal cords of pregnant mice. When mice with MS-like nerve damage were injected with the hormone, their myelin was repaired. The researchers found that pregnant mice had twice as many myelin-producing cells (oligodendrocytes) as virgin mice, and continued to generate new ones during pregnancy. More research needs to be done with prolactin before it is tested on humans with MS.[6]

❧ CHILDBIRTH

There is good news for any woman with MS who has had children or is thinking of becoming a mother: Once you already have MS, bearing children has a long-term protective effect, according to a study carried out in Belgium published in 2009. Researchers found that those women who had given birth since being diagnosed with MS took longer to reach level 6 on the disability scale (requiring a cane to walk), and that women with MS who had given birth at any time, whether before or after MS, had a reduced risk of severe disability. They conclude that there is a possible favorable long-term effect of childbirth on the course of MS.[7]

My book *Multiple Sclerosis and Having a Baby* goes into more detail about the risks and benefits of bearing a child when you have MS.

⸙ BREASTFEEDING

A California study published in 2009 found that breastfeeding exclusively, together with having suppressed menstruation, significantly reduced the risk of post-childbirth relapse.[8] They found that of the 52 percent of women with MS who did not breastfeed or began regular supplemental feedings within two months postpartum, 87 percent had a postpartum relapse, compared with 36 percent of the women with MS who breastfed exclusively for at least two months postpartum.

Since many women stop breastfeeding in order to be able to take disease-modifying drugs, researchers question the abandonment of breastfeeding.

⸙ MENSTRUATION, MENOPAUSE, AND MS SYMPTOMS

Both menstruation and menopause seem to aggravate MS symptoms such as weakness, loss of balance, fatigue, and depression. Women with MS can have worse MS symptoms during a period, and sometimes have erratic periods—or none—for a period of time. Disease activity can vary according to changes in hormones.[9]

A Dutch study published in 2002 found that 42 percent of women with MS had exacerbations of their MS symptoms in the premenstrual phase of their monthly cycle. The contraceptive pill did not give any protection against this.[10]

In a 2005 study at Tennessee's Vanderbilt University, researchers identified a PMS response, as well as chronic, severely depressed mood in women with MS as they approached menstruation.[11]

In a 1992 questionnaire, 54 percent of women with MS reported a worsening of their symptoms with menopause, but 75 percent of those who had tried hormone replacement therapy (HRT) reported an improvement.[12]

Lily: PMS De-stress with Natural Progesterone

I used to suffer from profound changes in MS symptoms ten to fourteen days before my period started: loss of mobility, vision, balance, and hearing; nausea; fatigue; spasms; slurred speech; and difficulty swallowing. I also ran a temperature and had typical PMS symptoms, all of which made work almost impossible. Even getting dressed was problematic.

Neurologists made me even more frustrated. I got comments like "You're a woman, what do you expect?" and "Just get on with it." Much more helpful were other women with MS, one of whom recommended natural progesterone cream.

At first I was pessimistic, because I had already tried synthetic progesterone tablets with no success. Even so, I began researching natural progesterone and talking to other people.

For the first few months things got worse. But now I am pleased to report real improvements in my vegetable-like status. I cannot say I breeze through my period, but at least I don't have MS exacerbations on top of everything else. Also, it shortened my periods by more than a week.

CAN ORAL CONTRACEPTIVES PROTECT AGAINST MS?

A study suggests that taking the oral contraceptive pill can cut a woman's short-term risk of MS. The Harvard School of Public Health research showed that the incidence of MS was 40 percent lower in those taking the pill, compared to those who were not. Women were also found to have a lower risk of MS during pregnancy, but a higher risk in the six months after having a baby, compared to those who were not pregnant.[13]

∞ TESTOSTERONE—CAN IT HELP COGNITIVE ABILITIES?

Dr. Voskuhl has also been investigating the possible use of testosterone to treat men with MS. Since testosterone converts to estrogen in the brain, it may have an impact, although not to the extent that estriol does in women.

One of Voskuhl's studies investigated ten men with MS. At the outset, the men showed testosterone levels in the low–normal range. With treatment the levels rose—but not above high–normal levels—and enhanced their cognitive abilities. The therapy also stabilized brain shrinkage. Blood analysis showed that testosterone modulates the immune system and enhances the production of brain-deprived protective factors.[14]

Do Women with MS Have Too Little Testosterone?

The Italian study mentioned earlier found that women with MS had significantly lower levels of serum testosterone compared to controls. They also found a clear link among women's testosterone levels, tissue damage shown on MRIs, and clinical disability. In men, there was a clear link between estradiol concentrations and brain damage.[15]

∞ DHEA

Dehydroepiandrosterone (DHEA) is an androgenic steroid hormone used by some doctors who practice integrative medicine in the treatment of MS and anti-aging. DHEA, produced in the adrenal glands, is a weak male hormone and a precursor to some other hormones, including testosterone and estrogen. It is being studied for its possible effects on selected aspects of aging, including immune system decline. I take it myself.

In a preliminary 1990 study by Roberts and Faubile, people with MS were found to have low DHEA levels that were improved by DHEA administration.[16] Most of these patients had noticeable improvement in their quality of life after taking DHEA, including increased energy levels, better dexterity, greater limb strength, decreased sensations of numbness, and increased libido. In a non-randomized 1990 study by Calabrese, it was concluded that DHEA administration helped to improve fatigue symptoms in those with MS.[17]

PART FOUR

Living a Healthy Life

16

Alleviating Specific Symptoms

The multipronged approach of giving up allergenic foods, changing your diet, taking supplements, doing regular exercise, detoxing, changing the way you think, and so on—all the things described in this book—is broadly aimed at getting rid of MS symptoms. However, certain therapies and lifestyle changes work especially well at alleviating specific symptoms.

ATTACKS

Some people have success in staving off attacks by avoiding humid heat, hot baths, overexertion, stressful events, overtiredness, and hunger; and by cooling off and resting deeply. Fasting and regular cleansing also help some people stave off attacks. LDN (page 209) and homeopathy (page 171) have both had some success in reducing the frequency of attacks, or relapses.

Attacks may be nipped in the bud by taking high doses of antioxidants and also LDN, omega-3 and omega-6 oils. Roy Strand, M.D., believes that since exacerbations are due to oxidative stress, the best treatment is high-dosage antioxidants. The antioxidants needed are zinc, copper, selenium, vitamins C and E, beta-carotene, OPCs (oligomeric proanthocyanidins), alpha-lipoic acid, acetyl-N-carnitine, and phosphatidyl serine. Dr. Bob Lawrence from Wales, who has MS himself, concurs. He says: "Used at high dosage these are as capable as steroids in reducing the intensity and development of relapses or exacerbations without the downside and adverse effects of steroids."[1] During an attack, double the usual dose to 2000 mg vitamin C, 800 IU vitamin E; 400 mcg selenium, and 30 mg beta-carotene.

The anthocyanidins, otherwise known as oligomeric pro-anthocyanidins, or OPCs, are plant-derived flavonoids that have a powerful antioxidant activity. The recommended dose is between 250 and 500 mg daily, but during an attack this can be increased to 500 to 1000 mg daily. Examples of anthocyanidins include pine bark extract (pycnogenol), grape seed extract, green tea extract, and extracts from many dark-colored seeds, such as bilberries, blueberries, or blackberries. Vitamin D and EPA fish oil also should be taken.

Steroids are routinely used by neurologists to treat MS exacerbations, but Dr. Lawrence is opposed to using steroids to treat MS attacks. He says: "Steroid use in any auto-immune disease, such as MS, will have a strong adverse effect by suppressing both the immune system and adrenal function. Thus, when these drugs are stopped, these reactions will result in an increase in both the risk of further relapse and the rate of disease progression. In addition, when steroids are used it will become necessary to stop taking LDN, further disrupting the level of disease stability."[2] LDN (low dose naltrexone) can also be effective in preventing and stopping attacks, and can be taken during a relapse.

ࣿ BALANCE AND COORDINATION PROBLEMS
Balance and coordination problems can be helped by using exercise machines, such as vibration trainers, and also by strengthening your core and training your balance through Pilates, yoga, t'ai chi, qigong, or physical therapy. Also particularly helpful for balance problems are the Alexander Technique, the Bowen Technique, and conductive education.

ࣿ BLADDER PROBLEMS
(See also Urinary Tract Infections, page 247)

Incontinence, urgency, hesitancy, retention, and urinary spasm problems can be helped by reflexology, acupuncture, shiatsu, craniosacral therapy, herbal medicine, traditional Chinese medicine, homoeopathy, magnetic beds, cooling, cannabis, cannabis medicines, colloidal silver, hyperbaric oxygen treatment, and D-mannose.

More conventional treatments—which are recommended for bladder problems—are intermittent self-catheterization (ISC), the drugs Oxybutynin and Desmopressin, the Queen's Square bladder stimulator,[3] and Botox injections. Avoid caffeine, stimulants, and carbonated drinks. There are many anecdotal cases of bladder symptoms clearing up when people have detected their food allergies and eliminated the offending foods.

If bladder problems get too troublesome, a suprapubic operation can make a huge difference. The procedure involves making a small incision in the abdomen and inserting a catheter into the bladder, thus diverting the urine from the urethra into a leg bag, which can be emptied at your convenience. It is a quick, simple operation (generally an outpatient procedure) done under local anesthetic.

One of the most common problems with MS is bladder urgency, leading to incontinence. This is often caused by not completely voiding all the urine in your bladder when you go to the toilet. The remaining—known as residual —urine aggravates the bladder so you feel an urgent need to go soon after the previous bathroom visit. The problem of residual urine can be addressed by making sure you have emptied every last drop. This may mean staying on the toilet longer, until you get a second or even third voiding. There are tricks to make this easier, such as prodding your lower tummy. If that fails, intermittent self-catheterization does the trick by removing all the urine at each toilet visit. This can often revolutionize someone's daily life, allowing them to go out and about without fear of accidents and leakage. Using catheters may be the only answer if you have bladder retention and cannot pass water no matter how hard you try or how urgently you want to urinate.

Injections of Botox are highly successful at treating a bladder going into spasm.

....

Fiona: Success with Botox

Before I discovered Botox, I had tried everything for my bladder—drugs, intermittent self-catheterization, the lot. I used a bladder stimulator, which was helpful, and a Uribag when out in the car, but ultimately I was peeing more than thirty times a day and up to five times during the night, which made my fatigue even worse.

My bladder was really getting me down and limiting my social life.

Then a doctor at my local hospital said he'd heard great things about Botox treatment. I was referred to the National Hospital, London, where I saw Dr. Kalski. I nearly cried when he said he had treated more than one hundred patients with Botox with a 100 percent success rate! While they were doing the actual procedure I could feel some of the injections, but it was over quickly and on a pain scale of one to ten I would say the average was around five. I was in no pain or discomfort afterward.

I knew the treatment could take a while to take effect. It took two weeks for me, which is average. It really is a miracle and I would urge anyone to have it done and not continue suffering. I have to intermittently self-catheterize now as I cannot go to the toilet normally. This is common for patients who have had the treatment. I now sleep right through the night and can hold for at least fifteen to twenty minutes when I start to feel the need to go. My bladder feels calm and I no longer get awful spasms all the time. My self-esteem is great, I feel sexy again, and I'm definitely more confident about going out. I am also not so fatigued.

They told me treatment lasts an average of eleven months. The effect gradually wears off but will never go back to how serious it was before the Botox. Recently I went back for another urodynamics test. Before, I could only hold around 100 ml. Now it is up to 850 ml!

....

Some other low-tech solutions for bladder urgency and incontinence include carrying with you a plastic jug or urinal and/or using absorbent pads. Tena pads are unbelievably absorbent and are also odor-free.

Bladder infections can be a secondary complication of bladder problems. These can often be prevented and treated with D-mannose. It is most important to deal with retention and infection before they can lead to anything worse.

You might think cutting down on your fluid intake will reduce your need to rush to the toilet. Not so. The trouble with drinking very little is that the urine becomes concentrated and foul-smelling, which can create its own problems. Ideally you should drink at least five glasses of fluid a day, more (eight to ten) if possible. Drink more earlier in the day. Do not drink anything for a couple of hours before going to bed if you normally have to get up during the night to urinate. If you wear a catheter, it is very important to drink a lot of fluid; otherwise, the catheter may collect debris. A high fluid intake will prevent this.

Drinking a good amount is also essential for staying regular. In fact, constipation itself can be a cause of stress incontinence if the full bowel presses on the bladder (see Bowel Problems, below). Both coffee and red wine can irritate the bladder lining and make you feel an urge to pass water. Other alcoholic drinks could have a similar effect.

✎ BOWEL PROBLEMS

Bowel problems—constipation, diarrhea, or fecal incontinence—can affect two-thirds of people with MS. By doing the things in this book, bowel problems can hopefully be avoided and never reach the extreme stage. However, in extreme cases of fecal incontinence, an operation called an ileostomy—or stoma—can solve the problem. This brings the end of the bowel out on to the wall of the abdomen where stool is collected in a special bag.

Constipation

Constipation, a common complaint in MS, causes many problems: toxins accumulate, the full bowel presses on the bladder and makes you more likely to be incontinent, and you feel uncomfortable. Constipation is greatly helped by diet—eat plenty of fiber in fruit and vegetables. High-fiber foods include onions, parsnips, celery, and stringy vegetables—raw or lightly cooked; also fresh and dried fruits and fruit purees. Another tip is to chew whole fruit and dried fruit, especially prunes and figs, and eat flaxseed or stewed prunes before each meal.

An excellent source of fiber is psyllium seed husks, a nondigestible plant fiber widely available. As much as one tablespoon can be taken with each meal, stirred in water or juice, until bowel regulation occurs. The amount can then be reduced to one or two teaspoons three times a day, every fourth day (to rotate this fiber with other fiber foods on a four-day rotation basis).

When you are eating a high fiber diet, it is crucial to drink a lot of water. The fiber needs water in order to pass easily through the bowel. In fact, water is probably the most important anti-constipation agent. The first thing to do if you are not regular is to drink as much water as possible. Make a habit of drinking one glassful when you get up.

Pre- and probiotics are also useful for constipation. Research shows that bowel regularity has more to do with your intestinal flora than with the amount of fiber you eat. Many people swear by taking capsules of acidophilus, a friendly bacteria found in the gut that always needs to be replaced after taking antibiotics.

Exercise is another good way to help avoid constipation. If your posture is sagging and you're generally sluggish, you are more likely to be constipated. Toning your whole system will get you going in more ways than one.

Also helpful are reflexology, acupuncture, shiatsu, and colonic irrigation, as well as herbal remedies, aloe, cascara, flaxseed and oil, psyllium, senna, hemp seed, alder buckthorn, basil, buckthorn, rhubarb, chlorophyll, bladderwrack, dandelion, and fenugreek. Homeopathic remedies include Bryonia, Calcarea carbonica, Causticum, Graphites, Lycopodium, Nux vomica, Sepia, Silica, and sulphur. Many people have found their constipation relieved by evening primrose oil capsules, and frequent use of oils in salad dressing and cooking will also help.

A good intake of vitamin C helps keep the stool soft—as much as 2000 to 4000 mg, three times a day. The use of vitamin C as a bowel softener has considerable value beyond the retention of fluid in the colon; it also counteracts toxins formed by bacteria in the colon.

Do not take laxatives. This makes the bowel lazy and costs your body much-needed vitamins and minerals. Repeated use of laxatives can make you feel very unwell. Finally, allow enough unhurried time in the bathroom— keep interesting reading material and a pair of eyeglasses there, if needed.

BRAIN FOG, COGNITIVE DIFFICULTY, AND MEMORY PROBLEMS

All these can be helped by giving up allergenic foods, changing your diet, and taking ginkgo biloba, coenzyme Q_{10}, yamabushitake mushrooms (also called Lion's Mane), and fish oil supplements. The liberation procedure for CCSVI, qigong, craniosacral therapy, ayurvedic medicine, LDN, transcendental meditation, combined antibiotic protocol, and hyperbaric oxygen treatment can also help, as can brain training (see below). The prescription drug Provigil (modafinil) can also help you keep alert and better able to do brain work.

Ginkgo biloba, an extract from the leaves of the ginkgo tree, native to Asia, is especially helpful and has been used for centuries to improve memory. The active ingredients are *Ginkgoflavoneglycos bilobalide* and terpenelactones, including ginkgolides A, B, and C. It increases blood flow to the brain by regulating the tone and elasticity of blood vessels, thereby increasing oxygen supply to the brain. It also enhances the brain's utilization of glucose. Ginkgo flavonoids directly dilate the micro-capillaries all over the body. Ginkgo increases the body's ability to produce the universal energy molecule ATP (adenosine triphosphate) and is a highly important antioxidant that can scavenge free radicals. (See also chapter 8, page 68.)

Ross: Ginkgo Biloba Made Me Smart Again

Before I started taking ginkgo biloba, I was always forgetting names and details. While I don't mind too much the limping and tingling of MS, having my mind fade away was quite unbearable. Then I started a low dose of ginkgo biloba, and worked up to 960 mg a day. It's expensive, but cheaper than being stupid. At that dose my brain returned to college level in thinking, analysis, and memory. What joy! If I'm tired or stop the supplements for any reason, I have problems again.

A trial of ginkgo biloba showed that it helped improve attention span in MS patients with impaired cognitive function. In the trial, twenty MS patients were put on ginkgo biloba and nineteen received a placebo. Patients on ginkgo biloba had increased attention span and were four seconds—around 13 percent—faster in response time than the placebo group.[4]

Brain Training Tools

Various brain training tools may also help combat cognitive decline. The brain is a remarkably adaptable organ and it is possible to develop and improve connections between its various parts by better and more frequent use. There are now a number of gadgets, games, puzzles, and books that help sharpen mental skills. These include Dr. Kawashima's Brain Training, played on Nintendo DS Lite; Mindscape's Bigger Brain Trainer CD-ROM; and Lifemax Brain Exerciser, which uses a hand-held game console popular with children. Training games include remembering lists of unconnected words, or writing down answers to simple arithmetic tests. Playing Sudoku or similar games, or doing crossword puzzles can achieve the same results.

Ian: Younger through Brain Training

At first my "brain age" was the same as that of an eighty-year-old man! By the end of my first session with a brain training game I'd gotten the score down to forty years—ten years younger than my actual age.

∾ CIRCULATION PROBLEMS

Cold feet, hands, and legs are often due to poor circulation from lack of mobility and exercise. Also, in MS, a faulty hypothalamus can cause impaired heat regulation. Severe cold can bring on an MS attack. You can prevent heat loss by wearing warm socks, shoes, or slippers, or use products that can be warmed in the microwave, like therapeutically heated slippers, called CosySoles. Electric heat pads and blankets are also good. Other suggestions include soaking your feet and legs in warm water for thirty minutes, rubbing cold areas vigorously, being massaged with warm sesame oil to get the circulation going, and exercise.

You need to move your limbs to get your blood moving. Without anything to jumpstart the upward journey, blood pools and stagnates in the feet, causing them to turn a nasty shade of blue or purple. Any kind of exercise is fine. Also, yoga and stretching exercises help. Other effective therapies for circulation are massage and shiatsu. There are also some new electronic circulation booster machines on the market, which are effective in getting the blood in your feet and legs moving. You put each foot on the pads provided on the machine, and set it to the length and intensity of your choice. You can feel the machine pumping into your feet, getting the blood moving.

Helpful supplements for circulation include:

- Butcher's broom (particularly for vein health)
- Cannabis
- Coenzyme Q_{10}
- Organic germanium
- Ginkgo biloba (good for cold hands and feet since it dilates microcapillaries throughout the body)
- Horse chestnut
- Pycnogenol
- Seacure (a commercial product made from fish, minerals, and omega-3 essential fatty acids)

Foods that are beneficial for circulation, include:

- Black pepper
- Cardamom
- Chilies
- Cinnamon
- Cloves
- Garlic
- Ginger
- Nutmeg
- Rosemary
- Saffron

Each of these complementary therapies also has a way of treating coldness:

- Acupuncture
- Homeopathy
- Massage
- Reflexology
- Tibetan herbal medicine
- Traditional Chinese herbal medicine
- Low dose naltrexone, in some cases

∽ DEPRESSION AND LOW MOOD

Depression is particularly bad for someone with MS because it weakens an already weakened immune system. Because of the strong mind-body connection, your state of mind has a direct effect on your state of health. Depression can be caused by many things, including food sensitivities, so determine and eliminate any bothersome foods. Exercise creates endorphins, so keep moving, especially in the fresh air and sunshine. Get out and mix with other people, and do something to help others. Think positively and dwell on your achievements. Full-spectrum light boxes, cannabis, aromatherapy, magnet therapy, psychotherapy, counseling, and cognitive behavioral therapy can all help. One Australian woman I know succeeds in keeping depression at bay with a simple plan:

- Get plenty of sleep. Never get overtired. (Notice how much more depressed and irritable you feel when you are tired.)
- Eat often and plenty. Never allow yourself to get weak with hunger.
- Exercise at least once a day. Exercise boosts your circulation, gets oxygen into your brain, and stokes up the body chemistry so that endorphins are released.
- Always have something to look forward to. Having MS can be like living in a dark tunnel. Always have treats in store to bring some sunshine into your life.
- Be sociable. Take an interest in other people. This takes your mind off you and your troubles. Having MS is not a sentence to social isolation.
- Think positively.
- Take care to look good. Being happy with the way you look makes you feel good about yourself.
- Stick to as ordered a routine as you can and keep on top of things. That way you know where you are.
- Keep your mind active and interested.
- Do something that gives you a sense of achievement, for example, a creative hobby or helping other people in the community. Being proud of what you do is a great boost to the spirits.
- Live in the present and get the most out of each experience as it is actually happening. Don't dwell on the past or be fearful about the future.

Depression as well as other emotional issues can also be helped by the Emotional Freedom Technique, counseling, psychotherapy, cognitive behavioral therapy, and hypnotherapy.

DIZZINESS AND VERTIGO

The occasional bout of dizziness can sometimes be managed simply by lying down with your eyes closed and resting. Physical manipulation may be necessary to combat frequent dizziness. Cranial osteopathy and acupuncture can sometimes help, or physical therapy. A physical therapist will see whether certain positions of the head make symptoms worse, and then show you how to build up tolerance to the head being in these positions. Vestibular rehabilitation therapy (VRT) can help by retraining the brain to recognize and process signals from the vestibular system—related to the inner ear. Some physical therapists use a set of exercises, known as the Cawthorn-Cooksey exercises, to gradually retrain the eye and body musculature to compensate for the loss of vestibular signals, which may be causing the vertigo and imbalance. In most cases VRT is so successful that no other treatment is required.

Other ways include balance training, Pilates, and yoga. Herbal remedies include ginkgo biloba to increase blood flow to the brain, feverfew, and ginger capsules or ginger leaf tea. Homeopathic treatments helpful in vertigo include Gelsemium, Calcarea, and Cocculus.

EYE PROBLEMS

Eye problems such as double vision or blurred vision can sometimes be a sign of food sensitivity and are resolved when the offending foods are given up. They can also be brought on by overexertion and heat. Eye problems can be helped by acupuncture, reflexology, homeopathy, cooling therapies, and antioxidants in foods such as blueberries. Royal jelly also helps. Other useful supplements include Devil's Claw, bromelain, lutein, beta-carotene, zinc, selenium, copper, omegas-3 and -6, flaxseed oil, and evening primrose oil. Useful vitamins are A, B, and D, and vitamin E in high doses. Homoeopathic remedies: Phosphorus appears to be specific for optic neuritis, an inflammation of the optic nerve that can cause vision to blur or be lost. It is sometimes combined with Hypericum. Double vision can be helped with Gelsemium.

ᐳᕞ FATIGUE AND LACK OF ENERGY

Fatigue—one of the invisible symptoms of MS—can be one of the most disabling, as it knocks you out of living a normal life. Fatigue and lack of energy may also be major symptoms of food sensitivity, which is particularly likely if you feel desperately tired after eating.

To get back your energy, start by giving up allergenic foods, changing your diet, and eating foods that promote the health of mitochondria—the energy-producing cells (see chapter 6 and the glyconutrients section in chapter 8.)

You also generate more energy when you expend more in regular exercise. Other fatigue fighters include acupuncture, homeopathy, hyperbaric oxygen, Indian head massage, meditation, LDN, anthroposophical medicine, ayurvedic medicine, herbal medicine, the Bowen Technique, conductive education, craniosacral therapy, crystal therapy, combined antibiotic protocol, cooling techniques, royal jelly, sleeping on a magnetic bed, massage, and drinking plenty of water. Treating CCSVI with Liberation Techinque can also help.

Supplements that help combat fatigue are ginkgo biloba, coenzyme Q_{10}, ginseng, NADH (a type of vitamin B_3), and Reishi and yamabushitake mushrooms (Lion's Mane). Also helpful: Detox and fasting, probiotics, cooling, acupuncture, oxygen therapies, or anything that increases oxygen supply to the brain and muscles. Cognitive behavioral therapy also helps fatigue, according to research done at the University of Southampton in England.[5]

Lifestyle changes are vital to combat fatigue:

- Never push yourself too hard.
- Conserve your energy and pace yourself—plan your day so you have rest periods after exertion.
- Stop before you get tired.
- Avoid heat and humidity.
- Give up smoking.
- Get sufficient rest and sleep to recharge your batteries. Take a daytime nap.
- Don't get hungry, but avoid heavy meals. Keep blood sugar levels balanced.
- Don't overdo things and avoid overexertion.

- Try to reduce the stress in your life.
- Reconsider the kind of work you do, the number of hours you work, and the time and energy spent commuting.
- Ask others to share (or do) chores.
- Delegate tasks that require a lot of energy.
- Take a nap before going out in the evening.

To conserve my energy, I have had to impose limits on how long I can drive in one trip (currently around three hours), how many hours I can work, how late I can stay up, and so on. My own limited sphere of remaining well corresponds roughly with the small box in the figure to the right. The old me, pre-MS, could operate very well within the bigger box. I do find that I can remain stable as long as I stay within this small box; the trouble starts when I try to go beyond it. One solution I have found is to pay for household help so I don't drain my energy doing cleaning or laundry. I also get all my groceries delivered, not just to my door—but to my fridge! I know that this is a luxury and not everyone can afford paid help or have groceries delivered. My advice is to delegate such chores, and to keep life as simple as possible. Friends and neighbors are often willing to help if you ask them. In the United Kingdom, if you are sufficiently disabled, your local social services department may pay for a caregiver who will do cleaning and shopping for you.

Underactive Thyroid

Fatigue and lack of energy, common symptoms of MS, can also be a symptom of low thyroid function (hypothyroidism). Some people with MS have found that energy improves when low thyroid function is treated.

A Spanish study of ninety-three people with MS, published in the European Journal of Neurology, found antithyroid antibodies (antibodies against peroxidase and thyroglobulin) five times more prevalent than in controls. Since MS patients are more likely to have antithyroid antibodies than the general population, the researchers recommend that all MS patients have thyroid-stimulating hormone (TSH) and antithyroid antibodies tested.[6]

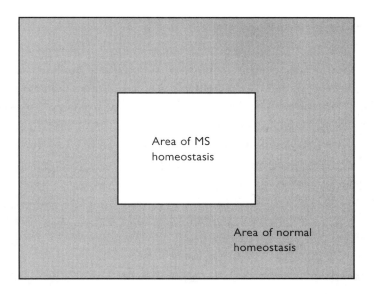

HEAT INTOLERANCE

Heat is a problem for many people with MS. It can be helped by avoiding humid heat and using cooling techniques, which include air conditioning or fans, sucking ice cubes, cooling down before and after any activity, and having a cold bath or shower—some people with MS add ice cubes. Use cooling products, such as Cool Ties (or Kool Ties), and drink plenty of fluids. Air conditioning is one of the most effective treatments for MS. (See also Cooling in chapter 14.)

IMMUNE SYSTEM DYSFUNCTION

If you are experiencing any MS symptoms, it is probable that your immune system in not functioning properly. Therefore, the aim of everything in this book is to normalize the immune system, especially through diet and supplements. There are also specific products containing plant sterols and sterolins commonly found in fruit and vegetables that can be particularly useful in restoring the immune system. Moducare, a pine extract product made by Thorne Research (see Resources), and Reishi mushrooms are both high in sterols. Yamabushitake mushrooms (Lion's Mane) modulate the immune system, boost the brain, and contain eninacines, which are strong nerve growth stimulators.

ᕫᔌ INFLAMMATION

Many of the diet and supplement recommendations in this book are anti-inflammatory, but there are some specific products designed to reduce inflammation. Proteases, or proteolytic enzymes, digest organic debris and neutralize the biochemicals of inflammation so that repair and regeneration can take place. Serrapeptase, a product used by the late Dr. Hans Nieper in Germany, is a brand of proteolytic enzyme that is produced in the intestines of silk worms to break down cocoon walls, and is said to digest non-living tissue, blood clots, and arterial plaque and inflammation.

Enzymes are naturally found in raw food but are diminished or destroyed by heat, so it's a good idea to take a digestive enzyme with meals.

Turmeric is also anti-inflammatory.

ᕫᔌ MOBILITY PROBLEMS AND MUSCLE WEAKNESS

Exercise, yoga, neurostimulation, Alexander Technique, and treatment of CCSVI with the Liberation Technique can be particularly helpful with mobility problems. Ayurvedic medicine, the Bowen Technique, conductive education, magnetic therapy, meditation, LDN, herbal medicine, Padma 28, and stem cells are also useful in this regard. Muscle weakness is helped by all forms of exercise. Eliminating foods to which you are sensitive and improving your diet can also have an effect.

Walking Aids

There are several products and procedures that can help with walking difficulties. Apart from canes, walkers, and rollators, these include Functional Electrical Stimulation and other products to help a dropped foot, such as MuSmate.

Functional Electrical Stimulation (FES)

Functional Electrical Stimulation (FES), the technology that drives the Odstock Dropped Foot Stimulator (ODFS), corrects a dropped or dragging foot by using electrical stimulation to produce contractions in paralyzed muscles. It should be obtained through a rehabilitation facility or doctor, so that it can be adjusted properly for you.

Self-adhesive electrodes attached to a control box are applied to the skin, and the electrical stimulation makes you lift your foot. It does this by causing a nerve impulse in the common peroneal nerve, which is situated below the knee. This impulse then travels along the nerve, causing the muscles that lift the foot to contract. The electrical impulse is timed to the patient's own walking rate via a small pressure pad (footswitch) placed inside the shoe under the heel. When weight is taken off the footswitch, the stimulation is turned on, causing the foot to lift as the leg is swung forward. When the heel strikes the ground, the stimulation is switched off. This makes walking safer because you are less likely to trip.

Several studies have shown that FES improves walking speed and efficiency, and can also relax spastic muscles and increase quality of life. Between January 1993 and September 1995, thirty-two MS patients took part in a controlled trial and were randomly allocated to treatment and control groups. Both groups received equal amounts of physiotherapy while the treatment group also used the FES device. Measurements showed that the treatment group had a statistically significant increase of 16 percent in walking speed and a 29 percent reduction in effort required to walk.[7]

In another study, forty-four people with secondary progressive MS and dropped foot were randomly divided into two groups, twenty getting FES and the remaining twenty-four receiving a physiotherapy home exercise program for a period of eighteen weeks.[8] The results were that the exercise group showed a statistically significant increase in the speed and distance they walked in three minutes. However, the FES group performed to a significantly higher level when fitted with the FES device than without it. The conclusion of this study was that, while exercise may provide a greater training effect on walking speed and endurance than FES, FES does provide an orthotic benefit. The researchers suggest that a combined therapy of exercise and FES may be best.

Other studies have also found that Functional Electrical Stimulation improves walking speed with less expenditure of energy. Most MS patients need to wear the device to get the effect—it generally does not carry over to when the device is taken off. However, a minority do increase their walking speed even when not using the device. In the United Kingdom, FES is now available on the National Health Service.

Further information and full references for all FES studies can be found at www.salisburyfes.com.

Kelsey: Kick-started with FES

When I found out about Functional Electrical Stimulation (FES), I couldn't believe that something so simple could make such a difference. The first appointment measured my general leg strength. It is at this hurdle that some people are eliminated—the leg cannot be too weak, nor too highly toned. At the second appointment some weeks later, I was fitted with the device. I have one electrode stimulating the nerve under the knee at the front (called the peroneal nerve). A second electrode is placed over the top of the fibula bone (the bone on the outside of my lower leg), and a current flows between them. The electrodes are thin, silver, circular sticky pads that need a lot of adjustments to get the position just right. The pulses are controlled by a foot switch in the inner sole of my shoe, so it's important that my shoes are flat and give a lot of support. Only a small amount of pressure needs to be taken off the switch to make it work. I raise my foot, the pulse kicks in, I lower my foot, and the pulse goes until the next time. Once I got the hang of it, it took an awful lot of energy out of the walking process.

Clipped to my belt or waistband is a little black box (easily camouflaged by clothing). This has a dial marked 1–10, which sets the level of electrical pulses. Depending on how I feel, I can turn the dial down or off, or use the pause button. I usually keep it set between 2 and 3. It feels like pins and needles or a very mild electric shock. If you've ever used a Slendertone or similar muscle-toning machine, it's a bit like that. If you turn up the power too high, it can hurt. Too low, and it won't work.

Be warned! Don't try to walk too much at first. I wasn't used to walking and overdid it, and it took me two days to recover. You don't really notice this contraption unless you wear short skirts, and with trousers it is nearly invisible. There's a wire coming out of your shoe, but it disappears up the back of your trouser leg. It takes less than a minute to put on, and about ten seconds to take off at night. Several weeks into its use, I'm finding the FES invaluable, not least because it forces me to use my right side. There is absolutely no doubt that this device can really be of benefit to anyone who has a dropped foot, and it's an invaluable way of giving the body a kick-start.

MuSmate

MuSmate lifts up a dragging or dropped foot. The MuSmate was tested on twenty volunteers with MS at the South West Therapy Centre in Exeter, United Kingdom. Over a ninety-day period, their walking speed increased by more than 100 percent. The volunteers also reported that the distance they were able to walk increased by up to 600 percent. Wearers reported that walking without the MuSmate also improved.

The device consists of a shoulder harness connected by an elastic cord to the wearer's shoe. The elasticated assembly—made from shock cord comprised of a bundle of elastic threads in a plastic coating—gently lifts the foot during the walking movement. One size fits all adults, and the length can be adjusted by moving a white rod up and down. This means that the person wearing it can not only adjust for leg length, but also vary the amount of lift and support as needed. For example, the lift can be increased so that stairs can be climbed or rough ground crossed without tripping.

The shoe harness goes around the back and underneath the shoe to form a more robust device for lifting the foot. This component is available in a variety of sizes and there are left and right versions. The elasticated assembly can be fitted to the shoe with a shoelace connector that goes around the shoelaces (or hook and loop fastenings) and has a hook or triangle to connect to the elastic cord.

Other Walking Aids

Most MS rehabilitation specialists are able to offer a brace or ankle foot orthosis to treat foot drop. The brace, usually made of plastic, is worn around the lower leg and foot. It supports the ankle and holds both foot and ankle in a flexed position.

᪐ PAIN

Pain can dominate the life of the person experiencing it, and left untreated, can affect every other aspect of the person's life. It can be helped by acupuncture, cannabis, Sativex cannabis spray, turmeric (curcumin), and exercise, and physical therapy may help to decrease spasticity and soreness of muscles. Regular stretching exercises help to release flexor spasms, and the magnetic bed can help relieve pain. Also helpful are anthroposophic medicine, crystal therapy, hypnotherapy, Reiki, shiatsu, relaxation techniques, meditation and deep breathing, massage, ultrasound, chiropractic treatments, hydrotherapy, transcutaneous nerve stimulation (TENS), moist heat and ice, and GABA—gamma amino butyric acid—an inhibitory neurotransmitter. Pain psychology—talking about your pain—is also offered in some hospital pain clinics, in addition to injections of local anesthetics such as novocaine, with or without cortisone-like medications.

੭੪ POSTURE

It's tempting to slump when you are in pain, or when some part of your body seems numb. However, slumping will impair your breathing and compromise your digestion and other bodily functions. Strengthening your core muscles, the internal and superficial muscles in your trunk, will help keep you stabilized and aligned, with good, upright posture. Pilates is a brilliant way to do this. Posture can also be helped with physical therapy, Alexander Technique, conductive education, yoga, t'ai chi, and qigong. You can also try imagining a string being pulled up from beneath the earth, through the back of your body and on up through the back of your head, and looping above you around a cloud.

੭੪ SEX ISSUES

There are excellent drugs to help overcome impotence, diminished libido, and inability to orgasm, and sexual aids are easily available to make satisfying lovemaking easier. Natural options such as noni juice can sometimes help a woman reach orgasm. However, your relationship and particularly open communication with your partner is also vital in making sex work well.

If you are the one with MS, it is very important that your partner continue seeing you as a sexually attractive person, and you must do everything to keep yourself that way. MS is not an excuse to be slobby and not take good care of your appearance. If you think you are unattractive or doubt your ability to attract or keep a partner, this will have a devastating effect on your self-image and self-esteem. It is vital to accept and love yourself so that others can feel that way about you too.

In order to overcome sex problems, you must communicate openly and honestly with your partner. If you do not share your feelings, your partner may not be aware of your needs. Love and patience on the part of both partners seldom fails to solve problems.

The worst thing you can do is avoid sexual contact. Some couples have a tendency to do this because they are afraid that sex will worsen the condition of the one with MS. On the other hand, they may avoid sex because they do not want it to end in disappointment or frustration, if this has been the outcome of previous encounters.

The danger is that if you become too watchful or worried about what might go wrong, "spectatoring" in itself becomes a problem. Performance anxieties always interfere with relaxation and enjoyment, and can inhibit sexual functioning.

Sex Drugs and Aids

Anything that gives mutual pleasure is positive, including oral sex, masturbation, massaging, cuddling, fondling, or any other means of touching, stimulating, and mutual caressing. In a healthy sexual relationship, these would all be additions to sexual intercourse, and not alternatives.

Sexual aids can give pleasure and satisfaction in lovemaking, so you should not treat them with suspicion just because they are manufactured and not "natural." Anything that does not actually cause pain in sex and that gives pleasure to both partners should be welcomed. After all, no one with poor eyesight objects to wearing glasses; the same attitude should apply to sexual aids.

There is no need to suffer in silence. If you are having sexual difficulty for any reason, talk to your health professional. Sexual aids are available over the Internet and are delivered in unmarked packaging. Most good-sized cities have at least one sex shop, where sales people tend to be quite matter-of-fact about their products and are happy to show you what is available.

Vibrators

If a woman has difficulty reaching orgasm, there is a new generation of more powerful vibrators. Even women quite severely disabled by MS find these strong vibrators help them achieve orgasm. Vibrators can also transform a potentially awkward session with a partner into a delightful adventure.

Viagra and Cialis

Erectile dysfunction (impotence), low libido, and difficulty reaching orgasm can sometimes be helped by taking the drug Viagra or Cialis. These can be effective for both sexes, even though the medical research says they work only for men. There are anecdotal reports that some women with MS find the drugs increase blood flow to the genitals, increase libido, and make orgasm easier.[9] Men may need two or more 100 mg Viagra doses to get an erection. Cialis can be taken every day and does not need as much time to be effective as Viagra—usually from thirty minutes to an hour.

Vacuum Pumps

Vacuum pumps are another solution for erectile dysfunction.

....

Ian: Don't Let ED Keep You Down

There is really no reason why a man with MS should have to put up with erectile dysfunction (ED), as there are at least two solutions—pump and Viagra. When it comes to the question of "pump or pill," it really is possible to have the best of both worlds. Getting it up should never get you—or me—down again.

Earlier this year, I saw an ad for a new vacuum pump, called the SomaCorrect Xtra. It was a stylish-looking thing and the ad reminded me of one important advantage that vacuum pumps have—they can be used as often as required, unlike Viagra, which can't be used more than once a day. I was interested. To start, you choose the size of tube that fits, place the tube over the penis, apply sealing gel to the base of it, operate the pump to create a vacuum, and after a few minutes remove the tube. You then place a rubber erection mainte-nance ring—a thick rubber band—on the base of the penis, sealing in the blood and keeping the penis erect. It took just a few minutes to get a useable erection—far quicker than Viagra, where I normally have to wait half an hour for the drug to work.

I found it a bit fiddly to use at first—it required a little practice. The only other downside is that you have to stop using it after half an hour after which time you have to take off the erection maintenance ring and let the blood flow back out of the penis.

....

SPASMS AND TREMORS

Muscle cramp, due to spasm, may be caused by too little calcium. Calcium and magnesium are both essential for the muscles to contract and relax normally. The natural amino acid gamma amino butyric acid (GABA) can also reduce spasm. Niacin (vitamin B_3) is also effective in some individuals; try 500 mg three times daily with food. Niacin must be taken with a daily dose of vitamin B complex—an essential vitamin for use in the treatment of MS—to be fully effective. Methyl-sulphonyl-methane (MSM), a natural sulphur-containing compound, can also be effective in reducing spasm. The powerful antioxidants anthocyanidins, taken in sufficient dosage (approximately 250 mg daily, or more) can work in reducing muscle spasm, too. Spasms may also be helped by Sativex cannabis spray, herbal medicine, conductive education, acupuncture, homoepathy, and LDN.

Tremors are helped by exercise and stretching as well as taking supplements such as magnesium.

SPASTICITY AND STIFFNESS

Sativex cannabis spray has been shown in scientific trials to relieve spasticity, the muscular hypertonicity so common to MS. Spasticity can also be helped by exercise, physical therapy, conductive education, and the magnetic bed. Stiffness can be helped by daily stretching exercises, anthroposophic medicine, herbal medicine, and all the therapies that help you relax, including massage, meditation, hypnotherapy, and hydrotherapy.

Botox injections have been shown in clinical trials to relieve spasticity in individual muscles for up to three months, without any significant side effects.[10] Further, large-scale clinical trials are needed before FDA approval can be sought for Botox as a treatment of MS-related symptoms. The toxin can be delivered by injection directly into an overactive muscle that has not responded to first-line oral medications prescribed by orthodox doctors, such as baclofen (Lioresal) and tizanidine (Zanaflex). Botox is considered by many physicians to be an additional strategy for temporary management of severe spasticity in an isolated area. The U.S. National MS Society is helping to recruit participants for one such study, supported by Allergan.

For those with significant leg weakness, however, a certain amount of spasticity gives them enough rigidity to allow them to stand and walk. In this case the goals would be to ease the discomfort of spasticity while retaining enough rigidity to allow mobility.

STRESS, TENSION, AND ANXIETY

Many things can help reduce stress, tension, and anxiety but removing the stressful circumstance is the most obvious way to start. If that is not possible, try changing your reaction to the things you find stressful. Ways of dealing with stress include meditation, exercise (releases endorphins), and relaxation techniques. Particular therapies that work well at alleviating stress, tension, and anxiety include Integrative Body-Mind Training (IBMT), acupuncture, autogenic training, ayurvedic medicine, shiatsu, Alexander Technique, aromatherapy, Indian head massage (also known as champissage) and other types of massage, hypnotherapy, herbal medicine, laughter, craniosacral therapy, and qigong.

Meditation using IBMT for just twenty minutes a day for five days helps reduce stress. A small study using the IBMT method that comes from traditional Chinese medicine found that those using this technique reported better control of stress than those relying on Western relaxation training. While in a state of restful alertness, the IBMT group received instructions on breath and mental images from a coach, as soothing music played in the background.

The study, published in the *Proceedings of the National Academy of Sciences,* was carried out in China by psychology professor Michael Posner from the University of Oregon. He assigned forty Chinese undergraduates (not necessarily with MS) to either integrative meditation or relaxation therapy. The students who used integrative meditation for twenty minutes a day for just five days showed less stress, anxiety, depression, and anger. They also displayed more energy, less fatigue, a significant drop in levels of the stress hormone cortisol, and an increase in immunoreactivity.[11]

Pet Therapy

Our four-legged friends provide more than companionship. Stroking a pet is a good way to ease stress; calm anxiety; lift depression; increase happiness, empathy, and self-esteem; and make you laugh. They also take your

mind off the disease. Dogs are the most calming pets, and long-haired varieties, such as spaniels and setters, seem to be the most effective, but other
animals such as cats, rabbits, pigs, and horses are also effective. Although
there has been no specific research on pet therapy and multiple sclerosis,
research with geriatric patients in a psychiatric hospital showed statistically
significant reductions in anxiety after animal-assisted therapy sessions.[12]

✍ TEMPOROMANDIBULAR JOINT PAIN (TMJ)

Some holistic doctors have found that people with MS have problems
with the temporomandibular joint, the hinge joint in the jaw that articu-
lates the mandible and the temporal bones. With a temporomandibular
joint problem, the teeth are out of alignment. A cranial osteopath, or
craniosacral chiropractor, should be able to correct this. Some people with
MS have reported that once the temporomandibular joint problem was
corrected, there was an improvement in other MS symptoms.

✍ URINARY TRACT INFECTIONS

You can help prevent a urinary tract infection (UTI) by drinking plenty
of fluids, so urine does not stagnate in the bladder. Used hygienically,
intermittent self-catheterization completely empties the bladder and thus
helps prevent UTIs.

Research shows that D-mannose, a simple carbohydrate sugar similar in structure to glucose, supports the health of the urinary tract, and
some people find success with cranberry juice. Taking 1,000 mg of vitamin C a day will lower the PH of your urine, and probiotics will keep
the good bacteria count high. Maintain good hygiene and always wipe
front to back using unbleached, undyed, unscented toilet paper, if possible; avoid powders and perfumed soaps. Empty the bladder immediately
before and after sex. Avoid spermicides. Avoid constipation. Colloidal
silver may also be useful.

✍ OTHER MS SYMPTOMS: NUMBNESS, TINGLING, PARALYSIS, SLURRED SPEECH, THE MS "HUG"

Any or all of these symptoms come on when you experience an attack or
episode, which can range from mild to intense. Slurred speech, in particular, is often brought on by eating and drinking the wrong things for you

and/or getting overtired. It often can be avoided by giving up allergenic food and drinks.

The combined approach of changing your diet, giving up foods to which you are sensitive, taking many supplements, doing some form of regular exercise, complementary therapies, resting when needed, detox, and addressing emotional issues (see chapter 20) targets all MS symptoms as it reduces inflammation, and so lessens the chance of having an attack. If you have MS, being proactive and taking as much control of your life as you can is your best defense.

17

MS Triggers and
Exacerbating Factors

JUST AS THERE ARE MANY WAYS to alleviate MS symptoms, there are numerous factors that can trigger an MS attack or worsen the condition. These will affect different people differently. (This chapter does not include those factors implicated in the causes of MS, which were discussed in chapter 3. Nor does it include mercury, the subject of the next chapter.)

These triggers include:

- Reactive foods and beverages
- Chemicals in food
- Stress—physical, emotional, psychological
- Heat and humidity
- Overexertion
- Trauma
- Smoking
- Environmental toxins
- Prescription drugs
- Vaccinations

❧ REACTIVE FOODS AND BEVERAGES

Consuming foods and beverages to which you have sensitivities is often a major factor in triggering an attack and in the progression of MS. (See chapter 4). You need to find which particular foods you are sensitive to, and give them up. However, there are some foods that seem to badly affect everyone with MS. These are alcohol, chocolate, and refined sugar and carbohydrates.

Alcohol

Alcohol can aggravate MS symptoms, which can make you look like a drunk even if you're stone cold sober. Alcohol can make coordination worse and may affect standing, walking, finger movements, eye movements, speech, and bladder control. Far from being a stimulant, alcohol acts as a depressant. It could well make you feel low, rather than high.

If you have the yeast infection candida—which thrives on yeast, fermented products, and sugars—alcohol will make it worse.

In some diets for MS (for example, the low-fat Swank Diet), alcohol is allowed in *small* quantities. If a glass of wine or sherry does not make you feel ill, you may find that there is no harm in drinking one occasionally. But if any kind of alcohol makes you feel worse (as it does me), it's better to avoid it completely.

In any event, a lot of alcohol can do you harm. It inhibits the conversion process of essential fatty acids, and nothing should get in the way of this vital process. Alcohol causes the amount of saturated fat in the blood to increase, and increases the need for vitamin B_1, pantothenic acid, and choline.

Many people have allergies to some of the ingredients in alcoholic drinks. Sugar, yeast, sulfites, and dozens of other flavorings and additives can legally be added to wine and other alcoholic beverages without any indication on the label, and mixed drinks usually add more sugar.

Unfortunately, alcohol is one of the most difficult things to refuse socially. Everyone expects everyone else to drink, and a glass of something is always being shoved in your hand at parties. However, if drinking alcohol makes you feel ill, you'd be wise to resist this kind of pressure. Insist on noncarbonated mineral water or unsweetened fruit juice. If you add a sliver of fresh lime or lemon, your beverage will look like a mixed drink and you'll get less pressure.

Chocolate (Cocoa)

There is a hypothesis that cocoa products are one of the foodstuffs most likely to cause adverse reactions in MS. Others are cola, coffee, and tea.

The adverse reactions may occur because people with MS are not able to metabolize chocolate properly. The theobromine found in cocoa needs the particular enzyme P450 (CYP) in order to be metabolized. There is some evidence that the P450 enzyme is abnormal in people with MS.[1]

This hypothesis, put forward by Dutch doctor Anna Maas, M.D., suggests that MS may be caused by an allergic or other adverse reaction to certain foods, mostly cocoa products, cola, and coffee. Many MS patients have one or more manifestations of other reactions to those foods, such as migraine, urticaria, or gastrointestinal disturbances. Dr. Maas has been successfully treating MS patients in Holland by taking them off chocolate and a long list of other foods. More specific information and interesting links can be found at Maas's website: www.msdietannamaasmd.com.

There has also been research showing that the incidence of MS coincides with the consumption of cocoa. When cocoa is introduced in a geographical area, the incidence of MS rises. The Swank Diet forbids cocoa and chocolate. There are some interesting postings on the web from people with MS who are convinced that cocoa—above all other foods—made them worse, and who got better when they gave it up.

....

Pat: Giving up Chocolate Gave Me Back My Life

Within three weeks of diagnosis in 1989 I was paralyzed and in a wheelchair, but now I feel wonderfully well without taking any drugs. What did I do? I gave up eating chocolate. I used to love eating chocolate and was even a bit of a chocoholic. But the minute I ate a piece of chocolate my head went numb. The feeling was so horrible that I went to see my neurologist about it, but he couldn't see any harm in my eating chocolates and told me to go on eating them, since I liked them so much. Luckily I didn't do that. I stopped completely. It breaks my heart when I see so many very sick people with MS, because I know they don't need to be like that if only they stopped eating the foods that are making them ill—especially chocolate.

The particular foods making *you* ill may not be the same ones affecting the next person with MS. However, there is one thing that is bad for *everyone* with MS, and that is chocolate! Every sweet, every cookie, sauce, pudding, ice cream, or drink with cocoa in it is bad for you. There's also hidden cocoa in cigarettes and cola.

When I eat or drink any of the things to which I'm sensitive, my MS symptoms get worse. In addition to chocolate and cocoa products, for me these particular foods are oranges and their juice, red wine, cola, fish, nutmeg, and monosodium glutamate (MSG). For others, it will be different foods. But chocolate is the worst one for me, and for everyone else with MS. When I stopped eating these things, my symptoms went away.

Before I worked out which foods were making me ill, I was in a wheelchair and paralyzed below the waist. I couldn't walk, talk, or swallow; my eyesight was very bad, I was constantly fatigued; and my head shook all the time. But after giving up all the foods that were bad for me, all these MS symptoms reversed. I can now walk, talk, and swallow; I don't suffer from fatigue; and my head doesn't shake. I really feel great!

When you have eaten something you are sensitive to, you are likely to get immediate or delayed symptoms—perhaps your legs stiffen, you suddenly get very tired, your walking gets worse, you experience pain, your bladder goes wrong, or any number of other symptoms. When that happens, you must ask yourself, "What have I eaten that could have brought on this symptom?" You must listen carefully to your body.

Refined Sugar and Carbohydrates

In the last twenty years, annual sugar consumption in the United States has increased to 160 pounds per person. The most obvious result is obesity, but sugar can also do a lot of damage in MS, and may be a contributory cause. Sugar can:

- Weaken the immune system
- Increase inflammation

- Create a sugar imbalance
- Cause free radicals in the bloodstream
- Interfere with the absorption of calcium and magnesium
- Weaken eyesight
- Impair the structure of DNA
- Upset minerals in the body
- Produce a rise in triglycerides
- Weaken the body's defenses against bacterial infection
- Make the body too acidic
- Put enormous stress on your hormones
- Increase levels of glucose and insulin
- Cause candida

When you crash from a sugar high, your adrenal glands kick in and release cortisol, a steroid-like substance, to help rescue you. Over time, your adrenal glands exhaust themselves trying to regulate your sugar levels, leaving you feeling washed out. This is likely to be playing a role in MS fatigue. You will feel much healthier if you cut out sugar and artificial sweeteners. Instead, get the sweetness you crave from fruits and sweeter vegetables, such as carrots and beets.

Refined carbohydrates, such as white processed flour, behave like refined sugar and have the same effect. They give a fast release of sugar, followed by a dip. They should be eliminated and replaced by complex carbohydrates.[2]

ᐒ CHEMICALS IN FOODS

Read labels like a hawk when you go food shopping, and ask what's been added to the food when you eat at restaurants. Avoid "fast food," which often has numerous additives and cheap ingredients. Unnatural, degraded, processed food may be a cause of degenerative diseases.

Chemical fertilizers, pesticides, and insecticides applied to fruit, vegetables, and crops while they are growing not only covers the outside, but actually grows into the crop and can't be removed by washing. Steroids and antibiotics are given to intensively reared livestock.

In the manufacturing process, a whole range of additives may be added to foods, including artificial colorings, flavorings, and preservatives. In the past few years the public has been alerted to the additives in manufactured foods, and a link has been established between certain additives in foods and hyperactivity in children. However, the additives in foods may also be affecting people who have MS. Chemicals in food and drink can produce allergic-type responses.

Even food that you think looks perfectly "natural"may have been polluted before it reaches you, the consumer. In fact, the more perfect the specimen of fruit or vegetable, the more suspicious of it you should be. Only fruit and vegetables that have been successfully protected (often by chemicals) will be picture-perfect.

Acrylamide

Watch out for acrylamide, a potent neurotoxin that can form in fries, chips, and other plant-based food when it's exposed to high temperatures for a long period of time. In 2002, scientists at Sweden's Stockholm University found that acrylamide forms from a heat-induced reaction between sugars (such as glucose or fructose) and asparagine, an amino acid found in carbohydrate-rich foods, and that it can cause damage to the nervous system. A few of the top culprits are French fries, potato chips, coffee, and breakfast cereals. The amount of acrylamide found in the fries in typical fast food restaurants often exceeds the safe limit recommended by government and international health bodies, and the FDA is considering issuing industry guidelines on reduction of acrylamide in food products.[3]

Monosodium Glutamate and Aspartame

Two particularly harmful additives are monosodium glutamate (MSG), often used in Chinese food, and the artificial sweetener aspartame. Both these are excitotoxins—amino acids that, quite literally, excite the nervous system and cause neurological damage. They may be a bigger culprit in MS than anyone has ever suspected. Excluding MSG and aspartame are central to Sue Ellen Dickinson's protocol to recovering from MS, as described in her book, *No More MS*.

They are often hidden behind ingredients such as hydrolyzed proteins, hydrolyzed oat flour, sodium caseinate, calcium caseinate, and yeast extract. Soybean extract is also rich in glutamate. Neurosurgeon Russell

Blaylock and other researchers have suspected for a long time that exci-totoxins can cause autoimmune disease, and their concerns have recently been supported by a study from the Albert Einstein College of Medicine in New York.[4]

How to Avoid Chemicals in Foods

Don't buy anything that is processed, especially not junk food. Whenever you buy anything in a can or a packet, at least read the label. If there are any additives, preservatives, colorings, or flavorings—don't buy it.

As a rule, always try to buy pure, fresh things instead of processed foods, and prepare your own meals. Even if they don't have preservatives in them, frozen and packaged meals are notoriously high in sodium. The fresher the food, the more "alive" it is. Frozen food will have lost some of its goodness and may have coloring in it, such as the bright green used on frozen peas.

However, if you have to choose between frozen and canned, always choose frozen. Metal particles can seep into canned foods and contaminate them. In addition, don't use aluminum or nonstick pans for cooking. Minute particles of aluminum or a pan coating can get into food prepared with these utensils.

If you can, switch to organic food. It is getting easier all the time to find places that sell organic food—not just organically grown fruit and vegetables, but also meat, poultry, bread, and everything else. Certified organic foods are free of all chemical fertilizers, pesticides, and artificial flavoring and coloring. There is great emphasis now on organic, fresh food, so take advantage of it. Ask your grocer to stock organic produce, and seek out organic stands at farmers markets.

⤳ STRESS

Stress is harmful because it puts your body into a constant state of fight or flight. The adrenal glands, located above the kidneys, release the stress hormone adrenaline. This accelerates heart and breath rate and blood pressure, and causes the liver to release more sugar into the bloodstream. Another hormone, cortisol, is then released, keeping blood pressure and blood sugar rates high, and keeping you alert. Although the body can cope with sudden stress, raised levels of these hormones and other chemicals produced during stress can, over the longer term, be damaging to health.

Cortisol can suppress the immune system and put you more at risk for autoimmune diseases, such as MS, or aggravate the condition. Cortisol is the hormone associated with feeling helpless and hopeless. Stress, together with an impaired hypothalamus–pituitary axis, has long been discussed as a factor in MS, and now there is plenty of hard evidence that acute stress affects people with MS. Many people will tell you that they went through a period of severe stress before MS was diagnosed, and that stress is a major trigger of attacks.

One definition of stress is not having the resources to meet the demands made of you. The more feeble your resources, the more stressful the demands feel. Resources mean both practical resources, such as money and equipment, and inner resources, such as strength of will and health. Obviously if you are ill your inner resources will be depleted, and demands that would not feel like stress to a well person suddenly become stressful. The more you can retain or regain your health and well-being, the better you will be able to deal with stress.

Attitude is also very important; one person's stress is another person's challenge. Your personality, or how you respond to a particular situation, is perhaps more relevant than the stressor itself. For example, some people get a thrill from taking off in an airplane, while others find it stressful. Some people love working on deadlines, while others seize up at the thought. If you can gain some insight into yourself and see what stress may be aggravating your symptoms, you could set about removing these stressors from your life and/or changing your attitude about them. Many people with MS identify themselves as having very short fuses, with a diminished ability to withstand even minor stress. If you can see that your reaction to stress is pronounced, you might benefit from counseling or psychotherapy.

✍ HEAT AND HUMIDITY

Many people with MS experience a temporary worsening of their symptoms when the weather is very hot or humid or they're running a fever, sunbathe, get overheated from exercise, or take very hot showers or baths. These temporary changes can result from a very slight rise in core body temperature, even as little as one-quarter to one-half of a degree, because an elevated temperature further impairs the ability of a demyelinated nerve to conduct electrical impulses. Heat intolerance can quickly bring on symptoms of fatigue, tremor, impaired cognitive function and memory, and blurred vision, known as Uhthoff's Symptom. All these can be reversed by getting cool.[5]

OVEREXERTION

One problem with MS is that many people—particularly the young and energetic—still want to do all the things they did previously, so they overcompensate and make themselves ill by overexertion.

Women with MS have, in my view, the toughest time because they are often expected to do three full-time jobs: go out to work, run the household, and be a mother. It's difficult enough for someone with MS to fulfill even one of these roles properly, let alone three. I've received letters from women that have made my blood boil. Even though the wife has MS, some husbands still expect them to cook, clean, look after the children, and earn income. Often they are called "lazy" if they don't visibly do all the chores, yet a woman with MS may feel so weak after a day at work that she's fit for nothing more than slumping in an armchair. Still, many of these women force themselves to cook a meal, clean the house, do the laundry, and so forth. The most likely place to suffer from overexertion is in the home. Fatigue is the likely result.

Many women receive this kind of unfair treatment from their families because they appear perfectly okay. Symptoms of MS, such as fatigue, are not as obvious as a limp or a hacking cough. However, worsening symptoms are almost inevitable if there is no let-up in the constant strain. The workload simply has to be shared, lessened, or both. This kind of situation may need relationship counseling or help from a social services agency. MS will almost certainly mean altering the traditional roles in your household, and it will take time to make the adjustments.

Overexertion may also be tied up with your work. Many people find that their work is simply not compatible with having MS. For example, a surveyor may not be able to continue climbing up on roofs. Two journalists I know could not continue traveling and meeting tight deadlines; a pilot had to forget about flying planes. The list is endless.

Once you have MS, your energy supply is much more limited, and you'll need to choose the best way to use it. It probably means setting your sights lower. It may also mean watching your contemporaries being promoted ahead of you.

It is particularly painful when MS strikes young people in their prime, which it often does. This is the age when people complete their education or make important strides in their chosen career or walk of life. Even if the illness is successfully stabilized, there will probably be some sacrifice regarding work. If your present job is strenuous or stressful, you'll have to decide if the price you'll have to pay in fatigue is worth it. If you continue working full-time in a demanding job, you may be too tired to do anything else when you come home. Young people who have not told their employers, associates, or even family members are particularly at risk of overexertion.

You may prefer to find part-time work, or change to a less demanding full-time job, even if it means stepping down a few rungs in the career ladder. You don't have to give up work altogether because you have MS—and to do so would be unnecessarily damaging to your self-esteem and self-confidence—but it's important to find a healthy balance between work and personal life.

TRAUMA

Patients with MS frequently relate the onset of the disease or a worsening in their symptoms to a traumatic episode in their lives. This may be a physical injury, such as a blow to the head with concussion, or a time of excessive stress, such as a divorce or bereavement.

There is controversy about the extent to which trauma is connected with MS. One school of thought is that a traumatic injury, such as whiplash injury to the neck, can produce a temporary alteration or breakdown in the blood-brain barrier. The hypothesis is that when the blood-brain barrier is opened by such an injury, deranged cells, known as T-lymphocytes, are permitted free passage from the bloodstream into the central nervous system, where they contribute to the development of MS plaques.

A recently published case study showed that correction of upper neck injuries may reverse the progression of MS. The research was performed by Erin Elster, D.C., an upper cervical chiropractic specialist working in Boulder, Colorado. She corrected chronic upper neck injuries in an MS patient, which may have stimulated a reversal of his MS symptoms.

"According to medical research, head and neck injuries have long been considered a cause of multiple sclerosis," said Dr. Elster. "But this is the first research to show that correction of those injuries can have dramatic effects on reversing MS."[6]

☙ SMOKING

Smoking is *terrible* for anyone with MS. One study found that people who smoke run twice the risk of developing MS. In particular, smoking damages the endothelial cells that form part of the lining of blood vessels. When damaged, these cells can react in a number of ways. In some cases the immune system, which normally fights off such bad agents as bacteria and viruses, can become "overactive," turning against the healthy cells of our own bodies. This is what happens in autoimmune diseases, including MS.

Damage to these endothelial cells can also lead to the blood vessels in the brain becoming leaky, allowing toxic substances to pass into the brain and cause damage. Normally, endothelial cells form a very tight barrier around the blood vessels in the brain and prevent toxic substances from entering.

Studies have also demonstrated that once you develop MS, smoking can make it worse. Toxic substances (heavy metals, allergens, pesticides, petroleum products and so on—see list on page 261) in tobacco and cigarette smoke strain the immune system by reducing antioxidants. This allows free radicals to form and react with important cellular components, such as DNA or the cell membrane, causing cells to function poorly or die.

Free radicals are highly reactive radicals that can start a chain reaction. Their chief danger lies in the damage they can do when they react with important cellular components. To prevent free radical damage, the body has a defense system of antioxidants, molecules that can safely interact with free radicals and terminate the chain reaction before vital molecules are damaged, but smoking drastically reduces these antioxidants. The more we introduce toxic substances into our bodies, the stronger these free radicals become; and the more we smoke, the fewer antioxidants our body defenses possess. This exacerbates problems or symptoms associated with MS. Smoking may also be a risk factor for transforming a relapsing/remitting course of MS into a secondary progressive one.

An American study published in the journal *Neurology* in 2009 showed that anyone with MS who had *ever* smoked for as little as six months had more destruction of brain tissue and brain atrophy than MS patients who never smoked. The smokers had more brain lesions and greater loss of brain volume, as well as higher scores on the disability scale, than MS patients with no history of smoking. Nonsmokers recorded an average disability score of 2.5, compared to 3.0 for smokers. (The Expanded Disability Status Scale ranges from 0—meaning no symptoms, a normal neurologic examination—to 10, which is death).

"Cigarette smoking is one of the most compelling environmental risk factors linked to the development and worsening of MS," said Robert Zivadinov, M.D., director of the Buffalo Neuroimaging Analysis Center where the research was conducted, and first author on the study.

"The biological basis of the potential link between smoking and MS has not yet been fully elucidated," Zivadinov said. "In addition to nicotine, cigarette smoke contains hundreds of potentially toxic components, including tar, carbon monoxide, and polycyclic aromatic hydrocarbons.

"In MS patients, smoking was associated with higher increased lesion burden and greater brain atrophy. Our results indicate that a wide range of quantitative brain MRI markers are affected by smoking in MS patients."

Results showed that smokers with MS had a greater breakdown of the blood-brain barrier, with nearly 17 percent more brain lesions—patches of inflammation in the sheath surrounding the nerve fibers that impair their function—than nonsmokers with MS, and also had less brain volume. Smoking was also associated with increased physical disability.[7]

In another recent study, it was found that smoking increased the risk of getting MS, made MS worse, and accelerated the progression from relapsing/remitting to a progressive course.[8]

Young people who start smoking before age seventeen may increase their risk for developing MS. In a study involving eighty-seven people with MS, among more than thirty-thousand people in a larger study, those with MS were divided into three groups—nonsmokers, early smokers (began before age seventeen), and late smokers (started at age seventeen or older)—and matched by age, gender, and race to 435 people without MS. Early smokers were 2.7 times more likely to develop MS than nonsmokers. Late smokers did not have an increased risk for the disease. More than 32 percent of the MS patients were early smokers, compared to 19 percent of participants who did not have MS.[9]

A List of Nasties in Cigarettes

A brief look at some of the main substances found in cigarettes shows why smoking is not only addictive, but also very harmful to your health:

Nicotine. A powerful addictive drug. It stimulates the central nervous system, which increases the heart rate and blood pressure. Nicotine is also used as an insecticide.

Carbon monoxide. A gas that displaces oxygen in the blood, resulting in less oxygen being available for use in bodily processes. Carbon monoxide is the toxic gas found in car exhaust fumes.

Benzene. A carcinogen (cancer-causing chemical) found in gas fumes.

Nitrosamines. Carcinogenic.

Ammonia. Used in anti-personnel spray (an irritant used in defense) and in cleaning products.

Formaldehyde. An embalming fluid.

Hydrogen cyanide. An industrial pollutant, also used as a method of legal execution.

Polycyclic aromatic hydrocarbons. Carcinogens also found in diesel exhaust and other combustion products.

ENVIRONMENTAL TOXINS

Some doctors working in the field of environmental and integrative medicine believe that degenerative diseases are a sort of slow poisoning of the human system, which turns it into a polluted, stagnant pond. Everyday things in our environment prove particularly toxic to some susceptible people who have a poorer ability to adapt than others. Case histories of some MS patients show that if they are exposed to certain environmental toxins their symptoms get worse, but when those toxins are taken away, the symptoms are alleviated.

These toxins include: mercury, which is such a significant poison for MS that an entire chapter will be devoted to the topic (chapter 18); airborne toxins such as fumes from car exhaust; agricultural toxins from pesticides; solvents and other chemicals in the workplace; as well as a huge variety of toxins in your own home.

Air Pollution

In places where there is air pollution, the MS exacerbation rate is higher. Research done in Finland and presented in 2001[10] showed that exposure to airborne particulates increases the exacerbation rate in multiple sclerosis patients. Peripheral microbial infections are known to increase MS exacerbations, according to Mervi Oikonen of the Aerobiology Unit at the University of Turku. Susceptibility to such infections of the airways increases with a rise in airborne particulates, through a complex of immune system and respiratory tissue changes.

Chemical pollutants that are particularly harmful for someone with MS are diesel fumes and lead from gas exhaust. Therefore, living in a city or near traffic-clogged routes is not optimal. These pollutants can also affect food sold in produce shops on main roads near traffic lights. If the fruit and vegetables are displayed outside on the sidewalk, they are bound to be contaminated with the toxins given off by the traffic.

Agricultural Toxins

Crop pesticides are also implicated in MS, as are sheep dips and other agricultural toxins. A landmark study carried out by the Environmental Research Center at the University of North Dakota and funded by the U.S. Department of Health claimed that chemicals routinely used by farmers can result in neurological disease, including MS.[11] The preliminary findings in a four-year study (unfinished at time of writing) show a link between pesticide exposure and neurological diseases—laboratory rats given pesticides developed brain damage and gut problems.

Researchers say they've also identified a disturbingly efficient way that pesticides may get into the human body. Dr. Patrick Carr, of the University of North Dakota, says there's clear evidence pesticide exposure at relatively low doses affects brain cells: "Some areas of the brain displayed physical changes—in other words, a loss of neurons in particular regions of the brain. In other regions of the brain you wouldn't notice a change in the number of cells present there, but now the cells that are present are expressing chemicals in different amounts, compared to normal rats." As an example, Carr found cells responsible for production of myelin were damaged or destroyed.

The researchers studied six common pesticides. Carr says some rats were given a single large dose, while others were injected with small doses over a nine-month period.

Workplace Toxins—Solvents and Other Chemicals

MS is more common among people who have worked with, or been exposed to degreasers, resins, solvents, and tannery chemicals.[12]

During the 1990s, Swedish researchers compared thirteen studies that evaluated the connection between solvents and autoimmune disease. The solvents included paint thinner and acetone, the substance used in nail polish remover. Ten of those studies indicated a significant relationship between organic solvent exposure and MS. All the analyses suggested that exposure to solvents increases the relative risk of developing MS.[13]

In 2002, a team of scientists in Norway analyzed the occupational health records of more than 57,000 workers over a sixteen-year period. They concluded that workers, such as painters, who were routinely exposed to solvents had a significantly greater incidence of MS than those not exposed to solvents in their jobs.[14] These results were compatible with the hypothesis that solvents are a possible risk factor for MS.

Acetaldehyde, used in the production of various products—mirrors, disinfectants, plastics, explosives, varnish, and food flavoring—can result in chemical poisoning. The type and severity of symptoms varies, depending on the amount of chemical involved and the nature of the exposure.

Toxins in Everyday Life

The place to find the most dangerous chemicals that can have an impact on your health is often your own home and backyard. Chances are that every single room in your home has things in it to which you could be reacting badly. Here are just some of the culprits:

- All solvents—for example, nail polish remover, correction fluid, glues, flip chart pens, dry cleaning fluid, gloss paint.
- Tap water contains chlorine, nitrates, fluoride, and polyphosphates.
- Aerosol sprays, such as furniture polish, air freshener, insect repellant,

perfume, and deodorant all use a liquid propellant. When you press the button, a spray of fine droplets of this propellant squirts out under the pressure of the gas in the can. This propellant liquid evaporates, leaving fine particles of the chemical in the air. The technical name for this kind of gas is halocarbon (carbon compounds that contain chlorine, fluorine, or bromine).

- Chemicals in cleaning agents, insect killers, and weed killers.
- Fumes from gas boiler, stove, or wood fires, if ventilation is poor.
- Particleboard and foam in furniture off-gas (slowly release) formaldehyde used in their composition. Formaldehyde is also found in the combustion products of natural gas, tobacco smoke, glossy magazines and books, and newspapers.
- Plastics off-gas toxins.
- Synthetic carpets and fabrics (carpets are also treated with insecticide in the manufacturing process).
- Cosmetics and toiletries made from coal tar products.
- Cosmetics and toiletries made with chemical colorants (beware of strong colors and scents).
- Toothpaste containing fluoride and coloring (fluoride interferes with a wide range of metabolic enzymes).

These chemicals can be inhaled through the airways, absorbed through the skin, or ingested. For example, undisolved dishwashing liquid on plates that haven't been rinsed properly can affect the stomach lining.

Unless you are obviously sensitive to these chemicals (for example, sneezing if someone uses aerosol hair spray), you may not be aware that the gases given off by these products are affecting you. In addition to the halocarbon vapor from aerosols and solvents, many common household products include acetone and ether. All of these gases dissolve into the air completely, leaving no haze. Even if you can't see them they may be having a toxic effect on you.

Other environmental pollutants include dust, house dust mites, mold spores, pollen, and cat and dog dander.

Nontoxic Alternatives

It is possible to find alternatives to all of the noxious chemicals mentioned. Organic produce retailers often offer household products, from biodegradable cleaning agents to beeswax candles. Your local natural foods store undoubtedly carries nonchemical cosmetics and toiletries, as do some pharmacies. Many household and bedding suppliers, even large retail chains, offer organic fibers and untreated products. An Internet search will reveal a wide assortment of options.

> *Water.* Install a water filter in your water supply system, either a whole-house system or one that functions as a designated tap on your sink. If you buy bottled spring water, try to purchase it bottled in glass or plastic #1, believed to be stable for single use. Although large plastic bottles used by water delivery companies are tempting as an environmentally sound reuse, the plastic they generally use is known to leach harmful bisphenol A, especially when exposed to heat from hot water and sun.
>
> *Cleaning agents.* Choose an ecological brand that is biodegradable. Or use ordinary baking soda or white vinegar.
>
> *Gas appliances.* Ideally, site the hot water heater outside the house; otherwise, house it in a casing that will prevent fumes from getting into the kitchen. If necessary, improve the ventilation.
>
> *Furniture.* Avoid particleboard, foam, and synthetic fabrics. Choose solid wood (unvarnished) and natural fibers in cushions, mattresses, décor, and furnishings.
>
> *Bedding.* Since you spend (hopefully) a third of your life in bed, it is important that your bedding be uncontaminated by chemical pollutants. Natural fiber mattresses can be quite expensive, so if that isn't an option, at least air your mattress (and box spring) with the windows open. Use a cotton, linen, silk, or bamboo mattress pad and bedding, organic if possible. Avoid foam pillows. Ideally, your bed frame should be metal or hardwood, although even a wood like pine gives off fumes, called terpenes, and foam and particleboard off-gas. Avoid polyester, which is a synthetic and part of the plastics family.
>
> *Clothes.* Avoid synthetic fabrics and wool, which is often treated

chemically. The best fabrics are untreated cotton, linen, silk, and bamboo. Avoid sending clothes to the dry cleaners, as dry cleaning fluid gives off fumes. If you have to dry clean certain garments, air them thoroughly outdoors before wearing them. You can probably safely ignore some "dry clean only" instructions on garment labels and wash by hand or on a machine's gentle cycle.

Cosmetics and toiletries. Use soap, shampoo, and personal care products without coloring or scent. Use non-chemical cosmetics with no additives (available at natural foods stores).

Toothpaste. Use bicarbonate of soda or a homeopathic brand.

PRESCRIPTION DRUGS

Your body is a living entity, so anything you put into it will have repercussions, positive and/or negative, visible and/or not. This is particularly true with prescription medications.

Oral Contraceptives

Dr. Ellen Grant, author of *The Bitter Pill,* believes that the increasing incidence of MS, especially among young women, can be linked to the pill, which has been in widespread use since the mid-1960s. The pill, among its many interactions with our systems, robs the body of zinc.

However, other studies indicate that the contraceptive pill may help protect against MS, finding that estrogen delays onset and eases the course of an MS-like disease in animals.[15] (See also chapter 15 on hormones.)

Overuse of Antibiotics

The overuse of antibiotics can deplete healthy gut flora and create a "perfect storm" for the formation of candida, very common in MS, which then needs to be treated. Some antibiotics, especially those for urinary tract infections, can bring on fatigue in MS as a side effect.

VACCINATIONS

There is considerable controversy over whether or not the mercury preservative, thimerosal, which was used in most vaccinations for many years and continues to be used in some, is a cause of chronic illness.

The view that vaccinations may be implicated in MS is shared by several holistic practitioners, including the late Dr. Robert S. Mendelsohn, editor of the journal *The People's Doctor*, who believed that MS is partly caused by doctor-produced (iatrogenic) procedures such as immunizations. Another practitioner who shares this view is Leon Chaitow, whose book *Vaccination and Immunization: Dangers, Delusions and Alternatives* was nominated as a book of the year by the U.K. *Journal of Alternative Medicine*.

It is probably safer to avoid any further vaccinations once MS is diagnosed, even though this may restrict visiting certain countries. If you can stand your ground against doctors, you might also consider saying no to all vaccinations for your children (except those for tetanus and polio).

HPV (Human Papillomavirus) Vaccine

Research in Australia has indicated that girls given the new human papillomavirus (HPV) vaccine, which protects against certain kinds of cervical cancer, might run a greater risk of getting MS or a similar demyelinating condition.

Doctors in Sydney reported five cases of "clinically isolated syndrome multiple sclerosis" that occurred within twenty-one days of vaccination with Gardasil. They suggest that this might be because the vaccine stimulates the immune system. However, they caution that no definitive conclusions can be drawn from this study about the risk of getting MS or any central nervous system disorder from being vaccinated with HPV, because teenage girls are at a susceptible age for getting MS in any event. The study did not find enough evidence to say whether or not adolescent girls with MS should have the HPV vaccine.[16]

Hepatitis B Vaccine

Some people with MS report that their first symptoms followed shortly after getting the hepatitis B vaccine. The scare began in France in the 1990s during the French government's hepatitis B vaccination campaign. Eight people were affected with MS-like symptoms following the hepatitis B vaccine, and proceded to sue the manufacturers. In 2001, a French court upheld a lower court ruling that found a link between hepatitis B vaccine and multiple sclerosis, and ordered the drug companies to pay an undisclosed amount of compensation to two women who contracted MS after receiving the vaccine.

The following year, a memo from the French General Directorate for

Health, dated February 15, stated that the hepatitis B campaign produced the "greatest series of side effects noted by pharmacovigilance since its creation in 1974." There was also testimony to the court from a Dr. Marc Girard claiming that crucial evidence on vaccine tolerance was withheld from doctors so as not to disrupt the vaccination drive.[17]

As reported in the journal *Neurology* in 2004, Boston-based researchers conducted a study of British patients that identified those who received the recombinant hepatitis B vaccine as three times more likely to develop MS. Out of 163 MS cases in the study, eleven developed symptoms of the disease within three years of getting the hepatitis B jab. The study's key finding was: "The proportion of cases that received at least one hepatitis B immunization during the thee years before the date of first symptoms was 6.7 percent, compared with 2.4 percent of controls. The odds ratio of MS for vaccination versus no vaccination was 3:1."[18]

Gemma: Hep B Theory Validated

I am convinced this happened to me, and have thought so almost since my diagnosis in '98, but unfortunately my theory has always been rubbished when suggested to anyone. Thank goodness someone in the medical profession has looked into the matter. I have gotten data from the Internet on the subject of recombinant hepatitis B vaccine that actually states one of the adverse effects can be MS.

Karen: Pursuing the Vaccination-MS Link

I used to be a nurse and first heard about the possible link between hep B vaccination and MS when learning how to give a vaccination. In 1997, I had full courses of hep B and tetanus concurrently over six months. Before that time I had been quite healthy, walking everywhere and riding my bike, but after that I kept getting infections. In 2000, I experienced rib/diaphragmatic spasms that were so excruciating I could hardly breathe. Looking back now, these spasms and the extreme fatigue I felt were probably my first symptoms of MS. Certainly more research into the possible connection between the hep B vaccination and the onset of MS symptoms is needed.

The U.S. Centers for Disease Control and Prevention lists numerous studies investigating the possible relationship between hep B vaccine and MS, and reports that the available evidence does not support it. Other studies have downplayed and denied any possible link between the hep B vaccine and MS. Most people with MS, and also in the general population, have not had the hepatitis B vaccination, so while it may be a factor in specific incidents, it's likely one of several.

Also, the World Health Organization (WHO) states there is no proven risk between the hepatitis B vaccine and MS. The following is from the National Center for Immunization Research in Australia, but the findings also apply elsewhere:

> The studies on hepatitis B vaccine and MS have been reviewed by the World Health Organization Global Advisory Committee on Vaccine Safety. They state that, "Multiple studies and review panels have concluded that there is no link between MS and hepatitis B vaccination." The WHO also affirm that the recent study by Hernán and colleagues does not provide sufficient evidence to link hepatitis B vaccination to MS, and does not justify discontinuation or modification of programs with hepatitis B vaccine. In addition, a review by the Institute of Medicine Immunization Safety Review Committee in 2003 found no link between hepatitis B vaccine and certain neurological disorders, such as MS. A systematic review from the Cochrane Vaccines Field in 2003 also found no evidence of an association between hepatitis B vaccine and MS. Recent statements by the U.S. Centers for Disease Control and the National Network for Immunization Information support this position.[19]

18

Mercury

MERCURY IS ONE of the most toxic metals on the planet. Of all the metals that can be toxic to someone with MS (and others), mercury is probably the worst. Yet mercury has been used in amalgam dental fillings for more than a century and continues to be used today. Norway, Sweden, and Denmark have banned mercury amalgam fillings.

There has been concern for some time that some of the mercury from dental fillings and other sources could be seeping into the body, causing serious health problems, including neurological ones.

Mercury does not get into our bodies only via dental fillings. Certain fish that have been swimming in contaminated waters—swordfish, shark, and king mackerel—contain high concentrations of mercury. Tuna, marlin, and red snapper are affected by intermediate concentrations of mercury. A study that looked at mercury levels in 1400 men from eight countries came to the conclusion that mercury counters the benefits of omega-3 if the fish source is contaminated. This study was in conjunction with cardiovascular disease but also has relevance to MS.[1]

Apart from fillings and contaminated fish, mercury can also get into the human body from air pollution, water, paint products, broken thermometers, coal-fired boilers, burning hazardous waste, and manufacturing processes. In agriculture, certain fungicides and weed killers contain mercury, perhaps explaining why MS is higher in farming, than fishing, areas. Mercury is also found in some industrial germicides. Some flu vaccines contained thimerosal, a mercury-based preservative, which has largely been withdrawn in the United States amid fears of a possible link to autism.

ᐛ DENTAL AMALGAM FILLINGS

Fillings combine pure elemental mercury (also known as quicksilver) with particles of silver, copper, and tin to form a putty-like mix. This mix—or amalgam—is placed in the tooth. The mercury hardens and holds these particles together, also stopping further decay in that particular area of the tooth.

Because mercury is mixed with these other metals, it was thought to be stable, but mercury in amalgam fillings is not stable. In emits vapor that can be breathed in, it can leak into the tooth or gum, and you can swallow minute particles of it with saliva.

Over the years, mercury seeps from fillings in minute amounts. How much mercury seeps out depends on how much dental plaque there is, the pH (acid-alkaline balance) inside the mouth, how old the filling is, how hard you chew, whether or not you grind your teeth, what food you eat, your individual body chemistry, and so on. There can be chronic low-level exposure for years.

There is also acute exposure to mercury vapor when you are having a filling put in or taken out. Elemental mercury gives off an easily breathed vapor when it is agitated, compressed, heated, or exposed to air at normal temperature. It goes through the thin bony plates at the top of the mouth, into the sinuses, into the orbit of the eye and the chambers of the inner ear where the body's balancing mechanism is situated. It also gets into the brain, which is so near the top of the mouth, and the temporomandibular joint, which controls the functions of the jaw. Mercury vapor also gets into the lungs.

Various biological processes inside the body transform mercury vapor into methylmercury, which is one hundred times more toxic than mercury vapor. Mercury vapor can mix with food. When it gets into the stomach, mercury can react with hydrochloric acid, resulting in the formation of mercuric chloride. This can create a shortage of hydrochloric acid, which means that food cannot be digested properly.

Even though your body will be excreting mercury, some mercury will remain in your system. How much mercury is there, where exactly it is, and what it is doing to you are far less easy to measure.

If you have several fillings in your mouth, you have a continuous source of mercury. Over time, there is a substantial loss, or leaching, of mercury from fillings, which means that mercury vapor is getting into the mouth and being ingested. This means that, in the course of a life span, mercury will accumulate in almost every organ.

All metals are reservoirs of energy called electrons, so if you have more than one kind of metal in your teeth, you have electricity in your mouth. If electrons can flow through some kind of conductor, then you have an electrical current. Saliva is an electrolyte (an aqueous solution with metal ions capable of transporting an electrical current). This electrical activity can cause corrosion of fillings. It can also affect the function of cranial nerves, which, in itself, can affect any system in the body.

WHERE DOES MERCURY INSIDE YOUR BODY GO?

Mercury can go everywhere, all over the body, upsetting intricate processes. Primarily mercury affects the central nervous system. In the immune system, mercury can inactivate the lymphocytes and alter the ratio between T-suppressor and T-helper cells.

Mercury can also accumulate in the kidneys, heart muscle, lungs, liver, brain, and red blood cells. Other areas where mercury can be stored are the thyroid gland, pituitary gland, adrenal glands, spleen, testes, bone marrow, and intestinal wall. Mercury can get through the blood-brain barrier and enter the nerve cells from the blood, destroying nerve tissue as it does so.

CONTROVERSY OVER AMALGAM FILLINGS

The people who have raised their voices against mercury in dental fillings and other sources have been a few brave dentists, nutritionists, environmentalists, and a handful of doctors in both the United States and the European Union. They have come up against the establishment line that mercury in dental fillings is safe.

For a long time, the official line on both sides of the Atlantic was that once the amalgam was in your mouth, the mercury was locked in and inert. However, many researchers have shown this not to be the case. The British

Dental Association now accepts that mercury vapor is released into the body from these fillings, but in such tiny amounts that the risk to health is insignificant. It does, though, accept that an estimated 3 percent of the population may be hypersensitive to amalgams and may have a reaction.

Recent FDA guidelines in the United States reclassified mercury amalgam fillings as safe for anyone who doesn't have mercury sensitivity, but that could likely be much of the population, and particularly those with MS. The FDA also cautioned that dental workers should use adequate ventilation to protect themselves from vapor, but did not mention the vapor danger to those who will inhale it daily in their mouths.

One leading British holistic dentist who strongly opposes the use of mercury fillings is Vicky Lee, who is also my own dentist and has removed all my amalgam fillings using a very careful protocol. Here, she sums up the case against mercury in fillings:

> The World Health Organization states that there is *no* safe level of mercury. All benchmark mercury doses are measured by the lowest amount of mercury present in the body that would present symptoms. Because mercury is a cumulative poison, very small doses will add up over many years to a much larger body burden of this toxic metal.

While the half life of mercury in the body is approximately one hundred days, its half life in the brain is at least twenty years. This is because both methyl mercury from fish and mercury vapor from fillings, being fat soluble, readily cross the blood-brain barrier. This then changes form and can no longer cross back into the blood to be detoxified. As a poison, mercury destroys the enzyme processes of neurotransmitters by locking on to the sulfhydryl ions and preventing them from working.

In 2003, researchers at the University of Rochester School of Medicine published a review of what is currently known about mercury toxicity. Among their findings:

- Mercury vapor, methyl mercury, and ethyl mercury all target the central nervous system and mercury vapor and ethyl mercury also target the kidneys. Inorganic (metallic) mercury primarily targets the kidneys and stomach.

- Chelators such as DMSA are effective in removing all forms of mercury from the body, but cannot reverse central nervous system damage.
- The allowable or safe intake of mercury has recently been reduced to 0.1 microgram/day per kilogram of body weight.
- The concentration of mercury in the brain, blood, and urine correlates with the number of amalgam fillings in one's mouth. The concentration increases markedly with increased chewing. Long-term use of nicotine gum by people with amalgam (silver) fillings may increase levels by a factor of 10, thus approaching occupational safety limits.
- There is concern, but no clear evidence, that mercury emitted from amalgam fillings may cause or worsen degenerative diseases such as ALS, Alzheimer's disease, multiple sclerosis, and Parkinson's disease.[2]

All of us have mercury in our bodies but some people are much more sensitive to it than others. Amalgam fillings contain approximately 50 percent mercury, most of which is bound to silver and tin, but some is present as metallic mercury, which vaporizes when exposed to the air.

Dentists are generally told that this is not released, but it is scientifically measurable. This mercury vapor is released in small amounts, but small amounts of a cumulative toxin become larger amounts over many years.

☙ SYMPTOMS OF MERCURY POISONING

Most people are not overtly affected by the mercury in their fillings, but there may be unseen consequences.

The symptoms of elemental mercury poisoning (the type of mercury in dental fillings) can include:

- Tremors
- Emotional changes (mood swings)
- Insomnia
- Neuromuscular changes (weakness, twitching)

- Headaches
- Disturbances in sensation
- Changes in nerve responses
- Performance deficits on tests of cognitive function

At higher exposures there may be kidney effects, respiratory failure, and death.

Effects of methylmercury poisoning (the type of mercury primarily found in fish) include:

- Impaired neurological development in children
- Impairment of peripheral vision
- Disturbances in sensations (pins and needles, numbness), usually in the hands and feet, and sometimes around the mouth
- Lack of coordination of movements, such as writing
- Impairment of speech, hearing, walking
- Muscle weakness

According to the many books and websites on the toxic effects of mercury (see Recommended Reading and Resources), mercury poisoning from any source can also bring on double vision, brain fog, tinnitus (ringing in the ears), chronic fatigue, and intense muscle spasms and tremors. As mercury is capable of damaging many tissues and organs, thereby disturbing their normal functions, it is not surprising that the list of symptoms also includes bleeding gums, increased salivation, a sour-metallic taste, facial paralysis, irregular heartbeat, depression, strong pains in the left part of the chest, retinal bleeding, dim vision, uncontrollable eye movement, irritability, vertigo, headaches, joint pains, pains in the lower back, stress intolerance, decreased sexual activity, and Bell's palsy.

In his book *Mercury Hazards to Living Organisms* Ronald Eisler writes: "Mercury is a known mutagen, teratogen (causes birth defects), and carcinogen (causes cancer). At comparatively low concentrations in vertebrate animals, it adversely affects reproduction, growth, development, behavior, blood and serum chemistry, motor coordination, vision, hearing, histology, and metabolism."[3]

URY AND MULTIPLE SCLEROSIS

for sure whether mercury triggers MS, or exacerbates MS, ...s MS. However, if it has triggered MS, this does not mean you can cure the patient by removing the mercury, but you can improve the symptoms by doing so.

Specific neurological symptoms include mild tremor; ataxia (lack of muscle coordination and irregular movement); sensory loss; visual problems; fatigue; numbness and tingling of hands, feet, or lips; muscle weakness progressing to paralysis; speech disorders; and general central nervous system dysfunction.

Mercury has a devastating effect on the body's immune system, particularly on the T cells, which have a vital part to play in cell-mediated immunity. This means that mercury can alter the body's defense mechanisms against infection and disease, and also make people more prone to allergy. In addition, mercury may cause vascular damage to the brain and spinal cord.

A study in Sweden involving thirty-four patients with central nervous system disorders indicated intoxication from dental amalgam. Tests showed pathological findings in 88 percent of these patients, of whom 60 percent showed an immune reaction to mercuric chloride. These findings support the view that chronic low level exposure to mercury can compromise or weaken the immune system and adversely affect the defense mechanisms of the body.[4]

Dr. Hal A. Huggins, an outspoken American opposed to mercury fillings (www.hugginsappliedhealing.com), states: "Should mercury attach to a nerve cell, the disease response could be called multiple sclerosis, Lou Gehrigs's disease, seizures, or several other things. If mercury attaches to an antibody in a nerve cell, it could result in lupus. If mercury attaches to a nerve fiber and causes the tau protein to disassemble and curl up in 'neurofibular tangles,' then the resultant autoimmune disease would be called diabetes."

Research into Mercury and MS

There has been a significant amount of research linking mercury with MS. In 1983, an article entitled "Epidemiology, Etiology, and Prevention of Multiple Sclerosis," written by Theodore H. Ingalls, M.D., of the Epidemiology Study Center in Framingham, Massachusetts, was published in the *Journal of Forensic Medicine and Pathology*.[5] It said, "Slow, retrograde seepage of ionic mercury from root canal or . . . amalgam fillings inserted many years previously, recurrent caries and corrosion around filling edges, and the oxidizing effect of the purulent response may lead to multiple sclerosis in middle age."

Dr. Ingalls, who has MS, went on to say that the world map of MS could be explained by the greater incidence of dental caries in the parts of the world where MS is high, and the lower incidence of dental caries in those parts of the world where MS is low. Obviously, the more dental caries there is, the more fillings there are. He suggested that perhaps dental caries is a precursor of MS. Dr. Ingalls thinks that lead (from car exhaust fumes and diesel fumes) may also be involved in MS.

A study in the late 1990s in the English county of Leicestershire backed up Dr. Ingalls's research. It found evidence of excessive dental caries among MS cases, compared with controls.[6]

In 1994, R. Siblerud and E. Kienholz of the Rocky Mountain Research Institute in Colorado investigated the hypothesis that mercury from amalgam fillings may be related to MS and came to the conclusion that these fillings may be a causal factor.[7] Dr. Siblerud also found a connection between depression and amalgam fillings.[8]

Another study in 1994 done in the Czech Republic found that the health of people with MS and other autoimmune conditions improved once their amalgam fillings were removed and concluded that mercury-containing amalgam may be an important risk factor for patients with autoimmune disease.[9]

However, it is only fair to add that several scientific studies have found no statistically significant evidence that mercury is implicated in MS, and some found only a mild connection. A thorough epidemiological study done in California in 2005 by Michael Bates concluded: "Limited evidence exists for an association with multiple sclerosis."[10]

❧ SHOULD YOU HAVE YOUR MERCURY FILLINGS REMOVED?

This question is not as simple as it seems. Some say you should, especially if you show a sensitivity to mercury. If you are sensitive to mercury, you should consider having your fillings out, but if you show no sensitivity to mercury, it wouldn't be worth the bother. Some dentists say leave the fillings in until you need dental work done on a particular tooth.

There are certain tests that can indicate whether you are hypersensitive to mercury. One, using an electrical meter, measures the electrical activity in the mouth. Other methods are the Vega test and applied kinesiology (see chapter 4, page 36). You would have to consult a private dentist or a clinical ecologist for these tests.

Hazards in the Removal of Fillings

The removal of fillings is not a simple matter, and the procedure can be hazardous. The danger with removing fillings is that mercury vapor is released into the air. There seems to be little disagreement that the highest levels of mercury vapor are reached during the insertion and removal of amalgam, with a potential danger to both the patient and the dental practitioner.

Some dentists are willing to place a full-mouth rubber dam in the mouth, which helps stop mercury vapor from escaping. As an extra precaution, they might take out only a few fillings at a time. This would make the removal process of a large number of fillings both lengthy and expensive.

However, there is no doubt that some people with MS have shown dramatic improvement after their fillings have been removed. Along with the more publicized cases of people with MS whose symptoms have disappeared after removal of mercury fillings, there are also cases where the MS has worsened after a full-scale removal of fillings.

The first thing to do is to find a sympathetic dentist, get yourself tested, and then make a decision. Even dentists who believe there is an overwhelming connection between mercury in your fillings and MS may think it is better to leave them alone if you show no sensitivity to mercury.

....

Tonya: Mercury Removal Brings Relief

A friend told me about a homeopathic dentist who could test for mercury leakage from fillings and then replace them safely. The testing involved placing a probe against each filling and taking a reading of the percentage of mercury leaking from it. Of my three offenders, two were extremely high (over 60 percent) and one not too bad.

This dentist prescribed various supplements to be taken two weeks before removal and a minimum of two weeks after. The essential ones were a multivitamin/mineral, vitamin C, glutathione, activated charcoal, and magnesium. I was also instructed to drink at least a gallon of water a day for four days after removal of amalgam.

The following month I was back to have the first filling removed. Now I was about to see for myself just how good my dentist was in the safe removal of mercury. I had been draped in a huge rubber bib, and now a tiny oxygen mask was placed over my nose, and my eyes were covered. I was told that the mercury was going to be drilled out, that there would be a lot of water and suction going on, and not to swallow. After about three minutes all the mercury was out.

Since then I have had all my mercury fillings removed. The effects on my MS have been a great improvement in energy levels, regular sleep patterns, a general sense of well-being that I didn't have before, and I no longer have that heavy legs feeling.

❧ MERCURY AND MICRONUTRIENTS

Many people with MS are low in zinc, manganese, chromium, selenium, and other trace elements. If you were to weigh the amount of mercury being placed in a large filling, there might be as much as one gram of mercury alone. There is potentially enough mercury in the mouth to interfere with the micronutrients in the body.

The amount of mercury released during the placement and removal of an amalgam filling is certainly enough to unbalance the very tiny amounts of micronutrients even in a healthy person, at least for a short time. When the body is short of essential micronutrients, it has a greater chance of being susceptible to mercury poisoning. If there is a shortage of zinc and selenium, mercury cannot bind to zinc/selenium protein complexes, and can rampage freely around the body, locked in because the mechanism for its removal is not there. The body may be attempting to rid itself of mercury through bile and sweat, but in fact may be reabsorbing mercury in the colon and through the skin, particularly if someone is not very physically active, cannot wash daily, or is constipated.

ᕯᕗ MERCURY AND CANDIDA

There seems to be a relationship between the presence of dental amalgam and the body's ability to cope with the yeast, *Candida albicans*. Candida is considered normal flora, but when the body's immune mechanisms are impaired, it can increase until it produces disease-like symptoms. If you have mercury in your body and are sensitive to it, candida organisms are resistant to treatment. Once you eliminate the mercury, however, candidiasis is more amenable to treatment.

ᕯᕗ GETTING RID OF MERCURY

If you have your amalgam fillings taken out, this will eliminate only 50 percent of the mercury in your system. Amalgam removal should definitely be followed up with one of the various nutritional protocols to get rid of the other 50 percent.

Oral Chelation Therapy

Oral chelation therapy can help detoxify the body and replace essential nutrients that may be inactivated by low level, chronic exposure to mercury and other metals. There is also an intravenous chelation therapy but it hasn't been approved by the FDA.

Chelation simply means latching on to something. Chelation agents chemically bond with heavy metals or toxins in the body and carry them out through its waste products. For this process you'll need a multivitamin and mineral product that also contains the amino acids cysteine and methionine, which are particularly effective at latching on to toxic minerals, such as lead or mercury. Once this latching-on process has happened, vitamin C (1,000 mg, three times daily) will help to excrete these toxic metals from the body. Onions and garlic are also valuable in detoxifying the body, but should be avoided if you are on homoeopathic remedies, because they'll act as an antidote.[11]

Chelation Protocol

There are different chelation protocols and ideally this should be done under the supervision of a trained practitioner.

The nutrients that play a part in oral chelation include:

- *Cysteine.* Has a specific affinity for mercury and will bind with it, allowing excretion from the body. Vitamin C must be taken with cysteine at a ratio of 3:1.
- *Glutathione.* A water-soluble antioxidant and free radical scavenger composed of the amino acids cysteine, glutamic acid, and glycine. Serves as storage and transport vehicle for cysteine. Suggested dose is 50 mg twice daily.
- *Vitamin C.* Scavenges free radicals caused by mercury. Suggested dose is 1,000 to 3,000 mg daily.
- *Vitamin E.* Scavenges free radicals and can reduce toxic effects of mercury. In lab tests reduced chromosomal breakage caused by mercury. Suggested dose is 100 to 400 IU daily.
- *Selenium and molybdenum.* Some studies have shown they reduce toxic effects of mercury. Do not exceed 2,000 mg of selenium a day, as it can be toxic. Take from 25 mcg up to 500 to 1,000 mcg of molybdenum a day, as your practitioner advises.
- *Zinc.* Can be displaced by mercury. A vital trace element that latches on to mercury and escorts it out of the body. Suggested dose is 20 to 50 mg a day.
- *Magnesium.* Supports activity of enzymes systems. Must be balanced with calcium in a ratio of approximately 2:1, calcium (most absorbable as calcium citrate) to magnesium. Suggested dose is 100 to 200 mg per day.
- *Rutin.* A bioflavonoid that has a specificity for binding to mercury and helping to remove it from the body.
- *Acidophilus.* Friendly bacteria in the intestinal flora that may play a significant part in determining the excretion rate of mercury.
- *Vitamin D.* Helps remove mercury safely by radically increasing the amount of intracellular glutathione. Can also inhibit the synthesis of nitric oxide synthase, suggesting a role in brain detoxification.
- *Vitamin B_6.* Helps with detoxification of mercury. Suggested dose is 50 to 200 mg daily. B vitamins should be taken in balance to each other.
- *Calcium pantothenate or pantothenic acid.* Also called vitamin B_5. Coenzyme A, which is also a cofactor in adrenal function, is synthesized from pantothenate and can be suppressed by mercury.

It is an acyl compound and very good at bonding with toxins for removal. Pantothenic acid is water soluble and should be taken if fillings are removed. Suggested dose is 100 to 400 mg daily.

- *Vitamin B₁* (thiamine). Important for cellular respiration and metabolism, and facilitates functioning of enzymes. Particularly useful in repairing the metabolic cycle so the body can more efficiently use coenzyme A and transport fatty acids to the mitochondria—the power centers of each cell. It is in the mitochondria that glucose and fatty acids are oxidized to generate the energy that powers us. Suggested dose of thiamine is 50 mg, morning and evening. However, if you find vitamin B stimulating, take the second dose in the afternoon. It should be taken in a B-complex tablet.

Top Ten Tips to Being Mercury Free

British holistic dentist Vicky Lee advises the following guidelines to help lower the burden of mercury in your body and increase its excretion rate:

1. *Don't take any more mercury into your body.* While there is no absolute evidence that mercury as a toxic metal is involved in the development of MS, it is common sense to keep away from this neuro-psychological toxin. This means no more amalgam fillings and no fish contaminated with mercury. At least 95 percent of the mercury in fish can go to the brain and neurological tissue. Choose Alaskan fish or sardines.

2. *Use caution when removing amalgam fillings.* Because mercury vapor is released when amalgam fillings are removed, fillings must be removed very carefully. There is a simple device that the dentist can slip over the tooth, called a clean-up. This sucks away all the fragments of amalgam, the water mist of the drilling, and mercury vapor. Without this device, the released mercury vapor would be inhaled, and 85 percent of inhaled mercury vapor enters the blood and crosses the blood-brain barrier.

   Alternatively, a rubber dam may be placed over the tooth, effectively externalizing the tooth from the mouth so no debris can enter the oral cavity. Be sure the nose is covered and you are not breathing this vapor.

3. *Maintain effective zinc levels.* This can easily be done by taking the zinc taste test,* which is cheap and effective. You need zinc and selenium to help eliminate mercury from the body, but zinc is easily lost from the body, or—depending on your diet—may not be absorbed properly. Both zinc and selenium bind with methionine and mercury to make mercury/zinc/seleno methionate, which is then excreted.

   Zinc and selenium should not be taken in excess. Do not take zinc supplements every day or the body will get used to getting zinc from supplements rather than from food. Some people may get sufficient zinc by eating zinc-rich foods, such as shellfish, meat, and pumpkin seeds.

   If very deficient, take 50 mg elemental zinc at night before sleep, only until the zinc taste test becomes normal. If mildly deficient, take 15 mg elemental zinc before sleep at night. Iron is preferentially absorbed over zinc, so taking zinc away from meals is most effective. Spinach, bran, and chocolate contain natural chemicals that bind to zinc and prevent its absorption.

4. *Maintain selenium levels.* Selenium levels can be self-monitored through hair analysis, which gives a good picture of nutrient status over a three-month period. A hair analysis will also monitor methylmercury, but only in the form it appears in fish, not dental fillings.

5. *Eat sulfur-rich foods.* Sulfur binds with mercury. Sulfur-rich foods, such as egg yolks and beans, are excellent sources of sulfur amino acids, which help detoxify the body of mercury. Onions and garlic also contain sulfur.

6. *Take MSM (methylsulfonylmethane) supplements (organic sulfur).* This compound used to be more present in foods and water. In its natural form, the precursor is made by ocean plankton. It evaporates into the atmosphere, changes to MSM, falls to earth in rain, is taken up by plant life, and consumed by us.

---

*For the zinc taste test, dissolve one gram of zinc sulphate in a quart of purified water and hold a sip in your mouth for ten seconds. How unpleasant, strong, and immediate the taste is will determine your degree of zinc deficiency, with zero taste sensation indicating the greatest deficiency. (Do not eat or drink for one hour before, as it could influence the results.)

7. *Take vitamin C.* Vitamin C combines with mercury to make mercury ascorbate, which is then excreted in the urine. Take 1000 mg a day, ideally as magnesium ascorbate.

8. *Take magnesium.* Magnesium levels are commonly deficient in MS, and the presence of mercury has been shown to disturb magnesium levels. Magnesium is needed for muscles to relax (calcium is needed for muscles to contract), and 70 percent of the body's enzymes need magnesium to work. Magnesium-rich foods are seeds, grains, and dark green vegetables. An excellent form is in juices and chlorella.

9. *Take epsom salts—magnesium sulphate.* Epsom salts are absorbed through the skin and help with detoxification. Use a cupful per bath, in tepid water. Soak for ten minutes and then rest for at least half an hour. This helps the detoxification process.

10. *Take chlorella.* The detoxification of mercury takes place in the liver, and mercury is then excreted in the bile. Unfortunately, however, it can be reabsorbed in the intestines on the way out. It is, therefore, important that the diet contains fiber or gels, such as pectin, seaweed, or chlorella, to bind to the excreted mercury and prevent its reabsorption.

19

Detoxing the Body

DETOXING WILL NOT ONLY HELP to reverse the symptoms of MS, but also give you more energy, brighter eyes, a clearer brain, and greater zest for life. It will also improve your mood and sleep, improve your skin, and help you maintain your appropriate weight.

The aim of physical detoxing is to eliminate toxicity and inflammation. It involves cleansing your gut, colon, liver, and gallbladder; toning up the kidneys; and purifying the lymphatic system and blood.

This can be done via herbal cleanse, juice fasting, pure water fasting, supplements, and products that help cleanse the liver and kidneys, and colonic irrigation. It can be maintained by changing to a healthy, junk-free diet. Some health care systems, such as ayurveda and naturopathy, specify detoxification to bring your body back into balance so it can heal itself. During the first few days of a detox program, you may experience discomfort due to sudden withdrawal from the foods you are used to, and the mobilization of accumulated toxins in your body. Symptoms can range from headaches, fatigue, and sore muscles to skin eruptions. All of these subside.

CANDIDA CLEANSE

Naturopaths and others believe there is a correct order to detoxifying. Some believe that the first thing is to eliminate candida, and to do this you need to go on a candida cleanse. You may also be prescribed Nystatin by a physician, to get rid of any fungal infection. Natural products helpful in candida cleanse include pau d'arco tea, berberine sulfate, caprylic acid, and garlic. There are also commercial candida cleanse products, such as Rainbow Light, available at Amazon.com and elsewhere.

⇜ DIGESTIVE SYSTEM

Your digestive system is the next thing in line for an overhaul, and that means giving up junk foods and eating a healthy diet. Digestion starts in the mouth with the saliva and teeth, so be sure to chew all food properly. Digestive enzyme supplements will also help with digestion.

⇜ COLON CLEANSING

Colonic irrigation and enemas will clean out the colon and bowel of old fecal matter. Constipation is very unhealthy, and for good health, you need to have at least one bowel movement every day. Personally, I find that a good daily probiotic supplement does the trick. Recommended products to keep regular include Naturalax 2 or 3 (Nature's Way), magnesium citrate (Metagenics), aloe vera juice, and triphala, an intestinal stimulant high in vitamin C. Some formulas include combinations of these. Also helpful are psyllium husks and flax seed.

⇜ LIVER AND GALLBLADDER CLEANSING

The liver is the largest internal organ and works constantly to detoxify the body from external toxins, as well as those produced in normal metabolic processes, such as breathing and eating. If the liver is stressed, all other organs start to dysfunction. In order for the liver to detoxify efficiently, it is very important to have a clear colon. So it's essential to do the colon cleanse before the liver cleanse.

Cleansing herbs for the liver include milk thistle, dandelion root, artichoke leaf, beet root, and root ginger.

⇜ CLEANING THE BLOOD AND KIDNEYS

The kidneys' job is to process nearly forty-eight gallons of blood every day. They filter, cleanse, rid the body of toxic wastes, and reabsorb nutrients and water. What they cannot use they excrete in the roughly one to two quarts of urine produced every day. When kidney and liver function is sluggish, toxic waste cannot be fully flushed from the body and recirculates in the bloodstream.

Inadequate drainage of toxins through the liver and kidneys can cause a buildup of toxicity, which can cause extensive free-radical damage, poor cell function, and disrupted energy production by the mitochondria in the cells. This leads to increased lactic acid and more toxicity with symptoms of fatigue, pain, sickness, poor memory, brain fog, mood swings, tingling/ numbness, and balance problems. Also, the brain gets damaged by toxins and free radicals because it can't get enough oxygen.

An overload of toxins makes the entire urinary tract more prone to infection. Normal kidney function may be disrupted, resulting in water retention, kidney stones, and mineral deficiencies.

Symptoms of sluggish kidneys include fatigue; a need to urinate frequently, especially at night; a decrease in amount of urine, or hesitancy in urination; swelling of the ankles, feet, and legs; puffiness around the eyes; low mood and mood swings; agitation; tension; irritability; difficulty concentrating; slow, sluggish movements and restless, heavy legs; and decreased sexual interest and erectile dysfunction.

Protein increases metabolic waste, which is something the kidneys must remove from the body, so to improve kidney function, restrict protein. Identify your food sensitivities and avoid chemicals and food additives. Maintain calcium, iron, and magnesium levels. Magnesium deficiency can have a direct effect on kidney function because of its link to high blood pressure, so it's important to eat magnesium-rich foods. Good sources of magnesium are green vegetables, nuts, seeds, and whole grains. Also, chew food well—this helps digestive enzymes to break food down.

To help cleanse the blood, drink red clover tea. Red clover is recognized as a detoxification herb and blood cleanser.

∾ LYMPHATIC DRAINAGE

The main task of the lymphatic system is to remove waste, so it needs to be stimulated to keep garbage from accumulating. Inactivity makes lymph drainage sluggish.

Good ways to help stimulate lymphatic drainage are daily exercise, manual lymphatic massage, daily dry skin brushing with brush movements up toward the heart, and deep breathing exercises.

ᴥ IMPROVING BLOOD CIRCULATION

Blood circulation is improved by exercise, ginkgo biloba, ginger, hawthorn berry, and niacin; also, oxygen therapies like hyperbaric oxygen therapy. Liquid oxygen can also be taken.

ᴥ ELIMINATING PARASITES

Parasites are organisms that live within the gastrointestinal tract but can also get into the liver, stomach, and brain. Parasites feed off the food we eat, as well as bodily tissues and cells. The body can be host to more than one kind of parasite at a time, including pin worms and microscopic organisms called *Giardia lamblia*. Parasites are constantly coming in to us—from exotic foods, improperly washed produce and grains, raw food, undercooked meat, contaminated water, pets, insects, soil, open cuts, and chemical toxins and pollutants.

There is a paradox about parasite infection and MS. You might think that if you have parasites, you would be better if they were eliminated. However, a study done in 2007 found that parasites might actually benefit people with MS by decreasing the number of inflammatory T cells. The study authors say: "Parasites may lead to increased regulatory T cell numbers or activity, either by generating new cells or by activating/expanding existing cells."[1] Other scientists have also claimed that getting infected with such things as parasites might help protect people against autoimmune disease, whereas excessive cleanliness and hygiene (the Hygiene Hypothesis) can do the opposite.

However, some alternative health practitioners think that parasites are very harmful, may be a cause of MS, and need to be eradicated. The leading proponent for the eradication of parasites in MS was Canadian medical scientist Dr. Hulda Clark. Of MS, she said:

> It is caused by fluke parasites reaching the brain or spinal cord and attempting to multiply there. Any of the four common flukes may be responsible. Kill them immediately with your Zapper [see page 290] and the herbal parasite program. They cannot return unless you rein-

fect yourself. Stop eating meats, except fish and seafood. All meats are a source for fluke parasite stages, unless canned or very well cooked. . . .

The most important question you must be able to answer is, "Why did these parasites enter your brain and spinal cord?" When the brain contains solvents, it allows flukes to multiply there. The solvents xylene and toluene are common brain solvents always seen in MS cases. Evidently these solvents accumulate first in the motor and sensory regions of the brain, inviting the parasites to these locations.

Xylene and toluene are industrial solvents used in paint and thinners. [They are] also a pollutant of certain carbonated beverages (I found it in 7-Up, ginger ale, and others that I tested). Stop drinking them.

All MS cases I have seen also harbor Shigella bacteria in the brain and spinal cord. These come from dairy products. They are manure bacteria. Be absolutely meticulous about sterilizing dairy products. Even one teaspoon of unsterilized milk could reinfect you. Not even heavy whipped cream or butter is safe without boiling. Kill bacteria every day with a Zapper. Shigellas produce chemicals that are toxic to the brain and spinal cord. Eliminating Shigellas brings immediate improvement.[2]

Dr. Clark believed she eradicated parasites by using her Zapper. Other methods put forward to get rid of parasites include antiviral herbs or drugs, diet change, reduced contact with chemicals, and regular liver cleanses.

The diet must exclude all foods to which you show intolerance. Herbs used to combat parasites are artemesia (wormwood), berberine, grapefruit seed extract, gentian, black walnut, and garlic. These should be prescribed by a natural health practitioner. There are some anecdotal reports of people with MS reversing their symptoms with this protocol.

Those who believe that parasites are harmful to people with MS say that parasitic infection can irritate the lining of the intestines and be a cause of leaky gut syndrome, which enables toxins and undigested food molecules to get into the bloodstream. A particular believer of the parasite theory is Gina Kopera M.H., author of the book *Cure Yourself Naturally*. I have not tried the Zapper or the Dr. Clark protocol myself.

The Zapper

Hulda Clark believed parasites are most effectively and safely treated with a particular hertz sound frequency generated by a small machine she invented, called a Zapper. This is set at a 30 KHz frequency at a voltage of about 5 volts. This energizes the white blood cells to attack the parasites, which are then eliminated from the body.

To use the Zapper, you hold the copper rods in your hands (or use the optional wrist straps), turn on the power, select the desired frequency, and let it run for seven minutes. When the time is done, turn the power off, wait twenty minutes, and repeat twice. (This can vary slightly from patient to patient.) The harmless sound waves are passed through the body repeatedly over three months and eventually kill all the parasites without any damage or side effect, other than perhaps a slight tingling at first. The healing process after the parasites have gone may take up to two years. There is no test to prove if the parasites have died. For the very ill, Dr. Clark recommended zapping eight times a day, or even continuous zapping, over one month.

Some people with MS report improvements in many symptoms as inflammation and cell damage is repaired and parasites begin to die off: balance and sleeping patterns improve, numbness and tingling diminishes, and constipation is alleviated. Some practitioners recommend doing a liver cleanse after completion of treatment with the Zapper.

For more about Dr. Clark's work, please visit www.drclark.net. For more detailed information about, or to purchase, the Zapper, see www.huldaclarkzappers.com.

Patricia: Lightening My Toxic Burden

I called a nutritionist who put me on Hulda Clark's parasite cleanse. I had not been tested for parasites, but figured it couldn't hurt and might help. This cleanse is relatively simple, and involves taking black walnut tincture, along with ground clove and wormwood capsules three times a day on an empty stomach.

I also saw a naturopathic M.D. who tested me for toxicity. Results showed evidence of an increased toxic burden, though not specifically related to heavy metals. He put me on Zeolite, which removes heavy metals, such as lead and mercury; and other toxins, such as pesticides, which could be triggering and exacerbating the disease. Zeolites are a group of natural volcanic minerals with a very unique cage-like structure, allowing them to trap and safely eliminate toxins from the body.

Zeolite is an easy-to-take liquid. Ten drops are put into the mouth three times daily to start, and then the dose is lowered after a time determined by your health practitioner. I am presently down to five drops, three times a day.

ꙮ JON BARRON'S DETOX

Some people with MS have successfully followed the detox protocol set out by Jon Barron, whose formulas, including Detoxifier Formula, Metal Magic, Liver Tincture, Liver Tea, and Blood Support, are sold by Baseline Nutritionals. His detox program includes intestinal cleansing, detoxification, and rebuilding and cleansing the liver and blood. His overall health program also includes many of the techniques put forward in this book, including changing your diet; taking probiotics, enzymes, vitamins, minerals, antioxidants, and herbs; drinking plenty of water; exercising; correcting any hormonal imbalances; and switching your thoughts from negative to positive. More information is available at www.jonbarron.org.

Frances: Colon Cleanse for a Cleaner Machine

In 2007, I saw Sue Ellen Dickinson's website, www.NoMoreMS.com, and read her book. I had tried many alternative approaches without success and was feeling pretty desperate. Sue Ellen followed aspects of Jon Barron's book, *Lessons from The Miracle Doctors,* together with his Baseline Nutritionals recommendations for MS. This program was much more than a regular detox. Not only does it target specific bodily functions (such as those of the liver, colon, and blood) it also addresses problems such as viruses, inflammation, and a compromised immune system.

I started with Barron's Colon Detoxifier, Super Viragon, Metal Magic, Probiotics, Digestive Enzymes, and Colon Corrector capsules. Colon detoxing was very gentle and easy. I personally found Colon Corrector too strong and instead used triphala with rose from Maharishi ayurveda products—two to three tablets each evening before bed.

Next came the liver cleanse. Each day begins with eight fluid ounces of pure water. This is followed by a liver-flush drink made in a blender with citrus juice (I used grapefruit), water, lemon juice, garlic, ginger root, and olive oil. The olive oil is gradually increased each day. You follow this with Liver Flush Tea, which alleviates any slight feelings of nausea you may have. You are urged to drink as much of this pleasant herbal tea as you like during the day.

During the liver cleanse you avoid all oils (even flax seeds), other than the olive oil in the drink. You literally starve your body of oils and fats for around twenty-four hours. It's important to take Liver Tincture three times daily, in water or juice. Barron encourages taking Blood Support tincture (to cleanse the blood) at the same time.

Every day of the liver cleanse you drink a lot of vegetable and fruit juice, and on days one and five you can have a raw vegetable salad for lunch. I personally had exacerbated MS symptoms (incontinence, exhaustion, collapsing legs/torso) during the liver cleanse, but it was impossible to tell whether this was a healing crisis or part of my normal roller-coaster MS ride.

On days two to four of the liver cleanse you have potassium broth. The high level of potassium flushes the system of toxins, unwanted salts, and acids—while giving you a boost of minerals and vitamins. Potassium broth is very warming and sustaining, though I found it wiped me out MS-wise.

As yet there has been no dramatic change as there was for Sue Ellen, but as she says, "There isn't any one specific thing that's going to fix the problem. There's no magic bullet." My starting point was very different from hers.

Hopefully the detox program has benefited my health in general. Part of my rationale for doing this was that if my insides are functioning better, all the supplements and other products I take, all the good food I eat, will be more effective.*

---

*Now with a severe intention tremor, Frances reports that she would need even more help to prepare and juice all the organic vegetables, make the special broth, and measure out tinctures and drinks. Although invaluable for overall health, and one of the best things she feels she's done for her MS, she found it exhausting and time-consuming to implement. She looks forward to seeing if it has a tangible, long-term effect by repeating the cleanse, ideally at least several times a year.

ᐎ FASTING

Fasting (also called therapeutic fasting) reduces inflammation, stops the intake of food-derived toxins, and allows the digestive tract to rest and restore its structural integrity. Fasting leads to detoxification and improvement in organ function. It accelerates the healing process and allows the body to recover in a dramatically short period of time. Paradoxically, fasting boosts suppressed immune function but also suppresses overactive immune function. During a fast the body seems able to get the immune system back into balance.

Different types of fasting include juice fasting, limited to homemade fruit and vegetable juice and water, which has met with good results in some people with MS. Some prefer an absolute fast in which only pure water is taken. Fasting should ideally be done under professional supervision and in a healing environment. Short fasts of up to three days are ideal.

Crystal: Fantastic after Fasting

Fasting is the number one thing that gets me back on track when I make a mistake and feel like crap. It seems to stop things in their tracks. I like it as a general catchall treatment because fasting can help regardless of what the initial trigger is—stress, virus, mistakenly eating something wrong, and so on. I think it's partly the leaky gut issue, and partly the rest from digestion that it gives my body, so it can take care of other stuff.

I've gotten into a regular habit of doing short, water-only fasts and recently completed a ten-day master cleanse that had me literally on top of the world. Well, except for the couple of days when I hit heavy detox. That was pretty yucky, but as soon as my body caught up with clearing the toxins I felt great again. I had spent many months reading about fasting and debating with myself whether to try it. Sooooooo glad I did!

❧ OTHER METHODS OF CLEANSING

- *Ionic cleansing.* Feet are placed in a bowl of water with the ionic device between the feet and near your ankles. The device produces positive and negative ions that accelerate the speed by which toxins are drawn out of the body.
- *Infrared sauna and steam.* Steam baths and saunas are excellent, but infrared saunas are 20 percent more effective in removing toxins. These can be infused with cleansing oils or herbs. They open the pores and bring impurities to the skin's surface, where they can be washed away.
- *Products that detoxify metals and chemicals.* These include Bio-Chelat Heavy Metal Chelator and bentonite clay, which is used in a foot bath.
- *Juicing.* Freshly juiced organic fruits and vegetables not only help to rid the body of toxins, but also supply antioxidants. Fresh fruit and vegetable juices clean out dead cells and flush fatty deposits and toxins, allowing them to be washed out of the body via the liver and kidneys. Juice can energize the body and clear the mind. Vegetable and citrus juice restores the pH balance of the body, putting its basic biochemistry back in balance.

....

Isabelle: Daily Juice

My new partner and I have just started juicing and endeavor to have one to two glasses a day. In the next few months we plan to upgrade our centrifugal juicer to a masticating juicer. These machines retain the enzymes in the plants, providing a more medicinal, healing juice. I don't eat much fruit because of the high sugar content but vegetables are my lifeline! We're only eating organically grown produce now and sometimes I really can feel their powerful energy.

....

- *Pure water.* Drink about eight glasses a day. It is better to drink between meals, rather than with meals.
- *The water cure.* Some think that MS and some other conditions are caused by prolonged chronic dehydration, which will improve

once that situation is remedied. F. Batmanghelidj, M.D., wrote *Your Body's Many Cries for Water* on that subject.

The water cure involves drinking half your body weight of water in ounces daily. So if you weigh 180 pounds, you need to drink ninety ounces of water. Divide that into eight or ten units throughout the day. Use one-fourth teaspoon of sea salt for every quart of water you drink. Drink only pure water. Don't drink tea or coffee.

- *Master Cleanse.* The Master Cleanse involves drinking a lemon juice concoction made from freshly squeezed lemon juice, organic maple syrup, cayenne pepper, and filtered water. No solid food is allowed during this cleanse.

Becky: Feeling Great after a Master Cleanse

With the Master Cleanse, the difference was unbelievable. I had heard stories but thought it too good to be true. The amount of energy I had was unreal . . . I cleaned my carpets, got the laundry and cleaning all caught up, and never felt as if I was fasting. The only time I felt bad was days six and seven, when I hit a major stage of detox. Once my body caught up with clearing all the toxins, I felt great again. I did ten days this time, and I'm planning a twenty-day Master Cleanse in the fall. If you are having fatigue, you will probably feel better on it.

- *Sweating.* This is a good way to help eliminate toxins. Methods include sauna (see previous page), eating cayenne pepper, and exercising. Some industrial toxins and pesticides can leave your body only through the sweat glands.
- *Naturopathic cleanse.* Naturopathy includes regular fasting, and also moving away from acidic foods to an alkaline-rich diet, to normalize the pH of body fluids. It can also involve eating superfoods, such as green barley, wheat grass, and bee pollen. Nutrients that have detoxification properties include garlic, turmeric, and watercress. Supplements include milk thistle (silymarin).
- *The Revulsion Technique.* Dermot O'Connor, who was severely affected by MS but is now the picture of health and energy and

running his own Dublin clinic, agrees that toxic wastes must be cleared from the body in order to regain health.

He used the Revulsion Technique to conquer food cravings for things he knew he shouldn't eat. In 1998, O'Connor changed his diet overnight, giving up all foods that were bad for him and MS, by telling his mind and body that particular foods would do him harm. When you tell yourself that certain foods are like eating a dead rat, you become revolted by them to the point of nausea. You also need to clear your kitchen of all disallowed foods and your mind of negative thoughts and emotions before you can get well.

20

Clearing the Mind
of Negativity

DETOXING IS NOT just clearing junk out of the body, it also means clearing emotional, mental, and spiritual toxic matter.

Some people who have successfully reversed their MS, such as Ann Boroch, author of *Healing Multiple Sclerosis,* and Dermot O'Connor, author of *The Healing Code,* argue this point very strongly. Betty Iams, author of *From MS To Wellness,* also believes that healing is as much about the mind and spirit as the body. This element has often been left out of advice on how to reverse MS, but is crucial.

Boroch believes that, at a subconscious level, we contribute to creating our own MS with toxic emotions. She argues that no amount of right diet, supplements, and other such strategies can work on their own—you have to confront your emotional and mental demons and exorcize them. She insists that you have to take responsibility for your own health, increase your self-awareness, and take many practical steps to uncover and release those things that have made you ill. Boroch believes that doing all these things has kept her free of all MS symptoms for ten years.

➳ WHY NEGATIVE THOUGHTS AND EMOTIONS ARE BAD FOR YOU

Negative thoughts and feelings include fear, rage, anger, sorrow, grief, guilt, anxiety, worry, depression, fright, jealousy, despondency, frustration, feelings of helplessness and hopelessness, and low self-worth going back to childhood. O'Connor believes that the three most poisonous emotions are anger, sorrow, and fear. He says, "If we don't treat the core emotional issue, symptoms may linger at a deeper level."[1]

Negative thoughts and emotions have a deleterious effect on the immune system, brain, organs, and even cells.* Particular emotions have a connection with particular parts of the body. Fear, for example, is associated with the kidneys and bladder, worry with the spleen, and anger with the liver. Long-standing depression can contribute to cardiovascular and immune system disorders.

In emotionally stressful situations, the brain releases the stress hormones cortisol and adrenaline. When this happens, the feel-good chemicals, serotonin and dopamine, drop. This might be alright now and again, but when you are permanently flooded with stress and fight-or-flight hormones, and low in feel-good hormones, health problems will surely follow.

➳ SUPPRESSED EMOTIONS

Negative emotions are normal in daily life. But when they are unrelenting over a long period of time, they can cause serious health problems in a particular organ or body system. It works the other way around too: Problems in an organ can have emotional effects. The body and mind are inextricably linked.

Practitioner Dermot O'Connor tries to help patients release suppressed emotions. He says:

> Many people trap themselves in a chain of negative emotions. If someone feels unreasonably frustrated or angry towards someone else, whether they express or repress this emotion, they will often feel very

---

Psychoneuroimmunology is the study of the interaction between psychological processes and the nervous, endocrine, and immune systems of the body.

upset afterwards. This will often lead to feelings of guilt and low self-worth. Ultimately they redirect this anger towards themselves. If this chain of negative emotions happens continuously over time, it can often lead to severe anxiety or depression. So an initial negative emotion spirals into a whole series of lingering negative emotions—each one damaging to the person. Emotional repression can make you feel like you're living in a pressure cooker. Emotions need to be expressed, not repressed. When an emotion is suppressed, it just works harder to try to find expression.

Often these repressed emotions find unhealthy avenues of expression. The stronger the emotion is, the more potential danger there is when it is repressed.

∼ THE NEGATIVE PERSONALITY

A negative personality is one who is lacking in self-confidence and is filled with self-doubt. Negative people say "no" rather than "yes." They say "I can't" rather than "I can." They always imagine the most pessimistic outcome of any event. Some are afraid of everything, have no faith in their own powers, and always go to other people for help. Negative people tend to fail because they have an attitude of "It can't work." They tend to see the worst in everything and everybody. They are very good at complaining and at forecasting doom and gloom, always seeing the "glass half-empty."

Nobody wants to admit to even partial self-recognition in this portrait. A negative personality, dominated by negative thoughts and feelings, cannot be happy. Such a person will be not only unhappy, but also unwell, as this kind of negative programming is incompatible with good health. It can even make those around them unhappy.

∼ THE POWER OF THOUGHT

Thinking positive thoughts is much healthier than thinking negative thoughts. You may not realize it, but what you think is in your control. Some see MS as an opportunity to change the way they think and live. Like toxic substances, negative thoughts and emotions can be purged from the body, using both the conscious and unconscious mind.

The first thing is to become aware of what negative thoughts and emotions you have, and for this you may need professional help from psychotherapy, cognitive behavioral therapy, counseling, hypnotherapy, or other therapies. Uncovering and releasing these thoughts and emotions is as much a part of the healing process as taking supplements.

Positive Affirmations

One way to change your thought and behavior patterns is by positive affirmations, ideally spoken out loud every day. By constantly repeating statements with your conscious brain, you can train your unconscious brain. An example of a positive affirmation is: "I give myself permission to release all unconscious anger that I am carrying, easily and effortlessly."

Hypnotherapy

Another way to shift thought and behavior patterns is by hypnotherapy, which uses deep relaxation and focused attention. People with MS sometimes use hypnotherapy for chronic worry and fear about the future. First they are taken through a series of relaxation exercises—getting them accustomed to just switching off and allowing the unconscious mind to be accessed. Then they are helped with a series of visualizations that show them overcoming their particular problem. For example, if someone is lacking confidence, a visualization allows them to see themselves in a social situation in a very positive way. It's quicker and easier to get results by working with a hypnotherapist, but anyone can learn basic self-hypnosis.

Visualization

Visualization is also very helpful. With visualization you use your imagination to see yourself in a particular situation that hasn't yet happened. You might see yourself successfully being free of MS, doing the things you want to do, or having what you desire. Once you've rehearsed something carefully in your mind, it's much more likely to happen in real life. Don't make room in your head for pictures of yourself in worse condition than you're in now.

When you visualize, it's important to envision an event or circumstance as if it has already occurred.

Set goals. Focus on exactly what you want to achieve, then visualize
yourself having achieved those goals. Start small and expand, giving yourself rewards along the way.

Focus on the positive. You can make problems smaller or bigger by
imaging them resolved in a positive or negative way. Focus on
something positive.

The best position for visualization is sitting erect (if possible) and
breathing deeply. How you imagine your MS being overcome is up to you.
Always picture yourself happy, healthy, and active. You could imagine
yourself swimming, running along a beautiful beach, dancing, climbing
mountains, or whatever suits your fancy.

Visualization works best if you do it twice every day. Set aside around
fifteen minutes, find a quiet place, and decide what you are going to envision. Relax and unwind for five minutes before you start. Then spend ten
minutes envisioning yourself doing the things you'd like.

....

Trish: Visualizing Health

I picture myelin around my nerves regenerating. I work up my spinal
cord, then around the brain, visualizing all the scarred tissue disap-
pearing. I go to my eyes and clear the blurred vision. Lastly, I imagine
myself running down the beach to my waiting family and friends. The
more vivid the picture in my mind, the better. It does take time and
commitment, but then—what doesn't?

....

⤙ COUNSELING

Counseling really can help. Anxieties are brought out into the open and
can be addressed. People can be helped to feel and behave better. Working
with a counselor can help someone with MS in the following ways:

- Reestablish the ability to enjoy life. The counselor can help deal
  with the anger that is preventing recognition of real pleasures and
  remaining abilities.
- Uncover hidden love. Resentment and anger arising out of the MS

can cover real love and affection. Counseling can help people to find, recognize, and express their love again.

- Help lift depression and stop the person with MS from seeming to punish the family for his or her condition.

Even talking things over with a telephone counselor can help people sort things out and feel better. Sometimes talking to a completely anonymous person, just a voice on the telephone, is easier than talking to someone in the family.

In the United Kingdom, the MS 24-hour telephone counseling service number is 0800 783 0518, and press 1. Many chapters of the U.S. National MS Society have counselors.

....

Tracy: Finding Peace through the Grieving Process

When I was told I had MS, I entered a world I didn't know. I did not take the diagnosis well, and soon after had two relapses, each leaving me worse than I was before. My eyesight suffered and also my coordination. I dropped things and could not do the simplest tasks without getting so fatigued I would sleep for more than twenty-four hours. I have two teenage girls and felt inadequate as a wife and mother. I was offered support from medical specialists, support groups, family, and friends, but I ignored them all and—without fully realizing it—fell into a pit of depression. I would lie around all day, sometimes not even bothering to get dressed. What was the point? I slept most of the time anyway.

I went from being a successful businesswoman to what I felt was a worthless nothing, no longer useful to anyone. I verbally beat myself up about how useless I was, and how much weight I had put on. One day I went for a routine check-up with my doctor and burst into tears when she asked, "How are you?" I caught a reflection of myself in a mirror. "A wreck," I replied, and then something snapped. I cried for what felt like forever. She sat silent and listened to my ranting about how unfair it all was. I wanted my old life back. I wanted the bright lights, not the dim crusty corners that now cluttered the edges of my muddled mind. She advised me to see a counselor. I agreed begrudgingly, with no intention of taking her advice.

A few weeks later I received an appointment with the counselor my doctor had recommended. I told my husband in no uncertain terms that I was not going. "You selfish cow," came his angry reply. I was livid and retreated to the only place I felt safe—my bedroom. As I lay in the dark feeling sorry for myself, angry at him, at everyone, something stirred—a glimmer of light from somewhere in the depths of my soul. I wondered if he was right.

Six sessions into seeing my counselor I realized that I was not mad but going through a grieving process for the loss of what used to be.

My childhood was full of physical, sexual, and mental abuse. It was drummed into me from an early age that in order to be loved, you have to be useful; otherwise, no one will want you. You had to have worth. I now realize we all have worth, no matter who we are, what we do, or how much we earn.

This journey I am on is slow, sometimes painful, sometimes hard to travel, but mostly it is an extraordinary insight into the person I am. I am a woman who is loved and cared for by my family. I have been given the chance to discover me.

I am learning I have not lost my life, just changed it. With the change comes a whole new wealth of opportunity. Never be afraid or too proud to let someone in, share your individualism with someone who just maybe able to help you turn on the light in your own personal darkness.

I have always loved reading; I now read all the time. I have always loved writing, so have enrolled in a creative writing course. In the mornings I get up, I dress, I smile, I walk on the beach or in the forest, and I have coffee and lunch with friends. Now, I live to live and it's wonderful. My only regret is that I let my pride and past stop me from seeing a counselor sooner. Counseling has been an inspiration. If I had not had MS I may never have discovered the other me, the me that had been buried under years of neglect and abuse.

⁀ THE METAPHYSICS OF ILLNESS

Some psychologists think that each physical illness has a particular attitude or set of attitudes that make up the personality of the person who has that illness.

In the United States, the metaphysics of illness has quite a following. One of the handbooks of this approach is *Heal Your Body* by Louise L. Hay. For each physical condition, she lists a probable metaphysical cause, along with a new thought pattern that will overcome the problem.

Problem	Probable Cause	New Thought Pattern
Multiple sclerosis	Mental hardness, hard-heartedness, iron will, inflexibility	I no longer try to control; I flow along with the joy of life

Louise Hay also wrote *You Can Heal Your Life,* in which she describes how changing your thought patterns can, literally, heal you. One of her positive affirmations for MS is: "By choosing loving, joyous thoughts I create a loving and joyous world. I am safe and free."

A similar metaphysical approach is taken by Arthur Hastings, James Fadiman, and James S. Gordon, authors of *Health for the Whole Person.* A person with MS is described as having the following attitude: "This person feels forced to undertake some kind of physical activity and does not want to. He has to work without help, has to support himself and usually others. He does not want to, and wishes help or support."[2]

You might feel that neither of these states of mind accurately describes you. Even so, examining your thought processes and attitudes, to see whether they need changing, is likely to be a worthwhile thing to do.

21

Life Is for Living

THE SHOCK OF BEING TOLD that you have MS is made worse by the fact that people often think multiple sclerosis means an inevitable downward slide into paralysis and a wheelchair. That scenario is not necessarily true, but that is the one imbedded in the public's mind, partly by MS charities seeking to raise money.

Still working and walking after thirty-six years of MS, I do not match that stereotype at all, nor do many, many others.

It is possible that MS may cause some disability. However, everything in this book is based on the real possibility of being able to halt or reverse the downward progression of the disease. Knowing that there are self-help therapies that work, and knowing that there are countless numbers of people with MS who have improved rather than gotten worse as a result of following particular therapies should make you and those around you feel more positive—as long as you take swift and drastic action.

CHANGES IN ATTITUDE

MS no longer has the stigma it once had. The last thirty-five years have brought welcome and dramatic changes in attitudes toward people with disabilities, greatly helped by legislation outlawing discrimination. Nowadays people with disabilities are not hidden away in shame; they are out in the world, integrated with everyone else, doing things that everyone else does and going places other people go, thanks to better accessibility.

✑ REACTIONS TO A DIAGNOSIS

It's difficult not to be knocked for a loop by a diagnosis of MS, but it's important to hold on to the fact that you are no lesser a person.

Self-esteem is a vital asset. MS can dent it more visibly than a limp in your walk. The most off-putting thing to other people is not that you walk with a limp or drag your foot, but that you look downcast, grim-faced, embittered, or ready to bite the head off anyone who speaks to you. Of course, when you have MS, it is easy to feel like damaged goods, but this negative attitude is disabling and it is vital to fight it off.

Self-esteem is important because people always think of you the same way you think of yourself. If you lack self-respect, you will not win respect from other people. If you are filled with self-loathing, you can be sure of a few enemies. If you have no love for yourself, no one else will be able to love you either. This is one of the hardest facts of life, but true.

Denial

One common strategy in dealing with MS is denial—you pretend to yourself and the world around you that you haven't got MS. There may be justifiable reasons for denial—you fear losing your job, you don't want people to pity you, and you don't want the stigma of MS.

Once you declare that you have MS, you fear that your social status will drop. Even today, people can behave differently around disabled people. Few people like others to feel sorry for them, but if you use the strategies in this book and don't get worse, you may not need to tell people you have MS.

Of course, denial only works if you don't have visible symptoms. If you *do* have obvious symptoms of disability, such as a limp, it's tempting to lie that you have a twisted ankle. However, with this strategy there is always the risk of being found out.

Pretending that you haven't got MS is a difficult act to maintain because you're always under the strain of hiding something from other people. It is very stressful to always be putting on a pretense. Even so, there might be some good practical reasons to keep up the pretense until you absolutely must reveal the truth. It's a common strategy for the period after diagnosis, a sort of holding strategy, until you decide what will work best for you.

Many people with MS lead a sort of double life. They tell some people but not others. They are likely to confide everything to other people with MS and turn to them for support and advice, yet say nothing about their MS to their family members and employers.

MS as Identity

The other extreme is letting MS dominate your life. There are some people for whom multiple sclerosis becomes their whole identity. After diagnosis, such people succumb to MS completely. They may give up work, go on disability pension, apply for a disabled sticker, and join an MS club. They meet other people less and less, as they shift their whole life to a subculture of disabled people. MS becomes their hobby.

Needing to meet and talk to other people with MS may be very important, but making MS your whole life can create problems with families and friends. I vividly remember the story of a man with MS who lived, breathed, and slept MS. It was all he ever thought or talked about. One day his wife screamed at him, "If I ever hear the words MS again in this house I shall go stark staring mad!" This was a sufficient jolt for him to put MS into the context of his whole life and lead a more balanced existence. MS has become part of your life, but it is not your whole life. Dominate it before it dominates you.

MS as an Excuse

Another strategy is to use MS as an excuse for opting out of life as it should be lived. For example, a friend asks you to go out for a day in the country. You say, "Sorry, I can't, I've got MS." You really want to go, but you fear that your MS symptoms will make the day problematic.

MS symptoms can indeed get in the way. The symptoms are real, but some of the fears about symptoms make them more severe in your head than they are in reality. By using MS as an excuse, you deny yourself many opportunities to have a pleasurable or fun time. One woman I know who is among the most disabled with MS has traveled all around the world with her husband and her wheelchair.

MS as a Blessing

Some people have actually felt that getting MS was a blessing in disguise. Sometimes—but not necessarily—such people are spiritual, and having MS has made them truly appreciate things in life that they used to take for granted. These are the people who derive newfound joy from the scent of a flower or the beauty of a tree. They strip their lives of the nonsense that clutters up most people's daily existence, and instead concentrate on what is truly important. I know many people with MS who have made the decision to change their life for the better by moving to some quiet spot, downscaling and living a simpler life. They may have MS, but they are happy.

MS is likely to change you, but some people perceive this as a change for the better. "I'm not the person I used to be" is a common phrase from those with MS, meaning that they are now wiser, humbler, probably nicer, and with a different set of life values. Because of this, some even say that MS is the best thing that could have happened to them.

❧ RELATIONSHIPS

Some relationships do not survive one partner getting MS; others do. Some people just don't want to face the possible prospect of looking after someone who may become incapacitated and disabled. Statistics show that men are seven times more likely to leave a wife or partner who has MS than the other way around.

One man I know of left his formerly free-spirited wife who became disabled with MS, because she no longer fit what he wanted from a wife and he resented her lack of mobility. He seemed more concerned about his own life and image than meeting her needs for love and acceptance. Their values no longer matched and they divorced, leaving both embittered.

It is not always the fault of the unaffected partner that relationships break down—it can also be the anger, depression, resentment, and low self-esteem of the partner with MS that kills the relationship. Many, many, many people with MS—both male and female—go through the painful breakup of a relationship due to MS. But many of these same people have gone on to meet someone else, sometimes with MS or another condition, and live happy and fulfilled lives.

Many partners rise to the challenge when a spouse develops MS. Be assured that there are plenty of loving, caring men and women who make wonderful partners and want to support their partners with MS in having the best and happiest life possible. I meet people like this all the time: the husband who went to endless trouble to create a perfect accessible garden for his wife; the wife who goes to great lengths to make sure her husband has wonderful holidays; the husband who took his wife on a fantastic safari in Africa with special accommodations for her needs.

One man who found a new partner after the breakup of his first marriage is Chris Tatevosian, an American who wrote the book *Life Interrupted*. He took out all the anger and frustration of having MS on his first wife, driving her away with his appalling behavior. After their split, he took time to examine the way he had acted, so when he met the woman who became his new wife, he knew how to behave differently.

··

Chris: I Destroyed My Own Marriage

After ten years, my first marriage began dissolving when the "Monster" invited his friends to live in my house. If you have MS, I'm sure you've met the gang. There was the kingpin, Stress; his best friend, Anger; and his twin, Misdirected. Worthlessness was there with his brother, Inadequacy, who brought his best friend, Low Self-esteem, and side-kick, Depression. They all hung out with everybody's buddies, Worry and Anxiety. Communication was a no show, but sure enough, his sister Miss Communication popped in and overstayed her welcome. They never left, but my wife did. Sounds like a real nightmare, and I couldn't see myself ever waking up from it.

MS can destroy relationships between spouses, family members, even friends. I wrote the book *Life Interrupted, It's Not All about Me*, my real life story of a marriage interrupted by multiple sclerosis. It could have been any chronic illness or disability and it could have been anyone's relationship. Eventually, the combination of this physically debilitating disease and my quick-to-anger, "poor me" attitude was more than enough to confirm my wife's difficult decision to leave. This interruption to our once loving relationship had become too much for her to bear. I had lost sight of what was important in life.

My new bride, Jane, is fantastic, and even though my disease is worse now than during my first marriage, I could not ask for more. So what's changed? Why is my marriage working so well now, even though my MS has continued to progress over the past eight years? I can attribute this to two factors. First, Jane is truly a special person; and second, I wrote a book, which afforded me the opportunity to slow down and examine my life. The obvious fact is that we have the choice to go through life dealing with whatever trials and tribulations life throws at us with either a smile or a frown. Yes, we have an affliction, but that doesn't mean we have to spend the rest of our lives pissed off at everything and everyone, living in complete misery.

When I do begin to slip-up, it's so obvious that I can't help but catch myself. Jane has read the book, too, so when I slip up she's quick to point out, "Chris, I think you need to revisit page 76," and we have a good chuckle.

When my first marriage broke down, I never thought I would get married again. After all, who would marry damaged goods? At one point prior to my marriage I asked my wife-to-be, "Why would you marry someone with MS? That's like buying a vase with a hole in the bottom?" Her response was, "Maybe I want it to hold dried flowers." So these dried flowers are happily married and loving every minute of it.

......

Dating Websites

If you decide you'd like to find someone in the same boat as you, there are several disabled dating websites and clubs that make meeting someone easier. (These can be easily found through an Internet search.)

......

Fi: MS Led Me to My True Life Partner

I had what I thought was a good relationship until 2000, when I was diagnosed with MS. My partner of fifteen years said he wanted to support me, and in lots of ways he did, but in many ways he changed toward me. He looked at me differently and I think because of the MS he no longer found me attractive. He also felt embarrassed when I needed to use a wheelchair for long distances.

He sent me an e-mail saying he had been unhappy in the relationship for two years and had seen a counselor who advised him not to stay with me out of guilt. I had no choice but to leave the apartment that had been mine for twelve years and move back with my parents. I was also sick with stress and had to leave a job I loved as an office manager. I was very down and scared about my future.

Then a woman I met suggested I join some online disabled dating agencies to make new friends. This is what I posted with my photo: "Hi, my name is Fi and I am feeling down as my partner of fifteen years has ended our relationship. I have MS and I'm looking to make friends with someone who will make me laugh. Johnny Depp look-alike would be cool!"

"Dave from London" contacted me. There was no photo but he had typed masses about life and himself and how he was a regular guy with MS. Then began a courtship of e-mails and texting and talking on the phone. I fell for him. We eventually met on my fortieth birthday and had a wonderful time.

Three weeks later we met again and arranged to spend some time together, which quickly turned into two weeks. A week later I moved in with him.

We're now married and lead the most idyllic life. We've both taken medical retirement from work with a reasonable financial package and have a very relaxed time.

With Dave and me there's a complete understanding of each other and our MS, and the way symptoms, even invisible ones, can have an impact. Dave loves being out and pushing me in the wheelchair, and makes me feel so desirable. We both find it great to be with each other and with the same condition.

It doesn't faze us that our condition could deteriorate. You have to live life for now and not think too much about the future. If it weren't for the MS we would never have met. But both of us would rather have MS and have each other. I have found my soulmate, the love of my life.

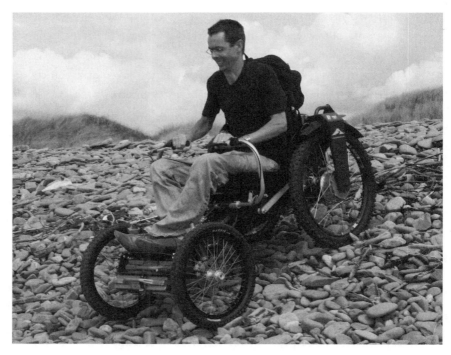

Chris enjoying a ride on his Boma off-road wheelchair

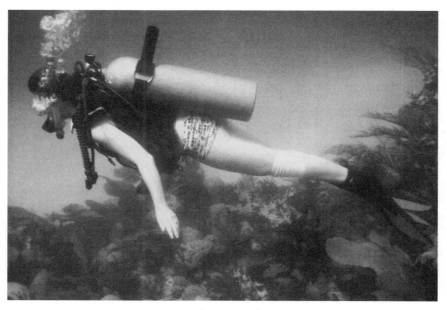

Louise exploring under water

❧ CONCENTRATE ON WHAT YOU CAN DO

With the right mental attitude you can do almost anything, regardless of having MS. It might mean taking up a new activity, learning something new, or going places you've never been before.

I personally know people with MS who have found joy in the new experiences of singing in a choir, writing novels or poetry, gardening, painting, or doing some kind of craft. And there are countless numbers who, by using equipment designed so that disabled people can be independent, enjoy the outdoors or a sport they thought was off limits. Here are a few of their stories.

❧ FOLLOW YOUR DREAMS

Chris: Romping in an Off-Road, All-Terrain Wheelchair

We go out as a family and take long walks over rugged ground—woods, forests, dunes, and beaches. I also have extraordinary fun when I go out by myself, when I tend to do mountain-bike trails. The off-road performance of the Boma all-terrain wheelchair is just wicked. It will go up, down, and through just about anything. Random teenagers have repeatedly exclaimed, "That's so cool!" It's fantastically liberating. And it's great in snow. I've now been able for the first time in years to join in throwing snowballs and pulling toboggans.

Louise: Under Water Freedom

I've discovered that—even with MS—I can still enjoy freedom of movement and balance in water. This summer I finally completed an Open Water Diver course, which was a dream come true. This achievement has given me some of my cherished freedom back and has opened up a whole new world of opportunity and excitement.

Fiona and David: MS Won't Stop Our Travel (and Romance!)

When I was diagnosed with MS in 2000, I never thought I would ever travel again. However, as both my husband and I have MS, we felt relaxed about traveling together and tackling any problems we might face. I also had Botox for my bladder, so that was not a problem.

When we arrived at our Amsterdam apartment, we were overjoyed. It was spacious, beautiful, very light and tranquil with big windows at the back of the living room that opened onto a patio. Our neighbors were locals, which made it feel very Dutch. It overlooked one of the canals so the setting was quite romantic!

We got around Amsterdam by Dave pushing me in my wheelchair. Also, the local people were very helpful in assisting us. You see a lot of mobility scooters in Amsterdam.

Amsterdam is such a romantic place. We chose to go in May as the temperature is ideal and not too hot. With the weather so perfect and cool, we could sit out at various cafes. We found the Dutch people and shop/café owners very helpful and accommodating.

Louise: Hitting the Slopes on a Ski-bike

Thanks to a ski-bike, I could once again experience the sheer joy of being able to ski alongside my family. In February, we returned for the third year running to the Austrian Alps for a week's skiing. However, since my MS diagnosis, I had to be content with off-piste activities while my family took to the slopes. Deep down, I battled with disappointment, while on the surface trying my best to keep positive. I used to be good at skiing. As a teenager I learned how to ski cross-country, and my sisters and I quickly progressed to downhill skiing with all the thrill of speed and spills. But with the progression of my MS, I no longer had the balance or coordination to handle speed. So, to begin with, I returned to cross-country skiing. My husband, Warren, and I would go out for daily traverses through the picturesque Austrian woods. It was a great help to have his encouragement as I picked myself up each time I fell. I was determined to keep going.

Unfortunately, during 2007, I suffered two bad relapses that exacerbated my symptoms, and this year I knew that skiing of any kind was out of the question. So I waved my husband and friends off on their ski adventures, took my son to ski school, and settled for a cup of tea, basking in the unbroken Austrian sunshine outside the cafés at the base of the slopes. Occasionally I would go up on a gondola to join my husband for lunch when he was skiing nearby. That was pretty thrilling, just to feel part of things, albeit in a passive sort of way. But most often I would watch my family grab onto the T-bar and disappear up into a magical kingdom of snow and ice I could but attempt to imagine.

However, things were about to change! Our wonderful host at Haus Salzburg in Hinterthal had other ideas. Carl Owen, ski-instructor extraordinaire, introduced me to the ski-bike, known in the sport as a "skibob," and hired some for all the family to try. The skibob is shaped like a bike with a seat and handlebars, but it has two skis in place of tires. The rider also wears short skis so that the feet stay in constant contact with the ground. Thus, I was able to maintain my balance.

The secret to successfully maneuvering is not to steer with the handlebars, but to turn by first heading downhill and then leaning the bike into the slope so as to weave back and forth across the slope at a gentle incline. Carl's careful coaching and practical tips made the whole process much more manageable, and the prospect of coasting downhill far less daunting. Over the course of an afternoon I was able to ski down the bunny slopes unaided.

Especially thrilling was being able to ski alongside my family and enjoy watching them all in action. It was also very gratifying to do something new that everyone else found just as challenging and adventurous as I did. My ten-year-old son Guy loved the ski-bike so much he just didn't want to stop. The second day, we went higher. There was the breathtaking view from the top of endless snow-capped peaks as far as the eye could see, and majestic pines opening out before us on the way down.

The piste was far more challenging than the beginner slopes of the day before, but ever watchful, Carl was there as my legs and balance whenever needed. As my confidence increased, he let me ski unaided down the gentler stretches, while catching me from behind to guide me and the bike down the more precipitous drops.

On arriving back at base I had to pinch myself to prove it hadn't all been a dream. Fortunately, we have video footage of the tremendous view from the summit, the two-thousand-foot descent (at times a white-knuckle ride), and the thrill of being able to ski downhill once more.

....

Judy: Flying and Free as a Bird

When it comes to daredevil antics, I am one of life's scaredy cats. So it was with some amazement that I found myself flying a light aircraft one sunny day. Admittedly, I was at the tiller for only ten minutes with ace pilot Bernd safely by my side at the dual controls, but I was flying nonetheless—just one of the hundreds of disabled people who can experience this thrill, thanks to the efforts of the British Disabled Flying Association. You don't feel your disability when you're flying.

....

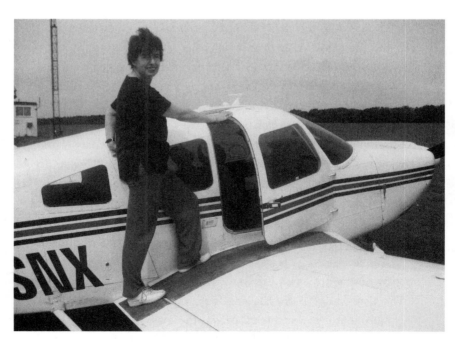

Judy preparing for flight

Linda: The Joy of Volunteering in Africa

It had always been my ambition to go on International Guiding, but when I was diagnosed with secondary progressive MS it looked as if my dream would be shattered. My dreams came alive again when I took over a local guide unit as Guider in charge. The SMILE (Supporting Mombasa in a Learning Experience) project was to build and refurnish the home in Mombasa, on the coast of Kenya, where all the children had, or were affected by, HIV/AIDS. I was excited about going but had my worries. How would I cope with the heat and fatigue? Would I be slowing up the others? Would I be able to cope with the work that would be given to us on the project? It was a huge commitment. I started to ask MS colleagues, friends, and my MS nurse: Was I mad to want to take part in such a challenge? The answer from everyone was, "Go for it, you'll never get another chance."

And so I did, and had a fantastic time helping orphans. What an amazing, fabulous experience I had on those fifteen days in Mombasa. I have memories that will be with me forever. If an opportunity comes up like this for anyone with MS, *go for it!* Think positively about what you can do, and not about what you can't do. I certainly achieved my dream!

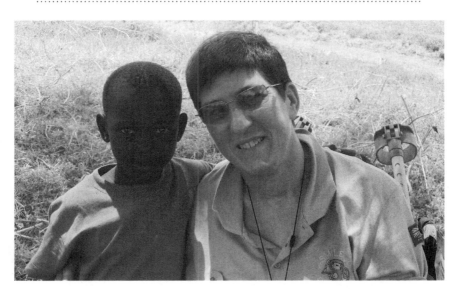

Linda living her dream—volunteering in Mombasa, Kenya

ᕙ LIVING LIFE TO THE FULLEST

MS can be a great spur to doing all the things you always wanted to do and living life to the fullest. Sometimes when people hear I have MS, they imagine that my life must have been severely limited by having the disease. Far from it! For twenty-five years—a full career—I worked as a TV producer for the BBC and other channels and traveled the world: North America, India, Pakistan, the Far East, and Australia, where I went bushwalking in the Outback. Above all, I have the most wonderful son, Pascal, who has rewarded me in every way by being kind, sensitive, clever, and handsome. As happens for many people, some relationships didn't stay the course, but I have been with my husband Sam—now disabled with Parkinson's disease—for more than twelve years. If you ask me how I've done it, I'd say I've just got on with it.

Among the hundreds of people with MS I have met over the years, I have heard the phrase "I just get on with it!" countless times from men and women who do not let MS get in the way of leading fulfilling lives.

The "just get on with it" philosophy is to make the most of life and enjoy it. A positive attitude sure beats wallowing in doom and gloom at the unfairness of your lot. MS is *not* a life sentence to being stuck at home. Rather, it can be an incentive to rethink your priorities, your life values, and do the things you want to do.

How you just get on with it is a personal decision. Some people decide to give up the stress of the rat race and downsize to a quiet life in some remote idyll; others move to another country where the pace of life and the climate are kinder. Some make a success of their chosen career regardless of MS, and others take early retirement and do the things they always wanted to do. There is no one prescription; we are all unique.

Concentrate on what you *can* do, not what you can't do. You may need to make some practical and mental adjustments to your symptoms, but you can still have fulfilling relationships and a family if you choose. You can still have adventure and travel, go wild and try new things, and take part in sports, hobbies, or any activities that strike your fancy.

Whatever you decide, have fun. Laugh! Love! And never let MS stop you from living life to the fullest.

Resources

ORGANIZATIONS AND WEBSITES FOR GENERAL MS SUPPORT

Betty's House . . . Life After MS
www.bettyshouselifeafterms.com
Website of Betty Iams, who has MS and believes in an alternative approach. Includes her newsletter "Journey to Wellness."

CureZone
www.curezone.com/diseases/ms
Testimonials, blogs, support groups, and resources focusing on alternative methods of treating MS.

IFM: The Institute for Functional Medicine
www.functionalmedicine.org/findfmphysician/index.asp
Information about physicians worldwide who believe MS is a result of food allergies, toxic exposures, infections, individual stressors, and genetics.

James S. Huggins' Refrigerator Door MS Page
www.jamesshuggins.com/h/ms-1/multiple-sclerosis.htm
Includes extensive list of resources and links to MS-related sites.

Mercola.com
www.mercola.com
Newsletter from alternative practitioner Dr. Joseph Mercola. Occasionally has items relevant to MS.

MS Crossroads

www.mscrossroads.org
Exhaustive list of MS resources compiled by Aapo Halko, a Finnish man with MS.

mscured MS Support Group

http://health.groups.yahoo.com/group/mscured/
An informative forum on all aspects of non-drug treatments for MS.

Multiple Sclerosis Information

www.msnews.org
General information about MS.

The Multiple Sclerosis Resource Centre

0 1206 505 444
24-hour Counselling Service: 0800 783 0518 (then press 1)
info@msrc.co.uk
www.msrc.co.uk
Based in the United Kingdom, but international in its scope, The Multiple Sclerosis Resource Centre provides excellent and comprehensive information about all aspects of MS. They also publish the widely acclaimed magazine, *New Pathways,* which focuses on alternative methods of treating MS and ways to continue living life to its fullest.

Multiple Sclerosis Society of Canada

www.mssociety.ca
The only national voluntary organization in Canada that supports MS research, as well as services for those with MS. Website includes information about regional chapters.

Multiple Sclerosis Trust

01 462 476700
info@mstrust.org.uk
www.mstrust.org.uk
Works with and for people in the United Kingdom with MS, providing information, education, research, and support. Extensive website.

National Multiple Sclerosis Society

www.nationalmssociety.org
The U.S. National Multiple Sclerosis Society has a 50-state network of chapters and a comprehensive website.

No More MS, A Journey Back to Life

www.nomorems.com

Website of Sue Ellen Dickinson, who says she has recovered from MS by following various complementary protocols.

Taking Control of Multiple Sclerosis

www.takingcontrolofmultiplesclerosis.org

Website of Dr. George Jelinek, an Australian doctor who reversed his MS with his Taking Control recovery program.

This Is MS

www.thisisms.com

Unbiased, unaffiliated site dedicated to eradicating MS. Information and forums on all aspects of treatment.

RESOURCES FOR CHAPTER 4:
FOOD SENSITIVITIES

Intestinal Permeability Test and Candida Analysis

Genova Diagnostics

63 Zillicoa Street

Asheville, NC 28806

(800) 522-4762

www.genovadiagnostics.com

ELISA Testing

Immuno Laboratories, Inc.

6801 Powerline Road

Fort Lauderdale, FL 33309

(888) 446-6866

www.BetterHealthUSA.com

Immunos

www.immunos.com

Meridian Valley Laboratory

801 SW 16th Suite 126

Renton, WA 98055

(425) 271-8689

www.meridianvalleylab.com

Optimum Health Resource Laboratories
419 South Federal Highway
Dania, FL 33004
(954) 926-8020
www.optimumhealthresource.com

Cambridge Nutritional Sciences Ltd
Eden Research Park
Henry Crabb Road
Littleport
Cambridgeshire
CB6 1SE
United Kingdom
0 1353 863279
www.food-detective.com

YorkTest Laboratories Ltd.
York Science Park
York
YO10 5DQ
United Kingdom
U.K. helpline: 0800 074 6185
www.yorktest.com

ALCAT Testing
Cell Science Systems
852 South Military Trail
Deerfield Beach, FL 33442
(800) US ALCAT (872-5228)
(954) 426-2304
www.alcat.com

For U.K.: 01708 44 11 43
www.alcattest.co.uk

Nutritional Profile: Hair Analysis
Doctor's Data, Inc.
3755 Illinois Avenue
St. Charles, IL 60174
(800) 323-2784
www.doctorsdata.com

Recommended U.K. Clinics

There are a few testing laboratories in the Harley Street area of London and elsewhere outside London. You have to be referred by a doctor who is treating you. To find one of the fifteen or so doctors who specialize in nutritional medicine to treat MS, contact:

British Society for Ecological Medicine
www.ecomed.org.uk/practitioners

The following clinics are ones that I have used myself and can therefore recommend:

Biolab Medical Unit
The Stone House
9 Weymouth Street
London
W1W 6DB
020 7636 5959
www.biolab.co.uk

The Diagnostic Clinic
50 New Cavendish Street
London
W1G 8TL
020 7009 4650
www.thediagnosticclinic.com

Dr. Georges Mouton
at the Hale Clinic
7 Park Crescent
London
W1B 1PF
Mobile: 0794 944 0893
gmouton@gmouton.com

RESOURCES FOR CHAPTER 5:
THE BEST BET DIET

Direct-MS
5119 Brockington Rd. NW
Calgary, AB, T2L 1R7
Canada
info@direct-ms.org
www.direct-ms.org
This is Ashton Embry's site and includes all his excellent essays on various aspects of MS, such as diet, supplements, and the importance of vitamin D. It also includes recipes, information on the latest research, and links to other resources that Embry recommends.

RESOURCES FOR CHAPTER 6:
FEED YOUR BODY, FEED YOUR BRAIN

Terry Wahls
terrywahls@gmail.com
www.terrywahls.com
This is a mine of information and also has links to her blog and other useful websites. The books Dr. Wahls mentions are: *The World's Healthiest Foods* by George Mateljan, available from the Mateljan Foundation (see www.whfoods.com), and *Eat to Live* and *Eat for Health*, both by Dr. Joel Fuhrman, available from Dr. Fuhrman's website (www.drfuhrman.com) and book outlets.

Instant Greens

Dr. Wahls says she mostly orders NSI brand instant greens. She advises to check the label of any instant greens product before you buy it to ensure it is free of gluten, dairy, and eggs. Instant greens may be ordered from the following websites:

www.bio-alternatives.net/greens.htm
www.purebulk.com
www.vitacost.com

RESOURCES FOR CHAPTER 7:
THE BODY'S DELICATE BALANCE

Robert Young and pH Miracle Living
16390 Dia Del Sol
Valley Center, CA 92082
(760) 751-8321
info@phmiracleliving.com
http://phmiracleliving.com

RESOURCES FOR CHAPTER 8:
NUTRITIONAL SUPPLEMENTS

Georges Mouton, M.D.
www.gmouton.com

Bee Pollen: Royal Cells and Nectar M
John Bazakis, The Royal Cells Institute
Kanakari 23
Patra, TK 26223
Greece
bazakis@otenet.gr

Dr. Tom Gilhooly's Recommended Supplements
The Essential Health Clinic
Unit 75, Mitchell Arcade
Rutherglen, Glasgow
G73 2LS
Phone (from U.K.): 0800 027 4969
www.essentialhealthclinic.com/website

Dermot O'Connor's Recommended Supplements
Dublin Clinic
33 Haddington Road
Ballsbridge
Dublin 4
01 667 2222

Hale Clinic (London)
7 Park Crescent
London
W1B 1PF
0871 218 0300

www.healing-code.com
info@healing-code.com

RESOURCES FOR CHAPTER 11:
EXERCISE AND EXERCISE MACHINES

Pilates
Fran Michelman
0 208 381 4061
Private Pilates teacher, northwest London

Belsize Studio
5 McCrone Mews
Belsize Lane
London
NW3 5BG
020 7431 6223
www.belsizestudio.com

Yoga

My MS Yoga
(800) 456-2255
www.mymsyoga.com/yoga
Classes led by Baron Baptiste in major cities across the country; free MS Yoga DVD offered through website.

Yoga for Multiple Sclerosis
www.naturalways.com/yoga-multiple-sclerosis.htm
Comprehensive yoga program designed to strengthen the nervous system and improve mental alertness.

Yoga for the Young at Heart
http://yogaheart.com
Offers chair yoga DVDs for people with limited mobility.

Rebounder, Vibration Trainers, and Resistance Chairs

Promolife
3656 Dead Horse Mtn. Rd.
Fayetteville, AR 72701
(479) 442-3404
(888) 742-3404
www.promolife.com
Sells rebounders, vibration training machines, resistance chairs, and several other products that may be useful for those with MS.

Neuromuscular Electrical Stimulation

Empi
www.empi.com
Empi devices are available only with a physician's prescription. The website provides further information on Empi products, so you can determine if the device might be a suitable option for you.

Tone-A-Matic
www.toneamatic.com
Provides product and ordering information.

RESOURCES FOR CHAPTER 12:
PHYSICAL THERAPY, PHYSIOTHERAPY, AND REHABILITATION

The National Rehabilitation Information Center
(301) 459-5900
(301) 459-5984 (for TTY users)
(800) 346-2742 (toll-free line)
www.naric.com
Provides an abundance of disability- and rehabilitation-oriented information and resources. Website has searchable databases and also allows for live chat with an information specialist during business hours.

RESOURCES FOR CHAPTER 13:
COMPLEMENTARY THERAPIES

National Institutes of Health: National Center for Complementary and Alternative Medicine
http://nccam.nih.gov
Research, training, and information about complementary and alternative medicine.

Anthroposophic Medicine
Rudolf Steiner Health Center (RSHC)
1422 W. Liberty
Ann Arbor, MI 48103
(734) 663-4365
rshc@steinerhealth.org
www.steinerhealth.org

RSHC for Outpatients:
Community Supported Anthroposophical Medicine
1825 W. Stadium Blvd.
Ann Arbor, MI 48103
(734) 222-1491
csam@steinerhealth.org

Raphael Medical Centre
01732 833924
www.raphaelmedicalcentre.co.uk

Camphill Medical Practice
www.camphillmedical.org.uk

Anthroposophic Health and Social Care
44 1224 869 621
www.ahasc.org.uk

Additional U.K. websites of interest:
www.anthroposphy.co.uk/
www.chisuk.org.uk/bodymind/whatis/anthroposophical.php
www.pafam.org.uk

Ayurvedic Medicine
Maharishi Ayurveda Health Centre
The Golden Dome
Woodley Park
Skelmersdale
Lancashire
WN8 6UQ
01695 51008
mahc@maharishi.co.uk
www.maharishiayurveda.co.uk

Maharishi Ayurveda Hospital
New Delhi, India
91 11 2747 1118
mahp@vsnl.net
www.maharishiayurvedaindia.org

National Institute of Ayurvedic Medicine
584 Milltown Road
Brewster, NY 10509
(845) 278-8700
ayurveda@niam.com
www.niam.com

Bowen Technique
Bowen Therapy Technique Practitioners
http://bowendirectory.com
An excellent resource for locating a local Bowen Technique Pracitioner in the
United States, Canada, United Kingdom, Europe, South Africa, Australia, or
New Zealand.

Bowen Therapists' European Register (BTER)
www.bowentherapists.com

The European College of Bowen Studies (ECBS)
The Corsley Centre
Old School, Deep Lane
Corsley, Wiltshire
BA12 7QF
0 1373 832 340
www.thebowentechnique.com

Conductive Education

Association for Conductive Education in North America (ACENA)
PO Box 7707
Grand Rapids, MI 49510
(616) 575-0575
acenaorg@acena.org
www.acena.org

**The National Institute of
Conductive Education**
Cannon Hill House
Russell Road
Moseley
Birmingham
B13 3RD
United Kingdom
0 121 449 1589
foundation@conductive-education.org.uk
www.conductive-education.org.uk

Hypnotherapy

American Society of Clinical Hypnosis
140 N. Bloomingdale Rd
Bloomingdale, IL 60108
(630) 980-4740
info@asch.net
www.asch.net

Hypnotherapy Practitioners Association U.K. Register
Wellbeing House
262 Spendmore Lane
Chorley
Lancashire
PR7 5DE
01257 795627
www.hypnotherapypractitioners.com

Magnetic Therapy
Viofor JPS System Products (Medica Health)
44 (0) 870 609 4583
info@medicahealth.org
www.medicahealth.org

EnerMed Therapy
Energy Medicine Developments
P.O. Box 10024, Suite 3000
700 West Georgia Street
Vancouver, BC, V7Y 1A1
(604) 602-0983
(888) ENERMED (363-7633)
info@enermed.com
www.enermed.com

Guided Imagery
Miriam Franco (Imagery Work)
Offices in Narberth and Phoenixville, PA
(610) 935-8330
info@imagerywork.com
www.imagerywork.com
Miriam Franco's guided imagery CD for MS (also available as an MP3), *Relaxation and Guided Imagery for Multiple Sclerosis*, is available from her website.

Speakeasier
01242 705681
speakeasier@blueyonder.co.uk
www.speakeasier.org
Steve Brisk, who has MS and is also a trained counselor, has recorded a number of guided imagery CDs, which are available through this U.K. website.

Naturopathy

American Association of Naturopathic Physicians
4435 Wisconsin Avenue, NW, Suite 403
Washington, DC 20016
(202) 237-8150
(866) 538-2267
www.naturopathic.org
The American Association of Naturopathic Physicians (AANP) is an organization of naturopathic doctors who hve completed four-year, accredited programs.

RESOURCES FOR CHAPTER 14:
OTHER MODALITIES THAT CAN HELP MS

Colostrum

For more information about Colostem, visit the following websites:
www.shaunamclean.com
www.stemcellcolostrum.co.nz

Combined Antibiotic Protocol

Dr. David Wheldon
dw@ms-treatment.org
www.davidwheldon.co.uk/ms-treatment.html

Support Network for CAP
www.cpnhelp.org

RESOURCES FOR CHAPTER 16:
ALLEVIATING SPECIFIC SYMPTOMS

Walking Aid: Functional Electrical Stimulation (FES)

National Clinical FES Centre
Dept. Medical Physics and Biomedical Engineering
Salisbury District Hospital
Salisbury, Wiltshire
SP2 8BJ
+44 (0) 1722 429065
enquiries@salisburyfes.com
www.salisburyfes.com

Odstock Medical Limited (OML)
+44 (0) 1722 439555
enquiries@odstockmedical.com
www.odstockmedical.com
For FES equipment, sales, and clinical service.

Bioness
www.bioness.com
Informational site for the Ness L300 Drop Foot System.

Innovative Neurotronics
3600 N. Capital of Texas Highway
Ste. B150
Austin, TX 78745
(512) 721-1900
(888) 884-6462
info@ininc.us
www.walkaide.com
Website for The WalkAide System for Treatment of Foot Drop.

Walking Aid: MuSmate
MuSmate Ltd.
P. O. Box 3976
Bath
BA1 0DF
United Kingdom
Phone and fax: (0845) 094 4674
www.musmate.co.uk

RESOURCES FOR CHAPTER 18:
MERCURY

The British Society for Mercury Free Dentistry
The Weathervane
22a Moorend Park Road
Cheltenham
GL53 OJY
01242 226 918
www.mercuryfreedentistry.org.uk

Consumers for Dental Choice
316 F Street, N.E., Suite 210
Washington, D.C. 20002
(202) 544-6333
info@toxicteeth.org
www.toxicteeth.org

Holistic Dental Association (HDA)
P.O. Box 151444
San Diego, CA 92175
(619) 923-3120
www.holisticdental.org

Huggins Applied Healing
5082 List Drive
Colorado Springs, CO 80919
(866) 948-4638
info@drhuggins.com
www.hugginsappliedhealing.com

Additional Informational Websites:
www.holisticmed.com/dental/amalgam
www.mercurypoisoned.com

RESOURCES FOR CHAPTER 19:
DETOXING THE BODY

Eliminating Parasites: Hulda Clark and the Zapper

Dr. Clark Information Center
info@drclark.net
www.drclark.net

Dr. Hulda Clark Zappers
411 Walnut Street, #7776
Green Cove Springs, FL 32043
drhuldaclark@gmail.com
www.huldaclarkzappers.com

Jon Barron's Detox

Baseline of Health Foundation
www.JonBarron.org
Jon Barron's informational website.

Baseline Nutritionals
www.BaselineNutritionals.com
Manufacturer of Jon Barron's detox formulas.

Recommended Reading

PARTS ONE AND TWO:
GENERAL MS SUPPORT, DIET, AND SUPPLEMENTS

Boroch, Ann. *Healing Multiple Sclerosis: Diet, Detox & Nutritional Makeover for Total Recovery.* Los Angeles: Quintessential Healing, 2007

Brostoff, J., and L. Gamlin. *Food Allergies and Food Intolerance: The Complete Guide to Their Identification and Treatment.* Rochester, Vt.: Healing Arts Press, 2000.

Buckley, Tessa. *The Multiple Sclerosis Diet Book.* London: Sheldon Press, 2007.

Clark, Hulda Regehr. *The Cure for All Diseases.* New Delhi, India: B. Jain Publishers Pvt. Ltd., 2008.

Cordain, Loren. *The Paleo Diet: Lose Weight and Get Healthy by Eating the Food You Were Designed to Eat.* Hoboken, N.J.: Wiley, 2002.

Courtier, Marie-Annick. *Cooking Well: Multiple Sclerosis: Over 75 Easy and Delicious Recipes for Nutritional Healing.* Long Island City, N.Y.: Hatherleigh Press, 2009.

Crook, William G. *The Yeast Connection Handbook.* Garden City Park, N.Y.: Square One Publishers, 1999.

Davies, Stephen, and Alan Stewart. *Nutritional Medicine: The Drug-Free Guide to Better Family Health.* London: Pan Macmillan, 1987.

Dickinson, Sue Ellen. *No More MS,* www.nomorems.com.

Elkins, Rita. *Miracle Sugars: The New Class of Missing Nutrients.* Salt Lake City, Utah: Woodland Publishing, 2003.

Erasmus, Udo. *Fats that Heal, Fats that Kill.* Burnaby, B.C.: Alive Books, 1993.

Fitzgerald, Geraldine, and Fenella Briscoe. *Special Diet Cook Books: Multiple Sclerosis: Healthy Menus to Help in the Management of Multiple Sclerosis*. London: Thorsons, 1989

———. *Multiple Sclerosis: Over 100 Recipes to Help Control Symptoms (Recipes for Health)*. London: Thorsons, 1998.

Holick, Michael, and Mark Jenkins. *The UV Advantage*. New York: iBooks, 2009.

Iams, Betty A. *From MS to Wellness: My Personal Story of Overcoming Multiple Sclerosis*. Davis, Calif.: Iams House, 1998.

Jelinek, George. *Taking Control of Multiple Sclerosis: Natural and Medical Therapies to Prevent its Progression*. Lancaster, U.K.: Fleetfoot Books, 2005.

———. *Overcoming Multiple Sclerosis: An Evidence-Based Guide to Recovery*: Crows Nest, NSW, Australia: Allen & Unwin, 2010.

Kopera, Gina. *Cure Yourself Naturally: What to Do When Your Doctor Cannot Heal You*. N.p.: CreateSpace, 2009.

MacDougall, Roger. *My Fight Against Multiple Sclerosis*. Mansfield, Ohio: Regenics, 1980. Also available online, http://www.direct-ms.org/rogermcdougall.html.

Mateljan, George. *The World's Healthiest Foods: Essential Guide for the Healthiest Way of Eating*. N.p.: World's Healthiest Foods, 2006.

O'Connor, Dermot. *The Healing Code: My Own Story and 5-Step Healing Programme*. London: Hodder & Stoughton, 2007.

Pageler, John. *New Hope, Real Help for Those Who Have Multiple Sclerosis*. N.p.: Multiple Sclerosis Foundation, 1986. Available online, www.infoonms.com.

Pepe, Celeste, and Lisa Hammond. *Reversing Multiple Sclerosis: 9 Effective Steps to Recover Your Health*. Newburyport, Mass.: Hampton Roads Publishing, 2001.

Sawyer, Ann D., and Judith E. Bachrach. *The MS Recovery Diet: Take Control of Your Health, Change What You Eat, and Live Symptom-Free*. New York: Avery, 2007.

Soll, Robert W., and Penelope B. Grenoble. *MS: Something Can Be Done and You Can Do It: A New Approach to Understanding and Managing Multiple Sclerosis*. Chicago: Contemporary Books, 1984.

Swank, Roy Laver, and Barbara Brewer Dugan. *The Multiple Sclerosis Diet Book: A Low-Fat Diet For The Treatment of MS*. New York: Doubleday, 1987.

Wahls, Terry. *Macronutrients, Micronutrients, Chronic Disease and the American Diet*. Iowa City, Iowa: TZ Press, n.d.

———. *Minding My Mitochondria*. TZ Press, 2009.

———. *Up From The Chair—My Defeat of Progressive Multiple Sclerosis*. www.terrywahls.com, n.d.

Werbach, Melvyn, with Jeffrey Moss, *Textbook of Nutritional Medicine* (Tarzana, Calif.: Third Line Press, 1999)

Williams, Montel, with William Doyle. *Living Well: 21 Days to Transform Your Life, Supercharge Your Health, and Feel Spectacular*. New York: NAL Trade, 2008.

Young, Robert O., and Shelley Redford Young. *Sick and Tired? Reclaim Your Inner Terrain*. Salt Lake City, Utah: Woodland Publishing, 2000.

———. *The pH Miracle: Balance Your Diet, Reclaim Your Health*. New York: Wellness Central, 2008.

PART THREE:
EXERCISE, PHYSICAL AND COMPLEMENTARY THERAPIES, AND HORMONES

Betts, Liz. *Exercises for People with MS*. Letchworth, Herts, UK: MS Trust, 2004.

Elkins, Rita. *Bee Pollen, Royal Jelly, Propolis and Honey*. Salt Lake City, Utah: Woodland Publishing, 2007.

Fishman, Loren Martin, and Eric L. Small. *Yoga and Multiple Sclerosis: A Journey to Health and Healing*: New York: Demos Medical Publishing, 2007

Fowler, Janine. *Everybody Stretch: A Physical Activity Workbook for People with Various Levels of Multiple Sclerosis* (Toronto: Multiple Sclerosis Society of Canada, 2003). Available at www.mssociety.ca/en/pdf/EverybodyStretch.pdf.

Gibson, Beth E. *Stretching with a Helper for People with MS: An Illustrated Manual* (n.p.: National Multiple Sclerosis Society, 2007). Available at www.nationalmssociety.org/download.aspx?id=332.

———. *Stretching for People with MS: An Illustrated Manual* (n.p.: National Multiple Sclerosis Society, 2007). Available at www.nationalmssociety.org/download.aspx?id=331.

Gingold, Jeffrey N. *Mental Sharpening Stones: Manage the Cognitive Challenges of Multiple Sclerosis*. New York: Demos Medical Publishing, 2009.

Grant, Ellen. *The Bitter Pill*. London: Thorsons, 1986.

Hamler, Brad. *Exercises for Multiple Sclerosis: A Safe and Effective Program to Fight Fatigue, Build Strength, and Improve Balance*. Long Island City, N.Y.: Hatherleigh Press, 2006.

Kent, Howard. *Yoga for the Disabled: A Practical Self-help Guide to a Happier Healthier Life*. London: Thorsons, 1985.

Lee, John R., with Virginia Hopkins. *What Your Doctor May Not Tell You about Menopause: The Breakthrough Book on Natural Hormone Balance*. New York: Grand Central Publishing, 2004.

Plowden, Judith, Ron Lawrence, and Paul Rosch. *Magnet Therapy: The Pain Cure Alternative*. Rocklin, Calif.: Prima Publishing, 1998.

Regelson, William, and Carol Colman. *The Superhormone Promise*. New York: Pocket Books, 1997.

PART FOUR:
TARGETING SYMPTOMS, TRIGGERS AND
EXACERBATING FACTORS, MERCURY, DETOXING,
LIVING LIFE TO THE FULLEST

Barron, Jon. *Lessons From The Miracle Doctors: A Step-by-Step Guide to Optimum Health and Relief from Catastrophic Illness.* Laguna Beach, Calif.: Basic Health Publications, 2008.

Blaylock, Russell L. *Excitotoxins: The Taste That Kills.* Santa Fe, N. Mex.: Health Press, 1996.

Chaitow, Leon. *Vaccination and Immunization: Dangers, Delusions and Alternatives.* London: C. W. Daniel Company, 2004.

Cleave, Thomas L. *Saccharine Disease: The Master Disease of Our Time.* New Canaan, Conn.: Keats Publishing, 1993.

Duffy, William. *Sugar Blues.* New York: Grand Central Publishing, 1986.

Eisler, Ronald. *Mercury Hazards to Living Organisms.* Boca Raton, Fla.: CRC Press/Taylor & Francis, 2006.

Graham, Judy. *Multiple Sclerosis and Having a Baby: Everything You Need to Know About Conception, Pregnancy, and Parenthood.* Rochester, Vt.: Healing Arts Press, 1999.

Hay, Louise L. *Heal Your Body: The Mental Causes for Physical Illness and the Metaphysical Way to Overcome Them.* Carlsbad, Calif.: Hay House, 2003.

———. *You Can Heal Your Life.* Carlsbad, Calif.: Hay House, 2004.

Huggins, Hal A. *It's All In Your Head: The Link Between Mercury Amalgams and Illness.* New York: Avery, 1993.

———. *Solving The MS Mystery: Help, Hope and Recovery.* York, Pa.: Matrix, 2002.

Tatevosian, Chris M. *Life Interrupted: It's Not All about Me.* Mustang, Okla.: Tate Publishing, 2008.

Williams, Montel, and William Doyle. *Living Well Emotionally: Break Through to a Life of Happiness.* New York: NAL Trade, 2010.

Yudkin, John. *Sweet and Dangerous.* New York: Bantam Books, 1973.

Ziff, Sam, Michael F. Ziff, and Mats Hanson. *Dental Mercury Detox (Health Information Guide Series).* Orlando, Fla.: Bio-Probe, 1997.

Ziff, Sam. *Silver Dental Fillings: The Toxic Time Bomb.* Santa Fe, N.Mex.: Aurora Press, 1984.

Notes

CHAPTER 3. POSSIBLE CAUSES OF MS

1. P. L. De Jager, K. C. Simon, K. L. Munger, et al., "Integrating Risk Factors: HLA-DRB1*1501 and Epstein-Barr Virus in Multiple Sclerosis," *Neurology* 70 (2008): 1113–18.

2. Michael F. Holick and Tai C. Chen, "Vitamin D: A Worldwide Problem with Health Consequences," *American Journal of Clinical Nutrition* 87 (2008): 1080S–86S.

3. C. A. Beck, L. M. Metz, L. W. Svenson, and S. B. Patten, "Regional Variation of Multiple Sclerosis Prevalence in Canada," *Multiple Sclerosis* 11, no. 5 (2005): 516–19.

4. C. W. Noonan, D. M. Williamson, J. P. Henry, et al., "The Prevalence of Multiple Sclerosis in 3 US Communities, " *Preventing Chronic Disease* 7, no. 1 (January 2010), www.cdc.gov/pcd/issues/2010/jan/08_0241.htm (accessed April 19, 2010).

5. P. Goldberg, "Multiple Sclerosis: Vitamin D and Calcium as Environmental Determinants of Prevalence (A Viewpoint). Part I: Sunlight, Dietary Factors and Epidemiology," International Journal of Environmental Studies 6 (1974): 19–27.

6. M. Rodríguez-Violante, G. Ordoñez, J. Bermudez, et al., "Association of a History of Varicella Virus Infection with Multiple Sclerosis," *Clinical Neurology and Neurosurgery* 111, no. 1 (2009): 54–56.

7. J. A. Lincoln, K. Hankiewicz, and S. D. Cook, "Could Epstein-Barr Virus or Canine Distemper Virus Cause Multiple Sclerosis?" *Neurologic Clinics* 26, no. 3 (2008): 699–715.

8. L. K. Munger, R. W. Peeling, M. A. Hernán, et al., "Infection with *Chlamydia pneumoniae* and the Risk of Multiple Sclerosis," *Epidemiology* 14, no. 2 (2003): 141–47.

9. R. H. S. Thompson, "A Biochemical Approach to the Problem of Multiple

Sclerosis," *Proceedings of the Royal Society of Medicine* 59 (1966): 269–76.

10. E. J. Field, B. K. Shenton, and Greta Joyce, "Specific Laboratory Test for Diagnosis of Multiple Sclerosis," *British Medical Journal* 1 (1974): 412–14.

11. R. L. Swank and B. B. Dugan, *The Multiple Sclerosis Diet Book: A Low-fat Diet for the Treatment of MS* (New York: Delacorte Press, 1987).

12. S. Winer, I. Astsaturov, R. K. Cheung, et al., "T Cells of Multiple Sclerosis Patients Target a Common Environmental Peptide that Causes Encephalitis in Mice," *Journal of Immunology* 166, no. 7 (2001): 4751–56.

13. Roberto di Marco, Katia Mangano, Cinzia Quattrocchi, et al., "Exacerbation of Protracted-Relapsing Experimental Allergic Encephalomyelitis in DA Rats by Gluten-Free Diet," *APMIS* 112 (2004): 651–55.

14. Philip James, "Hyperbaric Oxygen for Patients with Multiple Sclerosis," *British Medical Journal (Clinical Research Edition)* 288, no. 6433 (1984): 1831.

CHAPTER 4. FOOD SENSITIVITIES

1. W. G. Crook, *The Yeast Connection* (Jackson, Tenn.: Professional Books, 1986).

2. C. O. Truss, *The Missing Diagnosis* (Birmingham, Ala.: The Missing Diagnosis, 1982).

3. Stephen Davies and Alan Stewart, *Nutritional Medicine: The Drug-Free Guide to Better Family Health* (London: Pan Macmillan, 1987), 361–64.

4. See www.alcat.com/clinical_info.php (accessed April 19, 2010).

CHAPTER 7. THE BODY'S DELICATE BALANCE

1. Robert O. Young and Shelley Redford Young, *The PH Miracle* (Victoria, Australia: Warner Books, 2002).

2. Ibid., 142.

CHAPTER 8. NUTRITIONAL SUPPLEMENTS

1. Reinhold Vieth, "Why the Optimal Requirement for Vitamin D_3 Is Probably Much Higher Than What Is Officially Recommended for Adults," *Journal of Steroid Biochemistry and Molecular Biology* 89–90, nos. 1–5 (2004): 575–79.

2. G. E. Jensen, G. Gissel-Nielsen, and J. Clausen, "Leucocyte Glutathione Peroxidase Activity and Selenium Level in Multiple Sclerosis," *Journal of the Neurological Sciences* 48, no. 1 (1980): 61–67.

3. D. Bates, N. E. Cartlidge, J. M. French, et al., "A Double-Blind Controlled Trial of Long Chain N-3 Polyunsaturated Fatty Acids in the Treatment of Multiple Sclerosis," *Journal of Neurology, Neurosurgery & Psychiatry* 52, no. 1 (1989): 18–22.

4. "Multiple Sclerosis in the Orkney and Shetland Islands and in North-east Scotland," *British Medical Journal (Clinical Research Edition)* 282, no. 6263 (1981): 502–4.

5. B. Weinstock-Guttman, M. Baier, Y. Park, et al., "Low Fat Dietary Intervention with Omega-3 Fatty Acid Supplementation in Multiple Sclerosis Patients," *Prostaglandins, Leukotrienes and Essential Fatty Acids* 73 (2005): 397–404.

6. Udo Erasmus, *Fats That Heal, Fats That Kill* (Burnaby, B.C.: Alive Books, 1993); Erasmus's website, www.udoerasmus.com, also has many articles by him on flaxseed oil.

7. Judy Graham, *Evening Primrose Oil* (Rochester, Vt.: Healing Arts Press, 1989).

8. E. J. Field, G. Joyce, and B. M. Smith, "Erythrocyte-UFA (Eufa) Mobility Test for Multiple Sclerosis," *Journal of Neurology* 214, no. 2 (January 1977): 113–27; C. H. Tamblyn, R. L. Swank, G. V. Seaman, et al., "Red Cell Electrophoretic Mobility Test for Early Diagnosis of Multiple Sclerosis," *Neurological Research* 2, no. 1 (1980): 69–83.

9. Anthony J. Cichoke, *The Complete Book of Enzyme Therapy* (Garden City Park, N.Y.: Avery Publishing, 1999); A. J. Cichoke, "Natural Relief for Autoimmune Disorders," *Better Nutrition* 62, no. 6 (June 2000): 24.

10. P. Goldberg, M. C. Fleming, and E. H. Picard, "Multiple Sclerosis: Decreased Relapse Rate through Dietary Supplementation with Calcium, Magnesium, and Vitamin D," *Medical Hypotheses* 21 (1986): 193–200.

11. M. R. Werbach, *Foundations of Nutritional Medicine* (Tarzana, Calif.: Third Line Press, 1997), 210–11; V. Wynn, "Vitamins and Oral Contraceptive Use," *Lancet* 1, no. 7906 (1975): 561–64; G. A. Holt, *Food & Drug Interaction* (Chicago: Precept Press, 1998), 197–98.

12. S. Schwarz and H. Leweling, "Multiple Sclerosis and Nutrition," *Multiple Sclerosis* 11, no. 1 (February 2005): 24–32.

13. E. H. Reynolds, J. C. Linnell, and J. E. Faludy, "Multiple Sclerosis Associated with Vitamin B_{12} Deficiency," *Archives of Neurology* 48, no. 8 (August 1991): 808–11.

14. Ibid.

15. "Purported Link Between Vitamin B_{12} Deficiency and MS," What Doctors Don't Tell You, www.wddty.com/proported-link-between-vitamin-b12-deficiency-and-ms.html (accessed April 19, 2010).

16. T. Q. Nijst, R. A. Wevers, H. C. Schoonderwaldt, et al., "Vitamin B_{12} and Folate Concentrations in Serum and Cerebrospinal Fluid of Neurological Patients with Special Reference to Multiple Sclerosis and Dementia," *Journal of Neurology, Neurosurgery, and Psychiatry* 53 (1990): 951–54, doi: 10.1136/jnnp.53.11.951.

17. D. T. Wade, C. A. Young, K. R. Chaudhuri, et al., "A Randomized Placebo-controlled Exploratory Study of Vitamin B-12, Lofepramine, and L-phenylalanine (the 'Cari Loder Regimen') in the Treatment of Multiple Sclerosis," *Journal of Neurology, Neurosurgery, and Psychiatry* 73, no. 3 (September 2002): 246–49.

18. T. Korwin-Piotrowska, D. Nocoń, A. Stankowska-Chomicz, et al., "Experience of Padma 28 in Multiple Sclerosis," *Phytotherapy Research* 6 (1992): 133–36.

19. L. A. t'Hart, P. H. van Enckevort, H. van Dijk, et al., "Two Functionally and Chemically Distinct Immunomodulatory Compounds in the Gel of Aloe

Vera," *Journal of Ethnopharmacology* 23, no. 1 (1988): 661–71; L. A. t'Hart, A. J. van den Berg, L. Kuis, et al., "An Anti-complementary Polysaccharide with Immunological Adjuvant Activity from the Leaf Parenchyma Gel of Aloe Vera," *Planta Medica* 55, no. 6 (1989): 509–12; J. C. Pittman, "Immune Enhancing Effects of Aloe," *Health Conscious* 13, no. 1 (1992): 28–30.

20. I. Ofek, J. Goldhar, Y. Eshdat, et al., "The Importance of Mannose Specific Adhesins (Lectins) Infections Caused by *Escherichia coli,*" *Scandinavian Journal of Infectious Diseases,* Supplementum 33 (1982): 61–67.

21. See www.wellnessletter.com/html/ds/dsGlyconutrients.php (accessed April 19, 2010).

22. C. Natarajan and J. J. Bright, "Circumin and Autoimmune Disease," *Advances in Experimental Medicine and Biology* 595 (2007): 425–51; C. Natarajan and J. J. Bright, "Curcumin Inhibits Experimental Allergic Encephalomyelitis by Blocking IL-12 Signaling through Janus Kinase-STAT Pathway in T Lymphocytes," *The Journal of Immunology* 168 (2002): 6506–13; C. Natarajan and J. J. Bright, "Peroxisome Proliferator-Activated Receptor-Gamma Agonists Inhibit Experimental Allergic Encephalomyelitis by Blocking IL-12 Production, IL-12 Signaling and Th1 Differentiation," *Genes & Immunity* 3, no. 2 (2002): 59–70.

23. O. Aktas, S. Waiczies, and F. Zipp, "Neurodegeneration in Autoimmune Demyelination: Recent Mechanistic Insights Reveal Novel Therapeutic Targets," *Journal of Neuroimmunology* 184, nos. 1–2 (March 2007): 17–26.

24. Harald Tietze, *Kombucha: The Miracle Fungus* (Bermagui, NSW, Australia: Harald W. Tietze Publishing, 1996); Kaye D. Hooper, Michael P. Pender, Penny M. Webb, et al., "Use of Traditional and Complementary Medical Care by Patients with Multiple Sclerosis in South-east Queensland," *International Journal of MS Care* 3, no. 1 (2001).

Additional Studies of Interest: Probiotics

C. B. Maasen and E. Claasen, "Strain-Dependent Effects of Probiotic Lactobacilli on EAE Autoimmunity," *Vaccine* 26, no. 17 (2008): 2056–57.

I. J. Broekaert and W. A. Walker, "Probiotics as Flourishing Benefactors for the Human Body," *Gastroenterology Nursing: The Official Journal of the Society of Gastroenterology Nurses and Associates* 29, no. 1 (2006 Jan–Feb): 26–34.

T. Matsuzaki and J. Chin, "Modulating Immune Responses with Probiotic Bacteria," *Immunology and Cell Biology* 78 (2000): 67–73.

Jon Barron, "The Barron Report: The Probiotic Miracle," *The Barron Report* 7, no. 3 (1999), www.jonbarron.org (accessed April 19, 2010).

Additional Studies of Interest: Glyconutrients

A. N. Stancil and L. H. Hicks, "Glyconutrients and Perception, Cognition, and Memory," *Perceptual and Motor Skills* 10 (2009): 259–70.

R. K. Murray, R. Sinnott, J. Ramberg, et al., "Recent Dietary Carbohydrates Utilization Research Provides Insights into the Health Effects of Glyconutritional Supplements," Presented at the Scripps Center for Integrative Medicine's 3rd Annual Natural Supplements Conference, La Jolla, California (January 20–22, 2006).

"Carbohydrates and Glycobiology," *Science* 291, no. 5512 (March 2001): 2263–502.

D. L. Lefkowitz, R. Stuart, B. T. Gnade, et al., "Effects of a Glyconutrient on Macrophage Functions," *International Journal of Immunopharmacology* 4 (2000): 299–308.

Additional Studies of Interest: Noni Juice

A. Hirazumi and E. Furusawa, "An Immunomodulatory Polysaccharide-rich Substance from the Fruit Juice of *Morinda citrifolia* (Noni) with Antitumor Activity," *Phytotherapy Research* 13 (1999): 380–87.

A. Hirazumi, "Antitumor Studies of a Traditional Hawaiian Medicinal Plant, *Morinda citrifolia* (Noni), *In Vitro* and *In Vivo*," Ph.D. Thesis, University of Hawaii, Honolulu, Hawaii, 1997.

A. Hirazumi, E. Furusawa, S. C. Chou, et al., "Immunomodulation Contributes to the Anticancer Activity of *Morinda citrifolia* (Noni) Fruit Juice," *Proceedings of the Western Pharmacology Society* 39 (1996): 7–9.

CHAPTER 9. VITAMIN D

1. M. F. Holick, "Sunlight and Vitamin D for Bone Health and Prevention of Autoimmune Diseases, Cancers, and Cardiovascular Disease," *American Journal of Clinical Nutrition* 80 (December 2004): 1678S–88S.

2. Margheritia T. Cantora, "Vitamin D and Autoimmunity: Is Vitamin D Status an Environmental Factor Affecting Autoimmune Disease Prevalence?" *Experimental Biology and Medicine* 223, no. 3 (2000): 230–33.

3. R. Vieth, "Vitamin D Supplementation, 25-hydroxyvitamin D Concentrations, and Safety," *American Journal of Clinical Nutrition* 69, no. 5 (May 1999): 842–56.

4. K. L. Munger, S. M. Zhang, E. O'Reilly, et al., "Vitamin D Intake and Incidence of Multiple Sclerosis," *Neurology* 62, no. 1 (2004): 60–65.

5. K. L. Munger, L. I. Levin, B. W. Hollis, et al., "Serum 25-hydroxyvitamin D Levels and Risk of Multiple Sclerosis," *Journal of the American Medical Association* 296 (2006): 2832–38.

6. G. C. Ebers, A. D. Sadovnick, R. Vieth, et al., "Vitamin D Intake and Incidence of Multiple Sclerosis," *Neurology* 63, no. 5 (September 2004): 939.

7. M. T. Kampmann and M. Brustad, "Vitamin D: A Candidate for the Environmental Effect in Multiple Sclerosis—Observations from Norway," *Neuroepidemiology* 30, no. 3 (2008): 140–46.

8. I. A. van der Mei et al., "Vitamin D Levels in People with Multiple Sclerosis and Community Controls in Tasmania, Australia," *American Journal of Neurology* 254, no. 5 (May 2007): 581–90.

9. T. Holmoy, "Vitamin D Status Modulates the Immune Response to Epstein Barr Virus: Synergistic Effect of Risk Factors in Multiple Sclerosis," *Medical Hypotheses* 70, no. 1 (2008): 66–69.

10. S. Christakos, "Vitamin D May Protect against MS," *Journal of Cellular Biochemistry* 105, no. 2 (2008): 338–43.

11. S. V. Ramagopalan, N. J. Maugeri, L. Handunnetthi, et al., "Expression of the Multiple Sclerosis-associated MHC Class II Allele *HLA-DRB1*1501* Is Regulated by Vitamin D," *PLoS Genetics* 5, no. 2 (2009): e1000369, doi:10.1371/journal.pgen.1000369.

12. Presented at MS Research Australia, Progress in MS Research Scientific Conference 14–17, Sydney, Australia (October 17, 2009).

13. 61st Annual Meeting of the American Academy of Neurology in Seattle, Washington (April 25–May 2, 2009).

14. M. Soilu-Hänninen, "A Longitudinal Study of Serum 25-hydroxyvitamin D and Intact Parathyroid Hormone Levels Indicate the Importance of Vitamin D and Calcium Homeostasis Regulation in Multiple Sclerosis," *Journal of Neurology, Neurosurgery & Psychiatry* 79 (2008): 152–57, doi: 10.1136/jnnp.2006.105320.

15. J. A. Woolmore, "Studies of Associations Between Disability in Multiple Sclerosis, Skin Type, Gender, and Ultraviolet Radiation," *Multiple Sclerosis Journal* 13, no. 3 (2007): 369–75.

16. I. A. F. van der Mei, A. Ponsonby, L. Blizzard, et al., "Regional Variation in Multiple Sclerosis Prevalence in Australia and Its Association with Ambient Ultraviolet Radiation," *Neuroepidemiology* 20 (2001): 168–74, doi: 10.1159/000054783.

17. T. Islam, W. J. Gauderman, W. Cozen, et al., "Childhood Sun Exposure Influences Risk of Multiple Sclerosis in Monozygotic Twins," *Neurology* 69 (2007): 381–88.

18. A. D. Sadovnick and G. C. Ebers, "Epidemiology of Multiple Sclerosis: A Critical Overview," *The Canadian Journal of Neurological Sciences* 20, no. 1 (February 1993): 17–29.

19. M. Pugliatt, S. Sotgiu, G. Solinas, et al., "Multiple Sclerosis Prevalence among Sardinians: Further Evidence Against the Latitude Gradient Theory," *Neurological Sciences* 22, no. 2 (April 2001): 163–65.

20. Ashton Embry, "Vitamin D Supplementation in the Fight Against MS," www.msrc.co.uk/downloads/bbd_Vitamin_D_update_GP_Letter-4.pdf (accessed April 19, 2010); John N. Hathcock, Andrew Shao, Reinhold Vieth, et al. "Risk Assessment for Vitamin D," *The American Journal of Clinical Nutrition* 85, no. 1 (January 2007): 6–18.

21. R. Vieth, "Vitamin D Supplementation, 25-hydroxyvitamin D Concentrations, and Safety," *American Journal of Clinical Nutrition* 69 (1999): 842–56; Reinhold

Vieth, "Why the Optimal Requirement for Vitamin D_3 Is Probably Much Higher than What Is Officially Recommended for Adults," *Journal of Steroid Biochemistry and Molecular Biology* 89–90, nos. 1–5 (2004): 575–79.

22. M. T. Cantorna, C. E. Hayes, and H. F. DeLuca, "1,25-Dihydroxyvitamin D_3 Reversibly Blocks the Progression of Relapsing Encephalomyelitis," *Proceedings of the National Academy of Sciences* 93, no. 15 (1996): 7861–64; Hector Deluca and Margherita Cantorna, "Vitamin D: Its Role and Uses in Immunology," *The FASEB Journal* 15 (2001): 2579–85; M. T. Cantorna, "Vitamin D and Its Role in Immunology: Multiple Sclerosis and Inflammatory Bowel Disease," *Progress in Biophysics and Molecular Biology* 92, no. 1 (2006): 60–64.

23. C. Willer, D. Dyment, A. Sadovnick, et al., "Timing of Birth and Risk of Multiple Sclerosis: Population Based Study," *British Medical Journal* 330 (2005): 120.

24. C. J. Willer, D. A. Dyment, A. D. Sadovnick, et al., "Timing of Birth and Risk of Multiple Sclerosis: Population Based Study," *British Medical Journal* 327 (2003): 316.

25. "Low Vitamin D Levels in Children Might Predict Risk for MS," University of Toronto, presented to World Congress on Treatment and Research in Multiple Sclerosis, Montreal, Canada (June 2004).

26. Carol L. Wagner and Frank R. Greer, "Prevention of Rickets and Vitamin D Deficiency in Infants, Children, and Adolescents," *Pediatrics* 122, no. 5 (November 2008): 1142–52.

27. "Vitamin D: Recommendations and Review Status," Health Canada, www.hc-sc. gc.ca/fn-an/nutrition/vitamin/vita-d-eng.php (accessed April 19, 2010).

Additional Studies of Interest: Vitamin D

Jorge Correale, María Célica Ysrraelit, and María Inés Gaitán, "Immunomodulatory Effects of Vitamin D in Multiple Sclerosis," *Brain* 132, no. 5 (2009): 1146–60.

Justin Rubio, "Genome-wide Association Study Identifies New Multiple Sclerosis Susceptibility Loci on Chromosomes 12 and 20," *Nature Genetics* 41, no. 7 (June 15, 2009): 824–28.

Emily Smith, "Vitamin D Deficiency Related to Increased Inflammation in Healthy Women, MU Study Finds," http://munews.missouri.edu/news-releases/2009/0406-peterson-vitamin-d.php (accessed April 19, 2010).

"Higher Levels of 25-hydroxyvitamin D Are Associated with a Lower Incidence of Multiple Sclerosis Only in Women," *Medical Update Memo* (Toronto: Multiple Sclerosis Society of Canada, September 10, 2008).

K. L. Munger, S. M. Zhang, E. O'Reilly, et al., "Vitamin D Intake and Incidence of Multiple Sclerosis," *Neurology* 62 (2004): 60–65.

B. M. VanAmerongen, C. D. Dijkstra, P. Lips, et al., "Multiple Sclerosis and Vitamin D: An Update," *European Journal of Clinical Nutrition* 58, no. 8 (2004): 1095–109.

"Study Reports Possible Link Between Vitamin D and Reduced MS Risk," *Medical Update Memo* (Toronto: Multiple Sclerosis Society of Canada, January 16, 2004).

"Study Examines Exposure to Sunlight and Risk of Developing Multiple Sclerosis," *Medical Update Memo* (Toronto: Multiple Sclerosis Society of Canada, August 20 2003).

C. E. Hayes, M. T. Cantorna, and H. F. DeLuca, "Vitamin D and Multiple Sclerosis," *Proceedings of the Society for Experimental Biology and Medicine* 216 (1997): 21–27.

M. T. Cantorna, C. E. Hayes, and H. F. DeLuca, "1,25-Dihydroxyvitamin D_3 Reversibly Blocks the Progression of Relapsing Encephalomyelitis, a Model of Multiple Sclerosis," *Proceedings of the National Academy of Sciences of the United States of America* 93, no. 15 (1996): 7861–64.

J. Nieves, F. Cosman, J. Herbet, et al., "High Prevalence of Vitamin D Deficiency and Reduced Bone Mass in Multiple Sclerosis," *Neurology* 44 (1994): 1687.

CHAPTER 10. FATS AND OILS AND THEIR ROLE IN MS

1. R. H. S. Thompson, "A Biochemical Approach to the Problem of Multiple Sclerosis," *Proceedings of the Royal Society of Medicine* 59 (1966): 269–76.

2. E. J. Field, B. K. Shenton, and Greta Joyce, "Specific Laboratory Test for Diagnosis of Multiple Sclerosis," *British Medical Journal* 1 (1974): 412–14.

3. David F. Horrobin, *Omega-6 Essential Fatty Acids: Pathophysiology and Roles in Clinical Medicine* (New York: Wiley-Liss, 1990).

4. Roy Laver Swank and Barbara Brewer Dugan, *The Multiple Sclerosis Diet Book: A Low-fat Diet for the Treatment of MS* (New York: Delacorte Press, 1987); Roy Laver Swank, "Multiple Sclerosis: Twenty Years on Low Fat Diet," Archives of Neurology 23 (1970): 460–74; R. L. Swank and B. B. Dugan, "Effect of Low Saturated Fat Diet in Early and Late Cases of Multiple Sclerosis," *Lancet* 336 (1990): 37–39.

5. Roy Laver Swank and Barbara Brewer Dugan, *The Multiple Sclerosis Diet Book: A Low-fat Diet for the Treatment of MS* (New York: Delacorte Press, 1987).

6. Essays by Ashton Embry, www.ms-direct.org and www.msrc.co.uk (accessed April 19, 2010).

7. Loren Cordain, "The Paleo Diet," www.thepaleodiet.com (accessed April 19, 2010).

8. Udo Erasmus, *Fats That Heal, Fats That Kill* (Burnaby, B.C.: Alive Books, 1993), see www.udoerasmus.com (accessed April 19, 2010).

9. L. S. Harbige and M. K. Sharief, "Polyunsaturated Fatty Acids in the Pathogenesis and Treatment of Multiple Sclerosis," *British Journal of Nutrition* 98, suppl. 1 (2007): S46–S53.

10. Artemis P. Simopoulos and Jo Robinson, *The Omega Diet* (New York: HarperCollins Publishers, 1999).

Additional Studies of Interest: Essential Fatty Acids

Melvyn R. Werbach, "Nutritional Influences on Illness: Essential Fatty Acids in Multiple Sclerosis," *Townsend Letter for Doctors and Patients* (November 2003), http://findarticles.com/p/articles/mi_m0ISW/is_244/ai_111271914/ (accessed April 19, 2010).

V. Gallai, P. Sarchielli, A. Trequattrini, et al., "Cytokine Secretion and Eicosanoid Production in the Peripheral Blood Mononuclear Cells of MS Patients Undergoing Dietary Supplementation with n-3 Polyunsaturated Fatty Acids," *Journal of Neuroimmunology* 56 (1995): 143–53.

D. Bates, "Dietary Lipids and Multiple Sclerosis," *Upsala Journal of Medical Sciences, Supplement* 48 (1990): 173–87.

S. Nightingale, E. Woo, A. D. Smith, et al., "Red Blood Cell and Adipose Tissue Fatty Acids in Mild Inactive Multiple Sclerosis," *Acta Neurologica Scandinavica* 82 (1990): 43–50.

S. C. Cunnane, S. Y. Ho, P. Dore-Duffy, et al., "Essential Fatty Acid and Lipid Profiles in Plasma and Erythrocytes in Patients with Multiple Sclerosis," *American Journal of Clinical Nutrition* 50, no. 4 (October 1989): 801–6.

R. H. Dworkin, D. Bates, J. H. Millar, et al., "Linoleic Acid and Multiple Sclerosis: A Reanalysis of Three Double-blind Trials," *Neurology* 34 (1984): 1441–45.

E. J. Field and G. Joyce, "Multiple Sclerosis: Effect of Gamma Linolenate Administration Upon Membranes and the Need for Extended Clinical Trials of Unsaturated Fatty Acids," *European Neurology* 22 (1983): 78–83.

I. S. Neu, "Essential Fatty Acids in the Serum and Cerebrospinal Fluid of Multiple Sclerosis Patients," *Acta Neurologica Scandinavica* 67 (1983): 151–63.

R. H. Dworkin, "Linoleic Acid and Multiple Sclerosis," *Lancet* 1 (1981): 1153–54.

D. F. Horrobin, "Multiple Sclerosis: The Rational Basis for Treatment with Colchicine and Evening Primrose Oil," *Medical Hypotheses* 5 (1979): 365–78.

E. J. Field and G. Joyce, "Effect of Prolonged Ingestion of Gamma-linolenate by MS Patients," *European Neurology* (17) 1978: 67–76.

CHAPTER 11. EXERCISE AND EXERCISE MACHINES

1. U.K. Department of Health, *At Least Five a Week: Evidence on the Impact of Physical Activity and Its Relationship to Health* (London: Department of Health, 2004).

2. B. S. Oken, et al., "Randomized Controlled Trial of Yoga and Exercise in Multiple Sclerosis," *Neurology* 62, no. 11 (June 2004): 2058–64.

3. Howard Kent, *Yoga for the Disabled: A Practical Self-help Guide to a Happier Healthier Life* (London: Thorsons, 1985).

4. N. Mills and J. Allen, "Mindfulness of Movement as a Coping Strategy in Multiple Sclerosis. A Pilot Study," *General Hospital Psychiatry* 22 (2000): 425–31.

5. N. Mills, J. Allen, and S. Carey-Morgan, "Does T'ai Chi Help Patients with Multiple Sclerosis?" *Journal of Bodywork and Movement Therapy* 4, no. 1 (2000): 39–48.

6. Kaye D. Hooper, Michael P. Pender, Penny M. Webb, et al., "Use of Traditional and Complementary Medical Care by Patients with Multiple Sclerosis in Southeast Queensland," *International Journal of MS Care* 3, no. 1 (2001): 3.

7. O. Schuhfried, C. Mittermaier, and T. Jovanovic, "Effects of Whole Body Vibration in Patients with Multiple Sclerosis: A Pilot Study," *Clinical Rehabilitation* 19, no. 8 (2005): 834–42; Siv Ohlin and Edzard B. Zeinstra, "Whole-Body Vibration Training in Multiple Sclerosis Patients—A Pilot Study," Department of Neurological Physiotherapy, Malmo, Sweden, Power Plate International, Amsterdam, The Netherlands, 2007.

8. F. Schyns et al., "Vibration Therapy in Multiple Sclerosis: a Pilot Study Exploring Its Effects on Tone, Muscle Force, Sensation, and Functional Performance," *Clinical Rehabilitation* 23, no. 9 (September 2009): 771–81.

9. B. S. Oken, S. Kishiyama, D. Zajdel, et al., "Randomized Controlled Trial of Yoga and Exercise in Multiple Sclerosis," *Neurology* 62 (2004): 2058–64.

10. E. McAuley, K. S. Morris, L. Hu, et al., "Enhancing Physical Activity Adherence and Well-being in Multiple Sclerosis: A Randomized Controlled Trial," *Multiple Sclerosis* 13, no. 5 (2007): 652–59.

11. O. H. Bjarnadottir, "Multiple Sclerosis and Brief Moderate Exercise. A Randomised Study," *Multiple Sclerosis* 13, no. 6 (2007): 776–82.

12. Darpan Patel, et al., "Aerobic Exercise Influence on Coronary Artery Disease Risk Factors in Multiple Sclerosis," presented to the American Physiological Society, January 5, 2007.

Additional Studies of Interest: Exercise

A. Bowling, "Exercise, the Brain, and a Revolution in Neurology," *InforMS* 24, no. 2 (2008): 3–7.

U. Dalgas, E. Stenager, and T. Ingemann-Hansen, "Multiple Sclerosis and Physical Exercise: Recommendations for the Application of Resistance-, Endurance- and Combined Training," *Multiple Sclerosis* 14, no. 1 (2008): 35–53.

R. W. Motl and J. L. Gosney, "Effect of Exercise Training on Quality of Life in Multiple Sclerosis: A Meta-Analysis," *Mutliple Sclerosis* 14, no. 1 (2008): 129–35.

P. Gallien, B. Nicolas, S. Robineau, et al., "Physical Training and Multiple Sclerosis," *Annales de Réadaptation et de Médecine Physique* 50 (2007): 373–76.

E. E. Gulick and S. Goodman, "Physical Activity among People with Multiple Sclerosis," *International Journal of MS Care* 8 (2006): 121–29.

H. I. Karpatkin, "Multiple Sclerosis and Exercise: A Review of the Evidence," *International Journal of MS Care* 7 (2005): 36–41.

L. S. De Bolt and J. A. McCubbin, "The Effects of Home-based Resistance Exercise on Balance, Power, and Mobility in Adults with Multiple Sclerosis," *Archives of Physical Medicine Rehabilitation* 85 (2004): 290–97.

T. G. Roehrs, "Effects of Aquatics Exercise Program on Quality of Life Measures for

Individuals with Progressive Multiple Sclerosis," *Journal of Neurologic Physical Therapy* 28 (2004): 63–71.

A. Romberg, A. Virtanen, J. Ruutiainen, et al., "Effects of a Six-month Exercise Program on Patients with Multiple Sclerosis: A Randomized Study," *Neurology* 63 (2004): 2034–38.

L. J. White and R. H. Dressendorfer, "Exercise and Multiple Sclerosis," *Sports Medicine* 34 (2004): 1077–100.

S. Mostert and J. Kesselring, "Effects of a Short-Term Exercise Training Programme on Aerobic Fitness, Fatigue, Health Perception and Activity Levels of Subjects with Multiple Sclerosis," *Multiple Sclerosis* 8 (2002): 161–68.

L. Harvey, A. Davies-Smith, and R. Jones, "The Effect of Weighted Leg Exercises and Quadriceps Strength, EMG, and Functional Activities in People with Multiple Sclerosis," *Physiotherapy* 85 (1999): 154–61.

J. H. Petajan, E. Gappmeier, A. T. White, et al., "Impact of Aerobic Training on Fitness and Quality of Life in Multiple Sclerosis," *Annals of Neurology* 39 (1996): 432–41.

J. A. Ponichtera-Mulcare, "Exercise and Multiple Sclerosis," *Medicine and Science in Sports and Exercise* 25 (1993): 451–65.

CHAPTER 12. PHYSICAL THERAPY, PHYSIOTHERAPY, AND REHABILITATION

1. F. Khan, J. F. Pallant, C. Brand, et al., "Effectiveness of Rehabilitation Intervention in Persons with Multiple Sclerosis: A Randomised Controlled Trial," *Journal of Neurology, Neurosurgery & Psychiatry* 79 (2008): 1230–35.

2. M. Wiles, R. G. Newcombe, K. J. Fuller, et al., "Controlled Randomised Crossover Trial of the Effects of Physiotherapy on Mobility in Chronic Multiple Sclerosis," *Journal of Neurology, Neurosurgery & Psychiatry* 70, no. 2 (2001): 174–79.

3. Albert C. Lo and E. W. Triche, "Improving Gait in Multiple Sclerosis Using Robot-Assisted, Body Weight Supported Treadmill Training," *Neurorehabilitation and Neural Repair* 23, no. 2 (2009): 108–16.

Additional Studies of Interest: Rehabilitation

A. Giesser, J. Beres-Jones, A. Budovitch, et al., "Locomotor Training Using Body Weight Support on a Treadmill Improves Mobility in Persons with Multiple Sclerosis: A Pilot Study," *Multiple Sclerosis* 13, no. 2 (2007): 224–31.

Francesco Patti, Maria Rita Ciancio, Ester Reggio, et al., "The Impact of Outpatient Rehabilitation on Quality of Life in Multiple Sclerosis," *Journal of Neurology* 249, no. 8 (2002): 1027–33.

S. Mostert and J. Kesselring, "Fitness, Fatigue, Health Perception and Activity Levels of Subjects with Multiple Sclerosis," *Multiple Sclerosis* 8, no. 2 (2002): 161–68.

L. O'Hara, H. Cadbury, L. DeSouza, et al., "Physical Rehabilitation Has a Positive Effect on Disability in Multiple Sclerosis Patients," *Neurology* 54, no. 6 (2000): 1396–97.

A. J. Thompson, "The Effectiveness of Neurological Rehabilitation in Multiple Sclerosis," *Journal of Rehabilitation Research and Development* 37, no. 4 (2000): 455–61.

J. A. Freeman, D. W. Langdon, J. C. Hobart, et al., "Inpatient Rehabilitation in Multiple Sclerosis: Do the Benefits Carry Over into the Community?" *Neurology* 52, no. 1 (1999): 50–56.

G. H. Kraft, "Rehabilitation Still the Only Way to Improve Function in Multiple Sclerosis," *Lancet* 354, no. 9195 (1999): 2016–17.

A. Solari, G. Filippini, P. Gasco, et al., "Physical Rehabilitation Has a Positive Effect on Disability in Multiple Sclerosis Patients," *Neurology* 52, no. 1 (1999): 57–62.

J. A. Freeman, D. W. Langdon, J. C. Hobart, et al., "The Impact of Inpatient Rehabilitation on Progressive Multiple Sclerosis," *Annals of Neurology* 42, no. 2 (1997): 236–44.

A. Jonsson, J. Dock, and M. H. Ravnborg, "Quality of Life as a Measure of Rehabilitation Outcome in Patients with Multiple Sclerosis," *Acta Neurologica Scandinavica* 93, no. 4 (1996): 229–35.

CHAPTER 13. COMPLEMENTARY THERAPIES

1. Rosemary E. Miller, "An Investigation into the Management of the Spasticity Experienced by Some Patients with Multiple Sclerosis Using Acupuncture Based on Traditional Chinese Medicine," *Complementary Therapies in Medicine* 4, no. 1 (1996): 58–62; S. Brunham, et al., "A Single-Blinded, Randomised Controlled Trial of Acupuncture for Symptomatic Therapy of Bladder Dysfunction in Multiple Sclerosis," *Neurology* 60S (2003): A485; Jan M. Keppel Hesselink and D. J. Kopsky, "Acupuncture for Bladder Dysfunctions in Multiple Sclerosis," *Medical Acupuncture* 17, no. 1 (2005): 38–39.

2. C. P. Donnellan and J. Shanley, "Comparison of the Effect of Two Types of Acupuncture on Quality of Life in Secondary Progressive Multiple Sclerosis: A Preliminary Single-Blind Randomized Controlled Trial," *Clinical Rehabilitation* 22, no. 3 (2008): 195–205; Caroline McGuire, "Acupuncture in the Treatment of Fatigue in a Patient with Multiple Sclerosis: Case Study," *Physiotherapy* 89, no. 11 (2003): 637–40.

3. Rosemary E. Miller, "An Investigation into the Management of the Spasticity Experienced by Some Patients with Multiple Sclerosis Using Acupuncture Based on Traditional Chinese Medicine," *Complementary Therapies in Medicine* 4, no. 1 (1996): 58–62.

4. S. Brunham, et al., "A Single-blinded, Randomised Controlled Trial of Acupuncture for Symptomatic Therapy of Bladder Dysfunction in Multiple Sclerosis," *Neurology* 60S (2003): A485.

5. L. F. Haas, "Mistletoe," *Journal of Neurology, Neurosurgery & Psychiatry* 58 (1995): 6, doi:10.1136/jnnp.58.1.6.

6. Andrew Vickers and Catherine Zollman, "Unconventional Approaches to Nutritional Medicine," *British Medical Journal* 319 (1999): 1419–22.

7. Amanda L. Howarth, "Will Aromatherapy Be a Useful Treatment Strategy for People with Multiple Sclerosis Who Experience Pain?" *Complementary Therapies in Nursing and Midwifery* 8, no. 3 (2002): 138–41.

8. Georgina Sutherland, Mark B. Anderson, and Tony Morris, "Relaxation and Health-Related Quality of Life in Multiple Sclerosis: The Example of Autogenic Training," *Journal of Behavioral Medicine* 28, no. 3 (2005): 249–56.

9. Marc S. Micozzi, "Biophysically Based Diagnosis and Treatment," *Seminars in Integrative Medicine* 2, no. 2 (2004): 49–53.

10. T. Korwin-Piotrowska, D. Nocoń, A. Stankowska-Chomicz, et al., "Experience of Padma 28 in Multiple Sclerosis," *Phytotherapy Research* 6 (1992): 133–36.

11. B. Brochet, J. M. Orgogozo, P. Guinot, et al., "Pilot Study of Ginkgolide B, a PAF-acether Specific Inhibitor in the Treatment of Acute Outbreaks of Multiple Sclerosis," *Rev Neurol* (Paris) 148 (1992): 299–301 [in French].

12. Erin L. Elster, "Eighty-One Patients with Multiple Sclerosis and Parkinson's Disease Undergoing Upper Cervical Chiropractic Care to Correct Vertebral Subluxation: A Retrospective Analysis," *Journal of Vertebral Subluxation Research* (August 2004): 1–9.

13. David C. Mohr, Arne C. Boudewyn, Donald E. Goodkin, et al., "Comparative Outcomes for Individual Cognitive-Behavior Therapy, Supportive-Expressive Group Psychotherapy, and Sertraline for the Treatment of Depression in Multiple Sclerosis," *Journal of Consulting and Clinical Psychology* 69, no. 6 (December 2001): 942–49.

14. David C. Mohr, William Likosky, Andrew Bertagnolli, et al., "Telephone-administered Cognitive Behavioral Therapy for the Treatment of Depressive Symptoms in Multiple Sclerosis," *Journal of Consulting and Clinical Psychology* 68, no. 2 (April 2000): 356–61.

15. N. A. Larcombe and P. H. Wilson, "An Evaluation of Cognitive-behavior Therapy for Depression in Patients with Multiple Sclerosis," *The British Journal of Psychiatry* 145 (1984): 366–71.

16. Kirsten van Kessel, Rona Moss-Morris, et al., "A Randomized Controlled Trial of Cognitive Behavior Therapy for Multiple Sclerosis Fatigue," *Psychosomatic Medicine* 70 (2008): 205–13.

17. R. O. Robinson, G. T. McCarthy, and T. M. Little, "Conductive Education at the Peto Institute, Budapest," *British Medical Journal* 299 (1989): 1145–49.

18. The Craniosacral Institute, www.cranial.org (accessed April 19, 2010).

19. Gil Raviv, Shai Shefi, Dalia Nizani, et al., "Effect of Craniosacral Therapy on Lower Urinary Tract Signs and Symptoms in Multiple Sclerosis," *Complementary Therapies in Clinical Practice* 15, no. 2 (2009): 72–75.

20. Stephens et al., "Use of Awareness through Movement Improves Balance and Balance Confidence in People with Multiple Sclerosis: A Random Controlled Study," *Neurology Report* 25, no. 2 (2001): 39–49.

21. Thomas E. Whitmarsh, "Homeopathy in Multiple Sclerosis," *Complementary Therapies in Nursing and Midwifery* 9, no. 1 (2003): 5–9.

22. Ibid.

23. C. Peterson, "Exercise in 94 Degrees F Water for a Patient with Multiple Sclerosis," *Physical Therapy* 81, no. 4 (2001): 1049–58; Richard F. Edlich, Ralph M. Buschbacher, Mary Jude Cox, et al., "Strategies to Reduce Hyperthermia in Ambulatory Multiple Sclerosis Patients," *Journal of Long-term Effects of Medical Implants* 14, no. 6 (2004): 476–79; Somaiyeh Ghafari, Fazlolah Ahmadi, and Masood Nabavi, "Effects of Applying Hydrotherapy on Fatigue in Multiple Sclerosis Patients," *Journal of Mazandaran University of Medical Sciences* 18, no. 66 (2008): 71–81.

24. H. Sutcher, "Hypnosis as Adjunctive Therapy for Multiple Sclerosis—A Progress Report," *The American Journal of Clinical Hypnosis* 39, no. 4 (1997): 280–90; J. R. Dane, "Hypnosis for Pain and Neuromuscular Rehabilitation with Multiple Sclerosis," *International Journal of Clinical and Experimental Hypnosis* 44, no. 3 (1996): 208–31.

25. Robert R. Provine, "Laughter," *American Scientist* 84 (1996): 38–47, www.americanscientist.org/issues/feature/laughter/1 (accessed April 19, 2010); Quentin Skinner, "Hobbes and the Classical Theory of Laughter," http://fds.oup.com/www.oup.co.uk/pdf/0-19-926461-9.pdf (accessed April 19, 2010); Victor Raskin, *Semantic Mechanisms of Humor* (Norwell, Mass.: Kluwer Academic Publishers, 1985); C. MacDonald, "A Chuckle a Day Keeps the Doctor Away: Therapeutic Humor & Laughter," *Journal of Psychosocial Nursing and Mental Health Services* 42, no. 3 (2004): 18–25; Kiyobumi Kawakami, Kiyoko Takai-Kawakami, Masaki Tomonaga, et al., "Origins of Smile and Laughter: A Preliminary Study," *Early Human Development* 82 (2006): 61–66.

26. Reuven Sandyk, "The Pineal Gland and Multiple Sclerosis," *International Journal of Neuroscience* 63, nos. 3–4 (1992): 157–62.

27. T. L. Richards, M. S. Lappin, J. Acosta-Urquidi, et al., "Double-blind Study of Pulsing Magnetic Field Effects on Multiple Sclerosis," *Journal of Alternative and Complementary Medicine* 3, no. 1 (Spring 1997): 21–29.

28. T. L. Richards, M. S. Lappin, F. W. Lawrie, et al., "Bioelectromagnetic Applications for Multiple Sclerosis," *Physical Medicine Rehabilitation Clinics of North America* 9, no. 3 (August 1998): 659–74.

29. Sangeetha Nayak, "Use of Unconventional Therapies by Individuals with Multiple Sclerosis," *Clinical Rehabilitation* 17, no. 2 (2003): 181–91.

30. M. Hernandez-Reif, et al., "Multiple Sclerosis Patients Benefit from Massage Therapy," Journal of Bodywork and Movement Therapies 2, no. 3 (1998): 168–74.

31. J. Graydon and N. McKee, "Massage as Therapy in Multiple Sclerosis," *International Journal of Alternative and Complementary Medicine* 15, no. 7 (1997): 27–28.

32. Ruth Werner, "Working with Multiple Sclerosis Patients," *Massage Today,* www.massagetoday.com/archives/2002/03/15.html (accessed April 19, 2010).

33. Richard J. Davidson, Jon Kabat-Zinn, Jessica Schumacher, et al., "Alterations in Brain and Immune Function Produced by Mindfulness Meditation," Journal of Psychosomatic Medicine 65, no. 4 (2003): 564–70.

34. B. L. Maguire, "The Effects of Guided Imagery Visualization on Attitudes and Moods for Multiple Sclerosis Patients," *Alternative Therapies in Health and Medicine* 2, no. 5 (1996): 75–79.

35. Multiple Sclerosis Association of America (MSAA), Research News, "Patient Education: Using Relaxation and Guided Imagery for MS: Lowering Anxiety Associated With MS & MS Injections," MSAA presentations at the 2008 Consortium of Multiple Sclerosis Centers (CMSC) Annual Meeting Summer 2008, www.msassociation.org/publications/summer08/research.asp (accessed April 19, 2010).

36. Lynne Shinto, Carlo Calabrese, Cynthia Morris, et al., "Complementary and Alternative Medicine in Multiple Sclerosis: Survey of Licensed Naturopaths," *The Journal of Alternative and Complementary Medicine* 10, no. 5 (2004): 891–97.

37. Andrew Vickers and Catherine Zollman, "Unconventional Approaches to Nutritional Medicine," *British Medical Journal* 319 (1999): 1419–22.

38. H. A. Yates, T. C. Vardy, M. L. Kuchera, et al., "Effects of Osteopathic Manipulative Treatment and Concentric and Eccentric Maximal-Effort Exercise on Women with Multiple Sclerosis: A Pilot Study," *Journal of the American Osteopathic Association* 102, no. 5 (2002): 267–75.

39. National Institute for Health and Clinical Excellence, "Multiple Sclerosis, Management of Multiple Sclerosis in Primary and Secondary Care," http://guidance.nice.org.uk/CG8 (accessed April 19, 2010).

40. I. Siev-Ner, "Reflexology Treatment Relieves Symptoms of Multiple Sclerosis—A Randomised Control Study," *Multiple Sclerosis* 9, no. 4 (2003): 356–61.

41. The Healing Pages, "Research into Reiki and Multiple Sclerosis," www.thehealingpages.com/Articles/ReikiAndMultipleSclerosis.html (accessed April 19, 2010).

42. P. A. Mackereth, K. Booth, V. F. Hillier, et al., "Reflexology and Progressive Muscle Relaxation Training for People with Multiple Sclerosis: A Crossover Trial," *Complementary Therapy & Clinical Practice* 1 (2009): 14–21; G. Sutherland, M. B. Andersen, and T. Morris, "Relaxation and Health-Related Quality of Life in Multiple Sclerosis: The Example of Autogenic Training," *Journal of Behavioral Medicine* 28, no. 3 (2005): 249–56.

43. Edythe Vickers and Subhuti Dharmananda, "Traditional Chinese Medicine and Multiple Sclerosis," www.itmonline.org/arts/ms&tcm.htm (accessed April 19, 2010).

44. Ibid.

45. Ibid.

46. Ibid.
47. Robert Groth, "How Montel Williams Conquers Multiple Sclerosis," www .articlesnatch.com/Article/How-Montel-Williams-Conquers-Multiple-Sclerosis/588581 (accessed April 19, 2010).

Additional Studies of Interest: Chiropractic

P. Dougherty and D. Lawrence, "Chiropractic Management of Musculoskeletal Pain in the Multiple Sclerosis Patient," *Clinical Chiropractic* 8, no. 2 (2005): 57–65

"Multiple Sclerosis Patient Helped with Chiropractic: A Case Report," *Journal of Vertebral Subluxation Research (JVSR)* 4, no. 2 (May 2001).

D. E. Stude and T. Mick, "Clinical Presentation of a Patient with Multiple Sclerosis and Response to Manual Chiropractic Adjustive Therapies," *Journal of Manipulative Physiol Therapies* 16, no. 9 (1993): 595–600.

Additional Studies of Interest: Craniosacral Therapy

M. J. Olek, "Multiple Sclerosis. Treatment Strategies," *Journal of the American Osteopathic Association* 99, no. 12 (1999): 611.

T. C. Vardy, *"Enhancing Homeostasis Using Osteopathic Techniques for Multiple Sclerosis,"* Australian Journal of Osteopathy 8, no. 2 (1997): 20–26.

Additional Studies of Interest: Feldenkrais Method

S. Jain, K. Janssen, and S. DeCelle, "Alexander Technique and Feldenkrais Method: A Critical Overview," *Physical Medicine & Rehabilitation Clinics of North America* 15, no. 4 (2004): 811–25.

S. K. Johnson, J. Frederick, M. Kaufman, et al., "A Controlled Investigation of Bodywork in Multiple Sclerosis," *The Journal of Alternative and Complementary Medicine* 5, no. 3 (1999): 237–43.

Additional Studies of Interest: Traditional Chinese Medicine

S. Dharmananda, "Chinese Herbal Treatment for Multiple Sclerosis," www.itmonline .org/arts/msalsmg.htm (accessed April 19, 2010).

Lu Xi, Li Zhi-wen, Wang Hua-yuan, et al., "A Study of the Chinese Medicine Prevention of Relapse of Multiple Sclerosis," *Journal of Chinese Medicine* (1995): 417–18.

CHAPTER 14. OTHER MODALITIES THAT CAN HELP MS

1. Omar Ghaffar and Anthony Feinstein, "Multiple Sclerosis and Cannabis: A Cognitive and Psychiatric Study," *Neurology* 71, no. 3 (2008): 164–69.
2. J. Zajicek, P. Fox, H. Sanders, et al., "Cannabinoids for Treatment of Spasticity and Other Symptoms Related to Multiple Sclerosis (CAMS study): Multicenter Randomized Placebo-controlled Trial," *Lancet* 362, no. 9395 (2003): 1517–26.

3. J. Zajicek et al., "Cannabinoids in Multiple Sclerosis (CAMS) Study: Safety and Efficacy Data for Twelve Months Follow-up," *Journal of Neurology, Neurosurgery & Psychiatry* 76 (2005): 1664–69.

4. D. Langdon, "The Effect of Cannabinoids on Psychological Factors in MS," Rehabilitation in Multiple Sclerosis (RIMS) 8th Annual Meeting (May 22–25, 2003).

5. P. Fox, P. G. Bain, S. Glickman, et al., "The Effect of Cannabis on Tremor in Participants with Multiple Sclerosis," *Neurology* 62, no. 7 (2004): 1105–9.

6. K. Maresz, G. Pryce, E. Ponomarev, et al., "Direct Suppression of CNS Autoimmune Inflammation via the Cannabinoid Receptor CB_1 on Neurons and CB_2 on Autoreactive T Cells," *Nature Medicine* 13 (April 2001): 492–97; Gareth Pryce, David Baker, et al., "*Cannabinoids* Inhibit Neurodegeneration in Models of Multiple Sclerosis," *Brain* 126, no. 10 (October 2003): 2191–202; David Baker and Gareth Pryce, "The Potential Role of the Endocannabinoid System in the Control of Multiple Sclerosis," *Current Medicinal Chemistry–Central Nervous System Agents* 4, no. 3 (September 2004): 195–202; David Baker and Gareth Pryce, "The Endocannabinoid System and Multiple Sclerosis," *Current Pharmaceutical Design* 14, no. 23 (August 2008): 2326–36.

7. C. M. Brady, R. Das Gupta, C. Dalton, et al., "An Open-label Pilot Study of Cannabis Based Extracts for Bladder Dysfunction in Advanced Multiple Sclerosis," *Multiple Sclerosis* 10, no. 4 (2004): 425–33.

8. Sativex data presented at ECTRIMS European Multiple Sclerosis Congress, October 3, 2006.

9. C. Collin, P. Davies, I. K. Mutiboko, et al., "Randomized Controlled Trial of Cannabis-based Medicine in Spasticity Caused by Multiple Sclerosis," *European Journal of Neurology* 14, no. 3 (2007): 290–96.

10. D. J. Rog, T. J. Nurmikko, and C. A. Young, "Oromucosal Delta9-tetrahydrocannabinol/Cannabidiol for Neuropathic Pain Associated with Multiple Sclerosis: An Uncontrolled, Open-label, 2-year Extension Trial," *Clinical Therapeutics* 29, no. 9 (2007): 2068–79.

11. D. J. Rog, T. J. Nurmikko, T. Friede, et al., "Randomized, Controlled Trial of Cannabis-based Medicine in Central Pain in Multiple Sclerosis," *Neurology* 65, no. 6 (2005): 812–19.

12. D. T. Wade, P. Makela, H. House, et al., "Long-term Use of a Cannabis-based Medicine in the Treatment of Spasticity and Other Symptoms of Multiple Sclerosis," *Multiple Sclerosis* 12, no. 5 (2006): 639–45.

13. GW Pharmaceuticals press release March 11, 2009, www.gwpharma.com/Positive-Outcome-of-Sativex-Phase-III-MS-Study.aspx (accessed April 19, 2010).

14. Mark A. Farinha, "University of North Texas Time-Kill Study on SilverKare Colloidal Silver," www.silvermedicine.org/colloidalsilverstudytexas.html (accessed April 19, 2010).

15. Zoltan P. Rona, "Bovine Colostrum Emerges as Immune System Modulator," *The American Journal of Natural Medicine* (March 1998): 19–23.

16. David Wheldon, "Empirical Antibacterial Treatment of Infection with *Chlamydophila pneumoniae* in Multiple Sclerosis," www.davidwheldon.co.uk/ms-treatment.html (accessed April 19, 2010).

17. S. Sriram, C. W. Stratton, S. Yao, et al., "*Chlamydia pneumoniae* Infection of the Central Nervous System in Multiple Sclerosis," *Annals of Neurology* 46, no. 1 (July 1999): 6–14; D. Buljevac, R. P. Verkooyen, B. C. Jacobs, et al., "*Chlamydia pneumoniae* and the Risk for Exacerbation in Multiple Sclerosis Patients," *Annals of Neurology* 54, no. 6 (December 2003): 828–31.

18. Philip James, "Hyperbaric Oxygen for Patients with Multiple Sclerosis," *British Medical Journal* (Clin Res Ed) 288, no. 6433 (June 1984): 1831.

19. B. H. Fischer, M. Marks, and T. Reich, "Hyperbaric-oxygen Treatment of Multiple Sclerosis: A Randomized, Placebo-controlled, Double-blind Study," *New England Journal of Medicine* 308, no. 4 (January 1983): 181–86.

20. Paolo Zamboni, et al., "A Prospective Open-label Study of Endovascular Treatment of Chronic Cerebrospinal Venous Insufficiency," *Journal of Vascular Surgery* 50, no. 6 (December 2009): 1348–58.

21. R. N. Golden, B. N. Gaynes, R. D. Ekstrom, et al., "The Efficacy of Light Therapy in the Treatment of Mood Disorders: A Review and Meta-analysis of the Evidence," *American Journal of Psychiatry* 162, no. 4 (2005): 656–62.

22. Results presented to World Congress on Treatment and Research in Multiple Sclerosis, Montreal, Canada (September 2008).

23. G. Gillson, T. L. Richards, R. B. Smith, et al., "A Double-blind Pilot Study of the Effect of Prokarin™ on Fatigue in Multiple Sclerosis," *Multiple Sclerosis Journal* 8, no. 1 (2002): 30–35.

24. R. K. Burt, Y. Loh, B. Cohen, et al., "Autologous Non-myeloablative Haemopoietic Stem Cell Transplantation in Relapsing-remitting Multiple Sclerosis: A Phase I/II Study," *The Lancet Neurology* 8, no. 3 (March 2009): 244–53.

25. Fereydoon Batmanghelidj, *Your Body's Many Cries for Water: You Are Not Sick, You Are Thirsty!* (Falls Church, Va.: Global Health Solutions, 1995); Fereydoon Batmanghelidj, *Water for Health, for Healing, for Life; You're Not Sick, You're Thirsty!* (New York: Grand Central Publishing, 2003).

Additional Studies of Interest: Cannabis

J. Croxford, G. Pryce, S. Jackson, et al., "Cannabinoid-mediated Neuroprotection, Not Immunosuppression, May Be More Relevant to Multiple Sclerosis," *Journal of Neuroimmunology* 193, nos. 1–2 (January 2008): 120–29.

P. F. Smith, "Symptomatic Treatment of Multiple Sclerosis Using Cannabinoids—Recent Advances," *Neurotherapeutics* 7, no. 9 (2007): 1157–63.

Lara Teare and John Zajicek, "The Use of Cannabinoids in Multiple Sclerosis," *Expert Opinion on Investigational Drugs* 14, no. 7 (July 2005): 859–69.

D. T. Wade, P. Makela, P. Robson, et al., "Do Cannabis-based Medicinal Extracts Have General or Specific Effects on Symptoms in Multiple Sclerosis? A Double-blind, Randomized, Placebo-controlled Study on 160 Patients," *Multiple Sclerosis* 10, no. 4 (2004): 434–41.

Additional Studies of Interest: Chlamydia pneumoniae

E. Fainardi, M. Castellazzi, I. Casetta, et al., "Intrathecal Production of *Chlamydia pneumoniae*-specific High-affinity Antibodies Is Significantly Associated with a Subset of Multiple Sclerosis Patients with Progressive Forms," *Journal of the Neurological Sciences* 217 (2004): 181–88.

S. Yao, C. W. Stratton, W. M. Mitchell, et al., "CSF Oligoclonal Bands in MS Include Antibodies against Chlamydophila Antigens," *Neurology* 56 (May 2001): 1168–76.

Additional Studies of Interest: Cooling

G. Flensner and C. Lindencrona, "The Cooling-suit: Case Studies of Its Influence on Fatigue among Eight Individuals with Multiple Sclerosis," *Journal of Advanced Nursing* 29 (2002): 1444–53.

E. A. C. Beenakker, T. I. Oparina, A. Hartgring, et al., "Cooling Garment Treatment in MS: Clinical Improvement and Decrease in Leukocyte Nitric Oxide (NO) Production," *Neurology* 57 (2001): 892–94.

J. Kinnman, U. A. Anderson, A. Anderson, et al., "Cooling Suit for Multiple Sclerosis: Functional Improvement in Daily Living," *Scandinavian Journal of Rehabilitation Medicine* 33 (2000): 20–24.

Y. E. Ku, L. D. Montgomery, H. Lee, et al., "Physiologic and Functional Responses of MS Patients to Body Cooling," *American Journal of Physical Medicine and Rehabilitation* 13 (2000): 8994–9115.

J. Kinnman, U. A. Anderson, and Y. Kinnman, "Temporary Improvement of Motor Function in Patient with Multiple Sclerosis after Treatment with a Cooling Suit," *Journal of Neurologic Rehabilitation* 11 (1997): 109–14.

G. Kraft and A. Alquist, "Effect of Microclimate Cooling on Physical Function in Multiple Sclerosis," *Cooling and Multiple Sclerosis* 1 (1997): 6–9.

L. D. Montgomery, R. W. Montgomery, and Y. E. Ku, "Enhancement of Cognitive Processing by Multiple Sclerosis Patients Using Liquid Cooling Technology: A Case Study," *Nasa Technical Reports Server* (1997).

R. G. Pellegrino, A. J. Roberts, and J. Harper-Bennie, "The Use of In-home Portable Conductive Cooling Units from the Study to Evaluate the Chronic Effects of Conductive Cooling in Multiple Sclerosis Patients," *Cooling and Multiple Sclerosis* 1 (1997): 9–10.

Y. E. Ku, L. D. Montgomery, and B. W. Webbon, "Hemodynamic and Thermal Responses to Head and Neck Cooling in Men and Women," *American Journal of Physical Medicine and Rehabilitation* 75 (1996): 443–50.

E. Capello, M. Gardella, M. Leandri, et al., "Lowering Body Temperature with a Cooling Suit as Symptomatic Treatment for Thermosensitive Multiple Sclerosis Patients," *Italian Journal of Neurological Sciences* 8 (November 16, 1995): 533–39.

Additional Studies of Interest: Hyperbaric Oxygen Therapy (HBOT)

M. H. Bennett and R. Heard, "Hyperbaric Oxygen Therapy for Multiple Sclerosis," *Cochrane Database of Systematic Reviews* 1 (2004).

R. M. Leach, P. J. Rees, and P. Wilmshurst, "ABC of Oxygen: Hyperbaric Oxygen Therapy," *British Medical Journal* 317 (1998): 1140–43.

M. P. Barnes, D. Bates, N. E. Cartlidge, et al., "Hyperbaric Oxygen and Multiple Sclerosis: Final Results of a Placebo-controlled, Double-blind Trial," *Journal of Neurology, Neurosurgery & Psychiatry* 50, no. 11 (November 1987): 1402–6.

J. Neiman, B. Y. Nilsson, P. O. Barr, et al., "Hyperbaric Oxygen in Chronic Progressive Multiple Sclerosis: Visual Evoked Potentials and Clinical Effects," *Journal of Neurology, Neurosurgery & Psychiatry* 48, no. 6 (June 1985): 497–500.

Additional Study of Interest: Low Dose Naltrexone (LDN)

M. Gironi, F. Martinelli-Boneschi, P. Sacerdote, et al., "A Pilot Trial of Low-dose Naltrexone in Primary Progressive Multiple Sclerosis," *Multiple Sclerosis* 14, no. 8 (2008): 1076–83.

CHAPTER 15. HORMONES AND MS

1. V. Tomassini, E. Onesti, C. Mainero, et al., "Sex Hormones Modulate Brain Damage in Multiple Sclerosis: MRI evidence," *Journal of Neurology, Neurosurgery & Psychiatry* 76 (2005): 272–75.

2. C. Confavreux, M. Hutchinson, M. M. Hours, et al., "Rate of Pregnancy-related Relapse in Multiple Sclerosis," *New England Journal of Medicine* 339, no. 5 (July 30, 1998): 285–91; J. N. Whitaker, "Effects of Pregnancy and Delivery on Disease Activity in Multiple Sclerosis," *New England Journal of Medicine* 339, no. 5 (July 30, 1998): 339–40.

3. S. M. Gold and R. R. Voskuhl, "Estrogen Treatment in Multiple Sclerosis," *Journal of Neurological Sciences* 286, nos. 1–2 (November 15, 2009): 99–103.

4. Donald G. Stein, "Is Progesterone Worth Consideration as a Treatment for Brain Injury?" *American Journal of Roentgenology* 194, no. 1 (January 2010): 20–22.

5. Michael Schumacher, Rachida Guennoun, Abdel Ghoumari, et al., "Novel Perspectives for Progesterone in Hormone Replacement Therapy, with Special Reference to the Nervous System," *Endocrine Reviews* 28, no. 4 (June 2007): 387–439.

6. University of Calgary, "Pregnancy Hormone Key to Repairing Nerve Cell Damage," news release, February 20, 2007.

7. M. B. D'hooghe, G. Nagels, and B. M. Uitdehaag, "Long-term Effects of

Childbirth in MS," *Journal of Neurology, Neurosurgery, and Psychiatry* 81 (November 2009): 38–41.

8. A. Langer-Gould, S. M. Huang, R. Gupta, et al., "Exclusive Breastfeeding and the Risk of Postpartum Relapses in Women with Multiple Sclerosis," *Archives of Neurology* 66, no. 8 (2009): 958–63, doi:10.1001/archneurol.2009.132.

9. C. Pozzilli, P. Falaschi, C. Mainero, et al., "MRI in Multiple Sclerosis During the Menstrual Cycle: Relationship with Sex Hormone Patterns," *Neurology* 53 (1999): 622.

10. Anneke Zorgdrager, "The Premenstrual Period and Exacerbations in Multiple Sclerosis," *European Neurology* 48 (2002): 204–6.

11. Maria K. Houtchens, "Understanding Fluctuations of Multiple Sclerosis across the Menstrual Cycle," *International Journal of MS Care* 2, no. 4 (2000): 2.

12. R. Smith and J. W. Studd, "A Pilot Study of the Effect upon Multiple Sclerosis of the Menopause, Hormone Replacement Therapy and the Menstrual Cycle," *Journal of the Royal Society of Medicine* 85, no. 10 (October 1992): 612–13.

13. Á. Alonso, S. S. Jick, M. J. Olek, et al., "Recent Use of Oral Contraceptives and the Risk of Multiple Sclerosis," *Archives of Neurology* 62 (2005): 1362–65.

14. Nancy L. Sicotte, Barbara S. Giesser, Vinita Tandon, et al., "Testosterone Treatment in Multiple Sclerosis, a Pilot Study," *Archives of Neurology* 64, no. 5 (2007): 683–88.

15. V. Tomassini, E. Onesti, C. Mainero, et al., "Sex Hormones Modulate Brain Damage in Multiple Sclerosis: MRI Evidence," *Journal of Neurology, Neurosurgery, and Psychiatry* 76 (2005): 272–75.

16. E. Roberts and T. J. Fauble, "Oral DHEA in Multiple Sclerosis: Results of a Phase One, Open Study," in *The Biologic Role of DHEA*, eds. M. Kalimi and W. Regelson, 81–93 (New York: Walter De Gruyter, 1990).

17. V. P. Calabrese, et al., "DHEA in Multiple Sclerosis: Positive Effects on the Fatigue Syndrome in a Non-randomized Study," in *The Biologic Role of DHEA*, eds. M. Kalimi and W. Regelson, 95–100 (New York: Walter De Gruyter, 1990).

Additional Studies of Interest: Estrogen

Rhonda R. Voskuhl, "Sex Hormones and Other Pregnancy-Related Factors with Therapeutic Potential in Multiple Sclerosis," in *Multiple Sclerosis Therapeutics*, eds. Jeffrey A. Cohen and Richard A. Rudick (London: Informa UK Ltd., 2007).

S. S. Soldan, A. I. Alvarez Retuerto, N. L. Sicotte, et al., "Immune Modulation in Multiple Sclerosis Patients Treated with the Pregnancy Hormone Estriol," *Journal of Immunology* 171, no. 11 (December 1, 2003): 6267–74.

N. L. Sicotte, S. M. Liva, R. Klutch, et al., "Treatment of Multiple Sclerosis with Pregnancy Hormone Estriol," *Annals of Neurology* 52, no. 4 (October 2002): 421–28.

CHAPTER 16. ALLEVIATING SPECIFIC SYMPTOMS

1. "Dr. Bob Lawrence," The Multiple Sclerosis Resource Center, http://www.msrc.co.uk/index.cfm?fuseaction=show&pageid=650 (accessed April 20, 2010).

2. Ibid.

3. A. Hextall, K. Boos, L. Cardozo, et al., "The 'Queen Square' Bladder Stimulator," *British Journal of Urology* 81, no. 1 (January 1998): 181.

4. Jesus Lovera, et al., Oregon Health & Science University, "OHSU Study Finds Ginkgo Beneficial For MS Symptoms," news release, April 27, 2005; S. K. Johnson, B. J. Diamond, S. Rausch, et al., "The Effect of Ginkgo biloba on Functional Measures in Multiple Sclerosis: A Pilot Randomized Controlled Trial," *Explore (NY)* 2, no. 1 (2006): 19–24; P. R. Solomon, F. Adams, A. Silver, et al., "Ginkgo for Memory Enhancement: A Randomized Controlled Trial," *Journal of the American Medical Association* 288, no. 7 (2002): 835–40; J. Lovera, B. Bagert, K. Smoot, et al., "Ginkgo Biloba for the Improvement of Cognitive Performance in Multiple Sclerosis: A Randomized, Placebo-controlled Trial," *Multiple Sclerosis* 13, no. 3 (2007): 376–85.

5. Kirsten van Kessel, Rona Moss-Morris, et al., "A Randomized Controlled Trial of Cognitive Behavior Therapy for Multiple Sclerosis Fatigue," *Psychosomatic Medicine* 70 (2008): 205–13.

6. E. Munteis, "Prevalence of Autoimmune Thyroid Disorders in a Spanish Multiple Sclerosis Cohort," *European Journal of Neurology* 14, no. 9 (2007): 1048–52.

7. I. D. Swain, P. N. Taylor, J. H. Burridge, et al., "Common Peroneal Stimulation for the Correction of Drop-foot," Report to the South and West Regional Development and Evaluation Committee, UK (1996), www.salisburyfes.com/dec.htm (accessed April 20, 2010).

8. C. L. Barrett, "A Randomized Trial to Investigate the Effects of Functional Electrical Stimulation and Therapeutic Exercise on Walking Performance for People with Multiple Sclerosis," *Multiple Sclerosis* 15, no. 4 (April 2009): 493–504.

9. R. Dasgupta, O. J. Wiseman, G. Kanabar, et al., "Efficacy of Sildenafil in the Treatment of Female Sexual Dysfunction Due to Multiple Sclerosis," *The Journal of Urology* 171, no. 3 (March 2004): 1189–93; I. F. Hussain, C. M. Brady, M. J. Swinn, et al., "Treatment of Erectile Dysfunction with Sildenafil Citrate (*Viagra*) in Parkinsonism due to Parkinson's Disease or Multiple System Atrophy with Observations on Orthostatic Hypotension," *Journal of Neurology, Neurosurgery, and Psychiatry* 71 (2001): 371–74.

10. J. Borg-Stein et al., "Botulism Toxin for the Treatment of Spasticity in Multiple Sclerosis: New Observations," *American Journal of Physical Medicine and Rehabilitation* 72, no. 6 (December 1993): 364–68.

11. Yi-Yuan Tang, Michael Posner, et al.,"Short-term Meditation Training Improves Attention and Self-regulation," *Proceedings of the National Academy of Sciences* 104, no. 43 (October 2007): 17152–56.

12. Sandra B. Barker and Kathryn S. Dawson, "The Effects of Animal-assisted Therapy on Anxiety Ratings of Hospitalized Psychiatric Patients," *Psychiatric Services* 49 (June 1998): 797–801.

CHAPTER 17. MS TRIGGERS AND EXACERBATING FACTORS

1. A. G. Maas and L. A. Hogenhuis, "Multiple Sclerosis and Intolerance for Xenobiotics," *Annals of Allergy* 59, no. 1 (July 1987): 76–79.
2. S. Scanto and J. Yudkin, "The Effect of Dietary Sucrose on Blood Lipids, Serum Insulin, Platelet Adhesiveness and Body Weight in Human Volunteers," *Postgraduate Medicine Journal* 45 (1969): 602–7; J. Yudkin, S. Kang, and K. B. Bruckdorfer, "Effects of High Dietary Sugar," *British Journal of Medicine* 281 (November 1960): 1396.
3. E. Tareke, P. Rydberg, P. Karlsson, et al., "Analysis of Acrylamide, a Carcinogen Formed in Heated Foodstuffs," *Journal of Agricultural and Food Chemistry* 50 (2002): 4998–5006.
4. "Multiple Sclerosis: Food Ingredient May Be Cause of Autoimmune Disease," *Townsend Letter* 304 (2008): 28–29; Russell Blaylock, *Excitotoxins: The Taste That Kills* (Santa Fe, N. Mex.: Health Press, 1996).
5. F. E. Marino, "Heat Reactions in Multiple Sclerosis: An Overlooked Paradigm in the Study of Comparative Fatigue," *International Journal of Hyperthermia* 1 (February 2009): 34–40.
6. Erin L. Elster, "Eighty-one Patients with Multiple Sclerosis and Parkinson's Disease Undergoing Upper Cervical Chiropractic Care to Correct Vertebral Subluxation: A Retrospective Analysis," *Journal of Vertebral Subluxation Research* 23, no. 8 (August 2004): 1–9.
7. R. Zivadinov, et al., "Smoking Linked to Lesions and Brain Shrinkage in Multiple Sclerosis," *Neurology* 73 (August 2009): 504–10.
8. B. C. Healy, E. N. Ali, C. R. Guttmann, et al., "Smoking and Disease Progression in Multiple Sclerosis," *Archives of Neurology* 66, no. 7 (July 2009): 858–64.
9. American Academy of Neurology's 61st Annual Meeting, Seattle, Washington (2009).
10. "17th World Congress of Neurology," *World Neurology* 16, no. 3 (September 2001).
11. University of North Dakota Energy & Environmental Research Center (EERC), "Study of Critical Potential Public Health Risks Related to Pesticide Exposure," news release, August 2006.
12. R. A. Marrie, "Environmental Risk Factors in Multiple Sclerosis Aetiology," *Lancet Neurology* 3, no. 12 (December 2004): 709–18.
13. A. M. Landtblom, U. Flodin, B. Söderfeldt, et al., "Organic Solvents and Multiple Sclerosis: A Synthesis of the Current Evidence," *Epidemiology* 7, no. 4 (July 1996): 429–33.
14. T. Riise, B. E. Moen, and K. R. Kyvik, "Organic Solvents and the Risk of Multiple Sclerosis," *Epidemiology* 13, no. 6 (November 2002): 718–20.

15. A. Alonso, "Oral Contraceptives Associated with Reduced Risk of Multiple Sclerosis," *Archives of Neurology* 65 (September 2005): 1362–65.
16. I. Sutton et al., "CNS Demyelination and Quadrivalent HPV Vaccination," *Multiple Sclerosis* 15 (2009): 116–19.
17. See www.vaccinetruth.org/france1.htm (accessed April 20, 2010).
18. Miguel A. Hernán, Susan S. Jick, Michael J. Olek, et al., "Recombinant Hepatitis B Vaccine and the Risk of Multiple Sclerosis. A Prospective Study," *Neurology* 63, no. 5 (September 2004): 838–42.
19. The National Centre for Immunisation Research and Surveillance of Vaccine Preventable Diseases (NCIRS), www.ncirs.usyd.edu.au/facts/f-hepb.html (accessed January 21, 2010).

Additional Studies of Interest: Stress

R. F. Brown, C. C. Tennant, M. Sharrock, et al., "Relationship between Stress and Relapse in Multiple Sclerosis: Part II," *Multiple Sclerosis* 12, no. 4 (August 2006): 453–64.

D. C. Mohr and D. Pelletier, "A Temporal Framework for Understanding the Effects of Stressful Life Events on Inflammation in Patients with Multiple Sclerosis," *Brain, Behavior, and Immunity* 20, no. 1 (January 2006): 27–36.

S. M. Gold, D. C. Mohr, I. Huitinga, et al., "The Role of Stress-response Systems for the Pathogenesis and Progression of MS," *Trends In Immunology* 26, no. 12 (December 2005): 644–52.

K. D. Ackerman, A. Stover, R. Heyman, et al., "Relationship of Cardiovascular Reactivity, Stressful Life Events, and Multiple Sclerosis Disease Activity," *Brain, Behavior, and Immunity* 17, no. 3 (June 2003): 141–51.

D. Buljevac, W. C. Hop, W. Reedeker, et al., "Self Reported Stressful Life Events and Exacerbations in Multiple Sclerosis: Prospective Study," *British Medical Journal* 327 (2003): 646.

P. Esposito, N. Chandler, K. Kandere, et al., "Corticotropin-releasing Hormone and Brain Mast Cells Regulate Blood-brain-barrier," *Journal of Pharmacology and Experimental Therapeutics* 303, no. 3 (December 2002): 1061–66.

P. H. Lalive, P. R. Burkhard, and M. Chofflon, "TNF-alpha and Psychologically Stressful Events in Healthy Subjects: Potential Relevance for Multiple Sclerosis Relapse," *Behavioral Neuroscience* 116, no. 6 (December 2002): 1093–97.

D. C. Mohr, D. E. Goodkin, S. Nelson, et al., "Moderating Effects of Coping on the Relationship between Stress and the Development of New Brain Lesions in Multiple Sclerosis," *Psychosomatic Medicine* 64, no. 5 (September–October, 2002): 803–9.

H. Strenge, "The Relationship between Psychological Stress and the Clinical Course of Multiple Sclerosis. An Update," *Psychotherapie, Psychosomatik, Medizinische Psychologie* 51, no. 3–4 (2001): 166–75.

D. C. Mohr, D. E. Goodkin, P. Bacchetti, et al., "Psychological Stress and the

Subsequent Appearance of New Brain MRI Lesions in MS," *Journal of Neurology* 55 (2000): 55–61.

Additional Studies of Interest: Heat

A. C. Fonseca, J. Costa, C. Cordeiro, et al., "Influence of Climatic Factors in the Incidence of Multiple Sclerosis Relapses in a Portuguese Population," *European Journal of Neurology: The Official Journal of the European Federation of Neurological Societies* 16, no. 4 (April 2009): 537–39.

D. A. Grahn, J. V. Murray, and H. C. Heller, "Cooling via One Hand Improves Physical Performance in Heat-Sensitive Individuals with Multiple Sclerosis: A Preliminary Study," *BioMedCentral Neurology* 8 (May 2008): 14.

R. K. Wexler, "Evaluation and Treatment of Heat-related Illnesses," *American Family Physician* 65, no. 11 (June 2002): 2307–14.

Additional Studies of Interest: Smoking

K. B. Friend, S. T. Mernoff, P. Block, et al., "Smoking Rates and Smoking Cessation among Individuals with Multiple Sclerosis," *Disability and Rehabilitation* 28, no. 18 (September 2006): 1135–41.

Iftah Biran, Israel Steiner, Trond Rüse, et al., "Smoking Is a Risk Factor for Multiple Sclerosis," *Neurology* 63, no. 4 (August 2004): 763.

Robin L. Brey, "Cigarette Smoking and MS: Yet Another Reason to Quit," *Neurology* 61 (2003): E11–E12

M. Riise, W. Nortvedt, and A. Ascherio, "Smoking Is a Risk Factor for Multiple Sclerosis," *Neurology* 61, no. 8 (October 2003): 1122–24.

M. Emre and C. de Decker, "Effects of Cigarette Smoking on Motor Functions in Patients with Multiple Sclerosis," *Archives of Neurology* 49, no. 12 (December 1992): 1243–47.

Additional Studies of Interest: Workplace Toxins

O. Axelson, A. M. Landtblom, and U. Flodin, "Multiple Sclerosis and Ionizing Radiation," *Neuroepidemiology* 20, no. 3 (August 2001): 175–78.

A. M. Landtblom, U. Flodin, M. Karlsson, et al., "Multiple Sclerosis and Exposure to Solvents, Ionizing Radiation, and Animals," *Scandinavian Journal of Work, Environment, and Health* 19, no. 6 (December 1993): 339–404.

Additional Study of Interest: Vaccinations

O. T. Rutschmann, D. C. McCrory, and D. B. Matchar, "Immunization and MS: A Summary of Published Evidence and Recommendations," *Neurology* 59, no. 12 (December 2002): 1837–43.

Additional Studies of Interest: Discounting the Link
between Hepatitis B Vaccine and MS

"Hepatitis B Vaccine and Multiple Sclerosis," National Network for Immunization Information, www.immunizationinfo.org/immunization_issues_detail. cfv?id=74 (accessed April 20, 2010).

"Hepatitis B Vaccination and Multiple Sclerosis (MS)," World Health Organization, www.who.int/vaccine_safety/topics/hepatitisb/multiple_sclerosis/en/ (accessed April 20, 2010).

"The Global Advisory Committee on Vaccine Safety Rejects Association between Hepatitis B Vaccination and Multiple Sclerosis (MS)," World Health Organization, www.who.int/vaccine_safety/topics/hepatitisb/ms/en/ (accessed April 20, 2010).

CHAPTER 18. MERCURY

1. E. Guallar, et al., "Mercury, Fish Oils, and the Risk of Myocardial Infarction," *The New England Journal of Medicine* 347, no. 22 (November 2002): 1747–54.

2. Thomas W. Clarkson, et al., "The Toxicology of Mercury—Current Exposures and Clinical Manifestations," *New England Journal of Medicine* 349 (October 30, 2003): 1731–37.

3. Ronald Eisler, *Mercury Hazards to Living Organisms* (Boca Raton, Fla.: CRC Press/Taylor & Francis, 2006).

4. Lita Tibbling, et al., "Immunological and Brain Changes in Patients with Suspected Metal Intoxication," *International Journal of Occupational Medicine and Toxicology* 4, no. 2 (1995): 285.

5. Theodore H. Ingalls, "Epidemiology, Etiology, and Prevention of Multiple Sclerosis," *The American Journal of Forensic Medicine and Pathology* 4, no. 1 (March 1983): 55–61.

6. C. W. McGrother, "Multiple Sclerosis, Dental Caries and Fillings: A Case-control Study," *British Dental Journal* 187 (1999): 261–64.

7. R. L. Siblerud and E. Kienholz, "Evidence that Mercury from Silver Dental Fillings May Be an Etiological Factor in Multiple Sclerosis," *Science of the Total Environment* 142, no. 3 (1994): 191–205.

8. R. L. Siblerud, "A Comparison of Mental Health of Multiple Sclerosis Patients with Silver/Mercury Dental Fillings and Those with Fillings Removed," *Psychological Reports* 70, no. 3 (June 1992): 1139–51.

9. Jarmila Prochazkova, et al., "The Beneficial Effect of Amalgam Replacement on Health in Patients with Autoimmunity," *Neuroendocrinology Letters* 25, no. 3 (June 2004): 211–18.

10. M. N. Bates, "Mercury Amalgam Dental Fillings: An Epidemiologic Assessment," *International Journal of Hygiene and Environmental Health* 209, no. 4 (July 2006): 309–16.

11. B. Hughes and L. Lawson, "Antimicrobial Effects of *Allium sativum* L. (Garlic), *Allium ampeloprasum* L. (Elephant Garlic), and *Allium cepa* L. (onion), Garlic Compounds and Commercial Garlic Supplement Products," *Phytotherapy Research* 5 (1991): 154–58; Majid Ali, "Integrative Management of Mercury Removal: A General Perspective," *Heavy Metal Overload and Toxicity: The Principles and Practice of Integrative Medicine* 7, see www.majidali.com/07.pdf (accessed April 20, 2010).

Additional Studies of Interest: Mercury

P. M. Bolger and B. A. Schwetz, "Perspective: Mercury and Health," *The New England Journal of Medicine* 347, no. 22 (November 2002): 1735–36.

K. Yoshizawa, et al., "Mercury and the Risk of Coronary Heart Disease in Men," *The New England Journal of Medicine* 347, no. 22 (November 2002): 1755–60.

CHAPTER 19. DETOXING THE BODY

1. Jorge Correale and Mauricio Farez, "Association between Parasite Infection and Immune Responses in MS," *Annals of Neurology* 61, no. 2 (2007): 97–108, doi: 10.1002/ana.21067.

2. Hulda Regehr Clark, *The Cure for All Diseases* (Chula Vista, Calif.: New Century Press, 1995), 240ff.

CHAPTER 20. CLEARING THE MIND OF NEGATIVITY

1. Dermot O'Connor, *The Healing Code: My Own Story and 5-Step Healing Programme* (London: Hodder & Stoughton, 2007).

2. Arthur Hastings, James Fadiman, and James S. Gordon, *Health for the Whole Person* (Boulder, Colo.: Westview Press, 1980).

Index

Page numbers in *italics* refer to illustrations.